Save Tin

Jones & Bartlett Learning Clinical Cards

These 4-color, 6-panel clinical cards measure 3.75 x 7.5 inches and present pertinent clinical information in a quick-reference format! Durable and compact, these cards are UV varnished for long life and are the perfect portable reference for busy healthcare professionals.

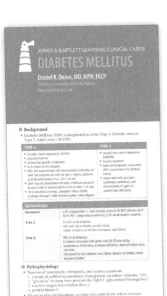

Acute Coronary Syndromes

Benign Prostatic Hyperplasia (BPH)

Crohn's Disease

Deep Vein Thrombosis and Pulmonary Embolism

Diabetes Mellitus

Erectile Dysfunction

Gastric Cancer

Gastroesophageal Reflux Disease (GERD)

Gout

Hematologic Emergencies

Myelodysplastic Syndromes

Non-Small Cell Lung Cancer

Oncologic Emergencies

Osteoarthritis

Overactive Bladder

Psoriatic Arthritis

Rheumatoid Arthritis

Secondary Depression, Mania, and Anxiety

Secondary Psychosis and Dementia

See www.jblearning.com for more details and ordering information.

The Little Black Book of
Hospital Medicine

Series Editor: Daniel K. Onion

Andrew J. Dionne, MD
Director, MaineGeneral Hospitalists
MaineGeneral Medical Center
Augusta and Waterville, Maine

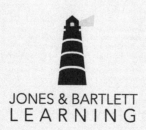

JONES & BARTLETT
LEARNING

World Headquarters
Jones & Bartlett Learning
40 Tall Pine Drive
Sudbury, MA 01776
978-443-5000
info@jblearning.com
www.jblearning.com

Jones & Bartlett Learning Canada
6339 Ormindale Way
Mississauga, Ontario L5V 1J2
Canada

Jones & Bartlett Learning
International
Barb House, Barb Mews
London W6 7PA
United Kingdom

Jones & Bartlett Learning books and products are available through most bookstores and online booksellers. To contact Jones & Bartlett Learning directly, call 800-832-0034, fax 978-443-8000, or visit our website, www.jblearning.com.

The authors, editor, and publisher have made every effort to provide accurate information. However, they are not responsible for errors, omissions, or for any outcomes related to the use of the contents of this book and take no responsibility for the use of the products and procedures described. Treatments and side effects described in this book may not be applicable to all people; likewise, some people may require a dose or experience a side effect that is not described herein. Drugs and medical devices are discussed that may have limited availability controlled by the Food and Drug Administration (FDA) for use only in a research study or clinical trial. Research, clinical practice, and government regulations often change the accepted standard in this field. When consideration is being given to use of any drug in the clinical setting, the healthcare provider or reader is responsible for determining FDA status of the drug, reading the package insert, and reviewing prescribing information for the most up-to-date recommendations on dose, precautions, and contraindications, and determining the appropriate usage for the product. This is especially important in the case of drugs that are new or seldom used.

Production Credits
Senior Acquisitions Editor: Nancy Duffy
Editorial Assistant: Sara Cameron
Production Director: Amy Rose
Associate Production Editor: Laura Almozara
Associate Marketing Manager: Katie Hennessy
V.P., Manufacturing and Inventory Control:
 Therese Connell

Project Management: Thistle Hill Publishing
 Services, LLC
Composition: Dedicated Business Solutions
Cover Design: Anne Spencer
Cover Image: © Photos.com
Printing and Binding: Malloy, Inc.
Cover Printing: Malloy, Inc.

Library of Congress Cataloging-in-Publication Data
Dionne, Andrew J.
 The little black book of hospital medicine / Andrew J. Dionne.
  p. ; cm. — (Little black book series)
Includes bibliographical references and index.
 ISBN-13: 978-0-7637-7370-0 (pbk.)
 ISBN-10: 0-7637-7370-0 (pbk.)
 1. Hospital care—Handbooks, manuals, etc. 2. Internal medicine—
Handbooks, manuals, etc. I. Title. II. Series: Little black book series.
  [DNLM: 1. Hospitalization—Handbooks. 2. Clinical Medicine—Handbooks. WX 39 D592L 2011]
 RA972.D56 2011
 362.11—dc22

                                                                    2010011801

6048
Printed in the United States of America
14 13 12 11 10   10 9 8 7 6 5 4 3 2 1

Dedication

This book is dedicated to my two favorite readers, Emily Rose and Drew.

Contents

Dedication   iii
Preface   ix
Acknowledgments   xiii
Medical Abbreviations   xv
Journal Abbreviations   xxvii
Notice   xxxv

Chapter 1 Cardiology   1

1.1 Acute Coronary Syndromes   1
1.2 Congestive Heart Failure   22
1.3 Arrhythmias   42
    Ventricular Ectopy and
        Tachycardia   42
    Supraventricular Tachycardia   46
    Atrial Fibrillation   50
1.4 Infectious and Inflammatory
    Cardiac Diseases   61
    Infective Endocarditis   61
    Acute Pericarditis   68
    Myocarditis   71
1.5 Hypertensive Crisis   73
1.6 Syncope   80

Chapter 2 Endocrinology   87

2.1 Adrenal Disorders   87
    Cushing's Syndrome   87
    Adrenal Insufficiency   90

2.2 Thyroid Disorders   94
    Myxedema (Severe
        Hypothyroidism)   94
    Thyrotoxicosis
        (Hyperthyroidism, Thyroid
        Storm)   96
2.3 Diabetic and Glucose
    Disorders   99
    Hyperglycemia, Inpatient
        (Including Diabetes
        Mellitus)   99
    Diabetic Ketoacidosis
        (DKA)   105
    Hyperosmolar Hyperglycemic
        State (HHS; Hyperosmolar
        Nonketotic Coma)   111
    Hypoglycemia   113
2.4 Mineral Disorders (Calcium/
    Magnesium/Phosphorus)   116
    Hypocalcemia   116
    Hypercalcemia   118
    Hypomagnesemia   121
    Hypermagnesemia   122
    Hypophosphatemia   123
    Hyperphosphatemia   124

Chapter 3 Gastroenterology 127

3.1 Abdominal Pain in Adults 127
3.2 Gastrointestinal Bleeding
    (Including Upper and Lower
    GI Sources) 129
3.3 Pancreaticobiliary Diseases 143
    Biliary Tract Disease
        (Including Cholecystitis,
        Bile Duct Obstruction,
        Cholangitis) 143
    Pancreatitis, Acute and
        Chronic 148
3.4 Infectious Diseases
    of the Gut 159
    Diverticulitis 159
    Appendicitis 163
3.5 Intestinal Obstruction and
    Pseudo-Obstruction 166
3.6 Intestinal Ischemia 174
3.7 Liver Disease and
    Complications 179
    Alcoholic Liver Disease
        (Including Hepatitis and
        Cirrhosis) 179
    Acute Liver Failure
        (Including Acetaminophen
        Overdose) 187
    Ascites and Spontaneous
        Bacterial Peritonitis
        (SBP) 192
    Hepatic Encephalopathy 198
    Hepatorenal Syndrome 201
    Evaluation of Abnormal
        LFTs 206

Chapter 4 Hematology 209

4.1 Anemia (Including
    Transfusion Practices) 209
4.2 Thrombocytopenia 222
    Heparin-Induced
        Thrombocytopenia
        (HIT) 231
4.3 Neutropenia 240
4.4 Multiple Myeloma 247

Chapter 5 Infectious Disease 257

5.1 Antimicrobial Medications 257
5.2 Gastrointestinal Infections 263
    Acute Diarrhea and
        Gastroenteritis 263
    Clostridium difficile Colitis 268
5.3 Systemic Infections 273
    Sepsis and Septic Shock 273
    Central Venous Catheters
        and Associated
        Infections 287
5.4 Soft Tissue Infections 292
    Cellulitis (Including
        Necrotizing Fasciitis
        and Gas Gangrene) 292
    Diabetic Foot Ulcers 299
5.5 Pulmonary Infections 302
    Pneumonia (Including
        Community-Acquired,
        Hospital-Acquired, and
        Ventilator-Associated) 302

5.6 Systemic Fungal Infections   319
    Antifungal Medications   319
    Aspergillosis   320
    Blastomycosis   322
    Coccidiomycosis (San
      Joaquin Valley Fever)   323
    Cryptococcosis   324
    Histoplasmosis   326
    Pneumocystis Pneumonia
      (PCP)   327
    Systemic Candidiasis   330
5.7 Urinary Tract Infections   331
    Complicated Urinary
      Tract Infections and
      Pyelonephritis   331
5.8 Central Nervous System
    Infections   336
    Meningitis   336
    Encephalitis   345

Chapter 6 Neurology   349

6.1 Stroke and Related
    Disorders   349
    Transient Ischemic
      Attack (TIA)   349
    Ischemic Stroke   351
6.2 Epilepsy and Seizure
    Disorders   360
6.3 Guillain-Barre Syndrome   367
6.4 Parkinson's Disease   369

Chapter 7 Pulmonary   373

7.1 Venous Thromboembolism
    (VTE)   373
    Pulmonary Embolism (PE)   373
    Deep Venous Thrombosis
      (DVT)   382
    VTE Prophylaxis in
      Hospitalized Patients   390
7.2 Diseases of the Airway   399
    Chronic Obstructive
      Pulmonary Disease
      (COPD) Exacerbations   399
    Asthma Exacerbations   411
7.3 Inflammatory Lung
    Disorders   417
    Acute Respiratory Distress
      Syndrome (ARDS)   417
    Interstitial Lung Diseases
      (ILDs)   429

Chapter 8 Renal/Urology   437

8.1 Acid-Base Disorders   437
8.2 Sodium and Potassium
    Disorders   443
    Hyponatremia   443
    Hypernatremia   451
    Hypokalemia   456
    Hyperkalemia   459
8.3 Acute Renal Failure   464
8.4 Nephrolithiasis   480

Index   487

Preface

Hospital medicine is the fastest-growing specialty in the United States. Some have interpreted this as further fracturing of patient care, splitting a patient's healthcare experiences between an outpatient and inpatient world. Others, myself included, argue that this new endeavor allows for comprehensive, patient-centered hospital care, with a team of physicians and other providers who have special expertise in hospital-based medicine.

This book is not meant to be an all-inclusive text of the medical issues encountered in the hospital. I'm sure that any text aimed at inpatient adult medicine would be deficient in some aspect of the depth and breadth of care provided by today's hospitalists. In addition, this is not a collection of algorithms to direct the care of individual problems. In my career as a hospitalist, I have found that not many inpatient decisions can be guided simply by an algorithm. There are too many competing interests of risks, benefits, patient and family wishes, local practice, and knowledge and comfort level of the physician. In *The Little Black Book of Hospital Medicine*, I have tried to provide a framework for managing the major problems we, as hospitalists, encounter every day. This includes thoughtful review of the issues and also an overview of the important clinical research that guides our decisions. When available, I have tried to summarize the best available evidence supporting a particular test or intervention, so that we may help our patients make an informed decision about their care. For more information about any of the subjects in this book, I would refer readers to the more than 1,500 reviews and clinical trials cited, as well as to other books in *The Little Black Book* series.

Although recognizing that inpatient care of children and adolescents is becoming a larger part of hospitalist care, the main content of this book centers on the care of adult inpatients. Sections are based on categories of disease, but as the reader knows, there is significant overlap with some clinical problems. When appropriate, I have provided cross-references to other sections for more details on a particular issue.

My hope is that this text will be useful to new learners of medicine, medical students, and resident physicians, but also to practicing hospitalists who wish to review the evidence behind the decisions we make every day. The specialty of hospital medicine is unique in that it draws people from many different medical backgrounds (internal medicine and medical subspecialties, family medicine, pediatrics, and a growing number of physician assistants and nurse practitioners), different points in their clinical careers (some coming right out of residency training, others returning to hospital work after years of outpatient primary care experience), and varying practice settings from large teaching centers to small community hospitals. My goal was to assist any one of those varied physicians and other medical providers.

In this text, I have cited many statistical calculations, especially in the review of pertinent clinical research. Here is a brief overview of the rationale behind some the terms you will encounter:

- In evaluations of diagnostic tests, true positives (TP) represent patients with a disease who also have a positive test; false positives (FP) are patients without the disease who have a positive test; true negatives (TN) are patients without the disease who have a negative test; false negatives (FN) are patients with the disease who have a negative test.
- Sensitivity = $TP/(TP + FN)$; a highly sensitive test has a low rate of false negatives, so a negative diagnostic test is very good at ruling out the disease.

- Specificity = TN/(TN + FP); a highly specific test has a low rate of false positives, so a positive test is very good at ruling in the disease.
- Positive predictive value (PPV) = TP/(TP + FP); a test with high PPV indicates that a positive test is most likely to represent true disease.
- Negative predictive value (NPV) = TN/(TN + FN); a test with high NPV indicates that a negative test is most likely to represent lack of the disease.
- Note that specificity and sensitivity are intrinsic to the diagnostic test, while PPV and NPV can vary based on the prevalence of the disease in the population studied.
- Relative risk reduction (RRR) represents the ratio of risk between two populations; e.g., if the risk of MI in the treatment arm of a study is 5%, and 10% in the placebo arm, the RRR = 10%/5%, or 50%.
- Absolute risk reduction (ARR) represents the mathematical difference between the two populations; e.g., using the same study cited above, the ARR = 10% − 5%, or 5%.

Number Needed to Treat (NNT) is the number of patients to whom the intervention must be given over a fixed time period to provide a benefit for one patient; NNT is the reciprocal value of ARR (or 1/ARR); e.g., in the above study, NNT = 1/0.05, or 20 (meaning that 20 patients need to be treated with the intervention for the time period studied in the trial for one patient to have the benefit of an averted MI). Number Needed to Harm (NNH) is calculated in a similar fashion, but applies to adverse events of therapy, such as bleeding risk in a trial of anticoagulant therapy.

Acknowledgments

The Little Black Book of Hospital Medicine would not have been possible without the assistance of many people.

Thanks to Dan Onion, MD, for his assistance, guidance, and terrific model in *The Little Black Book of Primary Care*; also, thanks for allowing me to borrow portions of his text in the chapters on Cardiology, Infectious Disease, Endocrinology, and Neurology.

Thanks to Barbara Harness and Cora Damon, MaineGeneral's fine medical librarians, for all their assistance in research; to my colleagues, James Schellenger, MD; John Smith, DO; Arun Ranganath, MD; Debra Nathan, MD; Dan Hammond, DO; and Lauren Labrecque, PA-C, for their review and thoughtful comments; to Steve Diaz, MD, author of *The Little Black Book of Emergency Medicine*, for his support and suggestions.

Thanks to my mentor and friend, Michael LaCombe, MD.

And thanks to my wife, Mary, for her love and support, with this project and always.

Medical Abbreviations

5-HIAA	5-hydroxyindoleacetic acid	ADA	American Diabetes Association
		ADEM	acute disseminated encephalomyelitis
AA	acetoacetate		
AAA	abdominal aortic aneurysm	ADH	antidiuretic hormone
		AEP	acute eosinophilic pneumonia
ab	antibody/ies		
ABC	airway, breathing, and circulation	AF	atrial fibrillation
		AFB	acid-fast bacillus
abd	abdominal	AHA	American Heart Association
ABG/s	arterial blood gas/es		
ABI	ankle-brachial index	AI	aortic insufficiency; or adrenal insufficiency
abx	antibiotics		
ACC	American College of Cardiology	AICD	automated implantable cardiodefibrillator
ACCP	American College of Chest Physicians	AIDP	acute inflammatory demyelinating polyradiculopathy
ACD	anemia of chronic disease		
		AIDS	acquired immunodeficiency syndrome
ACE	angiotensin-converting enzyme		
		AIN	acute interstitial nephritis
ACEI	ACE inhibitor		
ACLS	advanced cardiac life support	AIP	acute interstitial pneumonia
		aka	also known as
ACP	American College of Physicians	AKI	acute kidney injury
		AL	amyloid light chain
ACS	acute coronary syndrome	ALF	acute liver failure
ACTH	adrenocorticotropic hormone	alk phos	alkaline phosphatase

ALT	alanine transferase	BBB	bundle branch block; or blood–brain barrier
AMI	anterior myocardial infarction		
ANA	antinuclear antibody	BHB	beta-hydroxybutyrate
ANC	absolute neutrophil count	bid	2 times a day
		BiPAP	bilevel positive airway pressure
ANCA	antineutrophil cytoplasmic antibody/ies		
		biw	2 times a week
APA	antiphospholipid antibody	BM	basement membrane
		BMI	body mass index
APAP	acetaminophen	BMP	basic metabolic panel
ARB	angiotensin receptor blocker	BNP	brain natriuretic peptide
ARDS	acute respiratory distress syndrome	BOOP	bronchiolitis obliterans organizing pneumonia
ARF	acute renal failure		
ARR	absolute risk reduction	BP	blood pressure
ASA	aspirin	BPH	benign prostatic hypertrophy
asap	as soon as possible		
ASCVD	arteriosclerotic cardiovascular disease	bpm	beats per minute
		BS	blood sugar
AST	aspartate transferase	BUN	blood urea nitrogen
asx	asymptomatic	bx	biopsy/ies
AT-III	antithrombin III		
ATN	acute tubular necrosis	Ca	calcium; or cancer (depending on context)
ATP	adenosine triphosphate		
AV	arteriovenous; or atrioventricular		
		CABG	coronary artery bypass graft
avg	average		
AVM	arteriovenous malformation	CAD	coronary artery disease
		CA-MRSA	community-acquired MRSA
AVNRT	atrioventricular nodal reentrant tachycardia		
		CAP	community-acquired pneumonia
AVRT	atrioventricular reentrant tachycardia	cath	catheterization
		CBC	complete blood count
AXR	abdominal Xray	CBD	common bile duct

CBG	corticosteroid-binding globulin	CPT	Child-Pugh-Turcotte
cc	cubic centimeter	Cr	creatinine
CCB	calcium channel blocker	CrCl	creatinine clearance
CCU	critical care unit	CRF	corticotropin-releasing factor
CEA	carotid endarterectomy	CRH	corticotropin-releasing hormone
CF	cystic fibrosis	CRP	c-reactive protein
CHF	congestive heart failure	CRRT	continuous renal replacement therapy
CI-ARF	contrast-induced ARF	crs	course
CIWA	Clinical Institute Withdrawal Assessment	CRT	cardiac resynchronization therapy
CKD	chronic kidney disease	CSF	cerebrospinal fluid; or colony-stimulating factor
CK-MB	creatine kinase, myocardial bound	CSWS	cerebral salt-wasting syndrome
Cl	chloride	CT	computed tomography
cmplc	complications	CTA	computed tomography angiography
CMS	Centers for Medicare & Medicaid Services	CTPH	chronic thromboembolic pulmonary hypertension
CMV	cytomegalovirus		
CN	cranial nerve	CVA	cerebrovascular accident
CNS	central nervous system; or coagulase-negative staphylococcus	CVC	central venous catheter
		CVP	central venous pressure
CO	cardiac output	Cx	culture/s
COPD	chronic obstructive lung disease	CXR	chest Xray
cP	centipoise/s	d	day/s
CPAP	continuous positive airway pressure	D_5W	dextrose in water
CPK	creatine phosphokinase	DAH	diffuse alveolar hemorrhage
CPM	central pontine myelinolysis	DBP	diastolic blood pressure
CPR	cardiopulmonary resuscitation		

DI	diabetes insipidus	EPO	erythropoietin
DIC	disseminated intravascular coagulation	ERCP	endoscopic retrograde cholangiopancreatography
diff	differential		
dig	digoxin	ERDP	extended-release dipyridamole
DKA	diabetic ketoacidosis		
dL	deciliter/s	ER/ED	emergency room/ department
DLCO	diffusing capacity of the lung for carbon monoxide		
		ESC	European Society of Cardiology
DM	diabetes mellitus	ESR	erythrocyte sedimentation rate
DRGs	diagnosis-related groups		
		ESRD	end-stage renal disease
DST	dexamethasone suppression test	ESWL	extracorporeal shock wave lithotripsy
DTRs	deep tendon reflexes	ETOH	ethanol
DUD	duodenal ulcer disease	ETT	endotracheal tube
DVT	deep venous thrombosis	eval	evaluate; or evaluation
dx	diagnosis; or diagnostic		
		F	Fahrenheit
EBV	Epstein-Barr virus	f/u	follow up
ECF	extracellular fluid volume	FE_{Na}	fractional excretion of sodium
EEG	electroencephalogram	FEV_1	forced expiratory volume in 1 sec
EF	ejection fraction		
e.g.	for example	FFA	free fatty acids
EGD	esophagogastroduodenoscopy	FFP	fresh frozen plasma
		FiO_2	fraction of inspired oxygen
EGDT	early goal-directed therapy		
		fL	femtoliter/s
EKG	electrocardiogram	FLC	free light chain/s
ELISA	enzyme-linked immunosorbent assay	FOBT	fecal occult blood test
		FQ	fluoroquinolone
EMG	electromyogram	FRC	functional residual capacity
ENT	ear, nose, and throat		
Epidem	epidemiology	FSP	fibrin split products

FVC	forced vital capacity	HCl	hydrochloric acid
FVL	Factor V Leiden	HCO₃	bicarbonate
fx	fracture/s	Hct	hematocrit
		HD	hemodialysis
G6PD	glucose-6-phosphate dehydrogenase	HE	hypertensive emergency; or hepatic encephalopathy
GAVE	gastric antral vascular ectasia	HELLP	hemolysis, elevated liver enzymes, low platelets
GB	gall bladder		
GBM	glomerular basement membrane	hep	hepatitis
GBS	Guillain-Barre syndrome	Hg	mercury
		Hgb	hemoglobin
GCS	Glasgow coma scale	HH	hereditary hemochromatosis
GERD	gastroesophageal reflux disease	HHS	hyperosmolar hyperglycemic state
GFR	glomerular filtration rate	HHV	human herpes virus
GGTP	gamma-glutamyl transpeptidase	HIDA	hepatobiliary iminodiacetic acid
GI	gastrointestinal	HIT	heparin-induced thrombocytopenia
gm	gram/s		
GU	genitourinary	HITTS	HIT thrombotic syndrome
H. flu	*Haemophilus influenzae*	HIV	human immunodeficiency virus
h/o	history of		
H₂O	water	HLA	human leukocyte antigens
H2B	histamine receptor blocker/s	HOCM	hypertrophic obstructive cardiomyopathy
HAP	hospital-acquired pneumonia	HP	hypersensitivity pneumonitis
HAV	hepatitis A virus	hr	hour/s
HCAP	healthcare-associated pneumonia	HR	heart rate
		HRCT	high-resolution computed tomography
HCG	human chorionic gonadotropin		

HRS	hepatorenal syndrome	im	intramuscular
HSV	herpes simplex virus	IMA	inferior mesenteric artery
HTN	hypertension		
HU	hypertensive urgency	INR	international normalized ratio (PT)
HUS	hemolytic uremic syndrome		
hx	history	IPC	intermittent pneumatic compression
		IPF	idiopathic pulmonary fibrosis
I&D	incision and drainage		
i.e.	in other words	ITP	idiopathic thrombocytopenic purpura
I/O	intake/output		
IBD	inflammatory bowel disease	IU	international unit/s
		IV	intravenous
IBW	ideal body weight	IVC	inferior vena cava
ICH	intracerebral hemorrhage	IVCD	idioventricular conduction delay
ICP	intracranial pressure	IVDA	intravenous drug abuse
ICU	intensive care unit		
IDA	iron deficiency anemia	IVF	intravenous fluid
		IVIG	intravenous immunoglobulin
IDSA	Infectious Disease Society of America		
		IVP	intravenous pyelogram
IE	infective endocarditis		
IFA	indirect fluorescent antibody	J	joule
		JNC	Joint National Committee on Prevention, Detection, Evaluation, and Treatment of High Blood Pressure
Ig	immunoglobulin		
IgA	immunoglobulin A		
IgD	immunoglobulin D		
IgE	immunoglobulin E		
IgG	immunoglobulin G		
IgM	immunoglobulin M	JVP	jugular venous pressure/pulse
IHSS	idiopathic hypertrophic subaortic stenosis		
		K	potassium; or thousand
IJ	internal jugular	KCl	potassium chloride
ILD	interstitial lung disease	kg	kilogram/s

L	liter/s; or left	MDI	metered dose inhaler
LA	left atrium; or long act-	MDR	multidrug-resistant
	ing (if after a drug)	med(s)	medication(s)
LBBB	left bundle branch	mEq	milliequivalent/s
	block	MET(s)	metabolic equivalent(s)
LBO	large bowel obstruction	mets	metastases
LDH	lactate dehydrogenase	mg	milligram/s
LDL	low density	Mg	magnesium
	lipoproteins	mgt	management
LFTs	liver function tests	MGUS	monoclonal gammopa-
LGIB	lower gastrointestinal		thy of undetermined
	bleeding		significance
LLQ	left lower quadrant	MI	myocardial infarction
LMWH	low-molecular-weight	MIC	minimum inhibitory
	heparin		concentration
ln	natural log	min	minute/s
LOS	length of stay	mL	milliliter/s
LP	lumbar puncture	mm	millimeter/s
LPM	liters per minute	MM	multiple myeloma
LR	lactated ringer's	MMA	methylmalonic acid
	solution	mmol	millimole/s
LUQ	left upper quadrant	mo	month/s
LV	left ventricle	mOsm	milliosmole/s
LVEF	left ventricular ejec-	MRA	magnetic resonance
	tion fraction		angiography
LVH	left ventricular	MRCP	magnetic resonance
	hypertrophy		cholangiopancrea-
LVP	large-volume		tography
	paracentesis	MRI	magnetic resonance
			imaging
m	meter/s	MRSA	methicillin-resistant
MAP	mean arterial pressure		*Staph. aureus*
mcg	microgram/s	msec	millisecond/s
mcL	microliter	MSSA	methicillin-sensitive
MCV	mean corpuscular		*Staph. aureus*
	volume	MVI	multivitamin

N/V	nausea, vomiting	NSR	normal sinus rhythm
Na	sodium	NSTEMI	non-ST-elevation myo-cardial infarction
NAC	N-acetylcysteine		
NaCl	sodium chloride	NSVT	nonsustained ventricu-lar tachycardia
NAFLD	nonalcoholic fatty liver disease		
		NTG	nitroglycerin
NAPQI	N-acetyl-p-benzoquinone imine	NYHA	New York Heart Association
NASH	nonalcoholic steatohepatitis		
neg	negative	O$_2$	oxygen
neuro	neurological	OOB	out of bed
ng	nanogram/s	OR	odds ratio
NG	nasogastric	OSA	obstructive sleep apnea
NGT	nasogastric tube	osm	osmole/s
NH	nursing home	OTC	over-the-counter
NH$_3$	ammonia		
NIPPV	noninvasive positive pressure ventilation	PA	pulmonary artery
		PAC	premature atrial contraction
nmol	nanomole/s		
NMS	neuroleptic malignant syndrome	PaCO$_2$	partial pressure of carbon dioxide (arterial)
NNH	number needed to harm		
		PaO$_2$	partial pressure of oxygen (arterial)
NNT	number needed to treat		
NOMI	nonocclusive mesen-teric ischemia	Pathophys	pathophysiology
		PBC	primary biliary cirrhosis
noninv	noninvasive laboratory	PCI	percutaneous coronary intervention
NPH	neutral protamine Hagedorn (insulin)		
		PCN	penicillin
NPO	nothing by mouth	PCP	*Pneumocystis* pneumonia
NPV	negative predictive value		
		PCR	polymerase chain reaction
NS	normal saline		
NSAID	nonsteroidal anti-inflammatory drug	PCWP	pulmonary capillary wedge pressure

PD	Parkinson's disease	PSV	pressure support ventilation
PE	pulmonary embolism		
PEEP	positive end-expiratory pressure	PSVT	paroxysmal supra-ventricular tachycardia
PEF	peak expiratory flow		
PEG	polyethylene glycol	pt(s)	patient(s)
PF4	platelet-factor 4	PT	protime
PFO	patent foramen ovale	PTCA	percutaneous trans-luminal coronary angioplasty
PFT	pulmonary function test		
pg	picogram/s		
phos	phosphatase; or phosphate	PTH	parathyroid hormone
		PTHrp	parathormone-related protein
PICC	peripherally-inserted central catheter	PTT	partial thromboplastin time
plt	platelet/s		
PMI	point of maximum impulse	PTU	propylthiouracil
		PUD	peptic ulcer disease
PMNs	polymorphonuclear leukocytes	pulm	pulmonary
		PVC	premature ventricular contraction
PO	by mouth		
PO$_4$	phosphate	PVD	peripheral vascular disease
POMC	pro-opiomelanocortin		
pos	positive		
post-op	post-operative	q	every
ppd	pack(s) per day	qd	daily
PPI	proton pump inhibitor	qid	4 times a day
PPN	peripheral parenteral nutrition	qod	every other day
		QOL	quality of life
PPV	positive predictive value		
		r/o	rule out
PRBC(s)	packed red blood cell(s)	RA	rheumatoid arthritis
		RAA	renin-angiotensin-aldosterone
preop	pre-operative		
prep	preparation	RAD	reactive airway disease
PSC	primary sclerosing cholangitis	RBBB	right bundle branch block

RBC	red blood cell	SAH	subarachnoid hemorrhage
RCT	randomized controlled trial	SaO_2	arterial oxygen saturation
RDW	random distribution of width	SBE	subacute bacterial endocarditis
re	about	SBFT	small bowel follow-through
resp	respiratory; or respirations	SBO	small bowel obstruction
RF	rheumatoid factor	SBP	systolic blood pressure; or spontaneous bacterial peritonitis
rhAPC	recombinant human activated protein C		
RIA	radioimmunoassay		
RLQ	right lower quadrant		
RR	respiratory rate	SBT	spontaneous breathing trial
RRR	relative risk reduction		
RSBI	rapid shallow breathing index	SC	subclavian
		SCD	sequential compression device
RTA	renal tubular acidosis		
RUQ	right upper quadrant	SCT	stem cell transplantation
RV	right ventricle		
RVH	right ventricular hypertrophy	$ScvO_2$	central venous oxygen saturation
rx	treatment; or therapy		
		SDD	selective decontamination of the digestive tract
s/p	status post		
S_1	first heart sound		
S_2	second heart sound	sens	sensitivity
S_3	third heart sound, gallop	si	signs
		SIADH	syndrome of inappropriate ADH
S_4	fourth heart sound, gallop	SIMV	synchronous intermittent mandatory ventilation
SAAG	serum-ascites albumin gradient		
SAB	*Staph. aureus* bacteremia	SIRS	systemic inflammatory response syndrome

SLE	systemic lupus erythematosis	TIBC	total iron-binding capacity
SMA	superior mesenteric artery	tid	3 times a day
SOD	selective oral decontamination	TIPS	transjugular intrahepatic portosystemic shunt
specif	specificity	TMP	trimethoprim
SPEP	serum protein electrophoresis	TMP-SMX	trimethoprim-sulfamethoxazole
SQ	subcutaneous	TnI	troponin I
SSKI	saturated solution of potassium iodide	TnT	troponin T
		TPA	tissue plasminogen activator
SSRI	selective serotonin reuptake inhibitor	TPN	total parenteral nutrition
staph	*Staphylococcus*	TRALI	transfusion-related acute lung injury
STEMI	ST-elevation myocardial infarction	TRH	thyrotropin-releasing hormone
strep	*Streptococcus*		
SVC	superior vena cava	TSH	thyroid-stimulating hormone
SVR	systemic vascular resistance	TSI	transient symptoms associated with infarction
SVT	supraventricular tachycardia		
sx	symptom/s	TTE	transthoracic echocardiogram
T3	tri-iodothyronine	TTP	thrombotic thrombocytopenic purpura
T4	thyroxine		
TBW	total body water	TURP	transurethral resection of prostate
TCA	tricyclic antidepressant		
TEE	transesophageal echocardiogram	U	unit/s
		U/A	urinalysis
TEN	total enteral nutrition	UA	unstable angina
TIA	transient ischemic attack	UFH	unfractionated heparin

UGIB	upper gastrointestinal bleeding	vs	versus
		Vt	tidal volume/s
UPEP	urine protein electrophoresis	VT	ventricular tachycardia
		VTE	venous thromboembolism
URI	upper respiratory illness		
US	ultrasound	VZV	varicella zoster virus
UTI	urinary tract infection		
		w/	with
V/Q	ventilation/perfusion	w/u	work up
VAD	ventricular-assist device	WBC	white blood cell; or white blood count
VAP	ventilator-acquired pneumonia	WCT	wide complex tachycardia
VDRL	serologic test for syphilis ("Venereal Disease Research Lab")	wk	week/s
		WM	Waldenstrom's macroglobulinemia
		WPW	Wolff-Parkinson-White syndrome
VF	ventricular fibrillation		
vit	vitamin		
VRE	vancomycin-resistant *Enterococcus*	yo	years old
		yr	year/s

Journal Abbreviations

Abdom Imaging	Abdominal Imaging
Acad Emerg Med	Academic Emergency Medicine
Acta Neurol Scand	ACTA Neurologica Scandinavica
AIDS	AIDS
Aliment Pharmacol Ther	Alimentary Pharmacology and Therapeutics
Am Fam Phys	American Family Physician
Am Hrt J	American Heart Journal
Am J Cardiol	American Journal of Cardiology
Am J Cardiovasc Drugs	American Journal of Cardiovascular Drugs
Am J Clin Path	American Journal of Clinical Pathology
Am J Crit Care	American Journal of Critical Care
Am J Dig Dis	American Journal of Digestive Diseases
Am J Emerg Med	American Journal of Emergency Medicine
Am J Gastroenterol	American Journal of Gastroenterology
Am J Health Syst Pharm	American Journal of Health-System Pharmacy
Am J Kidney Dis	American Journal of Kidney Diseases
Am J Med	American Journal of Medicine
Am J Med Sci	American Journal of the Medical Sciences
Am J Neuroradiol	American Journal of Neuroradiology
Am J Ob Gyn	American Journal of Obstetrics and Gynecology
Am J Physiol	American Journal of Physiology
Am J Publ Hlth	American Journal of Public Health
Am J Respir Crit Care Med	American Journal of Respiratory and Critical Care Medicine
Am J Roentgenol	American Journal of Roentgenology

Am J Surg	American Journal of Surgery
Am Rev Respir Dis	American Review of Respiratory Disease
Anaesthesist	Anaesthesist
Anesthesiology	Anesthesiology
Ann EM	Annals of Emergency Medicine
Ann IM	Annals of Internal Medicine
Ann Neurol	Annals of Neurology
Ann Pharmacother	Annals of Pharmacotherapy
Ann Surg	Annals of Surgery
Ann Thorac Surg	Annals of Thoracic Surgery
Antimicrob Agents Chemother	Antimicrobial Agents and Chemotherapy
Arch Gerontol Geriatr	Archives of Gerontology and Geriatrics
Arch IM	Archives of Internal Medicine
Arch Neurol	Archives of Neurology
Arch Surg	Archives of Surgery
Arthritis Rheum	Arthritis and Rheumatism
Aust N Z J Surg	Australian and New Zealand Journal of Surgery
Biol Blood Marrow Transplant	Biology of Blood and Marrow Transplantation
Blood	Blood
Blood Coagul Fibrinolysis	Blood Coagulation and Fibrinolysis
Blood Rev	Blood Reviews
BMJ	British Medical Journal
Br J Clin Pract	British Journal of Clinical Practice
Br J Dis Chest	British Journal of Diseases of the Chest
Br J Haematol	British Journal of Haematology
Br J Radiol	British Journal of Radiology
Br J Surg	British Journal of Surgery
Calcif Tissue Int	Calcified Tissue International
Can Respir J	Canadian Respiratory Journal
Cancer	Cancer
Cardiol Rev	Cardiology in Review
Chest	Chest
Circ	Circulation

Circ Res	Circulation Research
Clin Cardiol	Clinical Cardiology
Clin Chem	Clinical Chemistry
Clin Chest Med	Clinics in Chest Medicine
Clin Geriatr Med	Clinics in Geriatric Medicine
Clin Infect Dis	Clinical Infectious Diseases
Clin Liver Dis	Clinics in Liver Disease
Clin Nephrol	Clinical Nephrology
Clin Radiol	Clinical Radiology
Clin Ther	Clinical Therapeutics
CMAJ	Canadian Medical Association Journal
Cochrane	Cochrane Database (Online)
Colorectal Dis	Colorectal Disease
Crit Care	Critical Care
Crit Care Med	Critical Care Medicine
Curr Hematol Rep	Current Hematology Reports
Curr Opin Neurol	Current Opinion in Neurology
Diab Care	Diabetes Care
Diab Med	Diabete et Metabolisme
Dig Dis Sci	Digestive Diseases and Sciences
Dis Colon Rectum	Diseases of the Colon and Rectum
Drug Saf	Drug Safety
Drugs	Drugs
Emerg Med J	Emergency Medicine Journal
Endo Metab Clin N Am	Endocrinology and Metabolism Clinics of North America
Endoscopy	Endoscopy
Epilepsia	Epilepsia
Epilepsy Res	Epilepsy Research
Eur Heart J	European Heart Journal
Eur J Clin Microbiol Infect Dis	European Journal of Clinical Microbiology and Infectious Diseases
Eur J Clin Pharmacol	European Journal of Clinical Pharmacology
Eur J Gastroenterol Hepatol	European Journal of Gastroenterology & Hepatology

Eur J Surg	European Journal of Surgery
Eur Radiol	European Journal of Radiology
Eur Respir J	European Respiratory Journal
Eur Spine J	European Spine Journal
Gastro Clin N Am	Gastroenterology Clinics of North America
Gastrointest Endosc	Gastrointestinal Endoscopy
Gastrointest Radiol	Gastrointestinal Radiology
GE	Gastroenterology
Geriatrics	Geriatrics
Gut	Gut
Gynecol Oncol	Gynecologic Oncology
Heart	Heart
Hepatol	Hepatology
Hosp Pract	Hospital Practice
HT	Hypertension
Inf Contr Hosp Epidem	Infection Control and Hospital Epidemiology
Int J Clin Pract	International Journal of Clinical Practice
Int J Surg	International Journal of Surgery
Intensive Care Med	Intensive Care Medicine
Ital J Gastroenterol Hepatol	Italian Journal of Gastroenterology and Hepatology
J Am Board Fam Pract	Journal of the American Board of Family Practice
J Am Coll Cardiol	Journal of the American College of Cardiology
J Am Coll Surg	Journal of the American College of Surgeons
J Am Ger Soc	Journal of the American Geriatrics Society
J Am Soc Nephrol	Journal of the American Society of Nephrology
J Antimicrob Chemother	Journal of Antimicrobial Chemotherapy

J Asthma	Journal of Asthma
J Cardiovasc Electrophysiol	Journal of Cardiovascular Electrophysiology
J Clin Endocrinol Metab	Journal of Clinical Endocrinology and Metabolism
J Clin Gastroenterol	Journal of Clinical Gastroenterology
J Clin Hypertens	Journal of Clinical Hypertension
J Clin Invest	Journal of Clinical Investigation
J Clin Microbiol	Journal of Clinical Microbiology
J Clin Oncol	Journal of Clinical Oncology
J Clin Pathol	Journal of Clinical Pathology
J Electrocardiol	Journal of Electrocardiology
J Emerg Med	Journal of Emergency Medicine
J Endocrinol	Journal of Endocrinology
J Endourol	Journal of Endourology
J Fam Pract	Journal of Family Practice
J Gastrointest Surg	Journal of Gastrointestinal Surgery
J Gen Intern Med	Journal of General Internal Medicine
J Hepatobiliary Pancreat	Journal of Hepato-Biliary-Pancreatic Surgery
J Hepatol	Journal of Hepatology
J Hosp Infect	Journal of Hospital Infection
J Hosp Med	Journal of Hospital Medicine
J Hypertens	Journal of Hypertension
J Infect Dis	Journal of Infectious Diseases
J Intensive Care Med	Journal of Intensive Care Medicine
J Intern Med	Journal of Internal Medicine
J Med Econ	Journal of Medical Economics
J Med Microbiol	Journal of Medical Microbiology
J Natl Compr Canc Netw	Journal of the National Comprehensive Cancer Network
J Neurol	Journal of Neurology
J Neurol Neurosurg	Journal of Neurology, Neurosurgery and Psychiatry
J Neurol Sci	Journal of the Neurological Sciences
J Thromb Haemost	Journal of Thrombosis and Haemostasis
J Trauma	Journal of Trauma

J Urol	Journal of Urology
J Vasc Surg	Journal of Vascular Surgery
JAMA	Journal of the American Medical Association
JPEN	Journal of Parenteral and Enteral Nutrition
Kidney Int	Kidney International
Lancet	Lancet
Lancet Infect Dis	Lancet Infectious Diseases
Lancet Neurol	Lancet Neurology
Liver Transpl	Liver Transplantation
Mayo Clin Proc	Mayo Clinic Proceedings
MCCVD	Modern Concepts of Cardiovascular Disease
Med	Medicine
Med Clin N Am	Medical Clinics of North America
Med J Aust	Medical Journal of Australia
Med Lett Drugs Ther	Medical Letter on Drugs and Therapeutics
MMWR Recomm Rep	MMWR Recommendations and Reports
Mov Disord	Movement Disorders
NEJM	New England Journal of Medicine
Nephron	Nephron
Neurol	Neurology
Neurosurg	Neurosurgery
Ob Gyn	Obstetrics and Gynecology
Pancreatology	Pancreatology
Parkinsonism Related Disord	Parkinsonism & Related Disorders
Pharmacoepidemiol Drug Saf	Pharmacoepidemiology and Drug Safety
Pharmacotherapy	Pharmacotherapy
Postgrad Med J	Postgraduate Medical Journal
QJM	Quarterly Journal of Medicine

Radiol	Radiology
Radiol Clin N Am	Radiologic Clinics of North America
Respir Med	Respiratory Medicine
Rev Infect Dis	Reviews of Infectious Diseases
Scand J Infect Dis	Scandinavian Journal of Infectious Diseases
Semin Gastrointest Dis	Seminars in Gastrointestinal Disease
Semin Hematol	Seminars in Hematology
Semin Nephrol	Seminars in Nephrology
Semin Respir Infect	Seminars in Respiratory Infections
Semin Thromb Hemost	Seminars in Thrombosis and Hemostasis
South Med J	Southern Medical Journal
Stroke	Stroke
Surg	Surgery
Surg Clin N Am	Surgical Clinics of North America
Surg Gyn Ob	Surgery, Gynecology & Obstetrics
Thorax	Thorax
Thromb Haemost	Thrombosis and Haemostasis
Thyroid	Thyroid
Transfusion	Transfusion
Treat Respir Med	Treatments in Respiratory Medicine
Urol	Urology
Urol Clin N Am	Urologic Clinics of North America

Notice

We have made every attempt to summarize accurately and concisely a multitude of references. However, the reader is reminded that times and medical knowledge change, transcription or understanding error is always possible, and crucial details are omitted whenever such a comprehensive distillation as this is attempted in limited space. And the primary purpose of this compilation is to cite literature on various sides of controversial issues; knowing where "truth" lies is usually difficult. We cannot, therefore, guarantee that every bit of information is absolutely accurate or complete. The reader should affirm that cited recommendations are reasonable still, by reading the original articles and checking other sources, including local consultants as well as recent literature, before applying them.

Drugs and medical devices are discussed that may have limited availability controlled by the Food and Drug Administration (FDA) for use only in research study or clinical trial. The drug information presented has been derived from reference sources, recently published data, and pharmaceutical tests. Research, clinical practice, and government regulations often change the accepted standard in this field. When consideration is being given to use of any drug in the clinical setting, the clinician or reader is responsible for determining FDA status of the drug, reading the package insert, and prescribing information for the most up-to-date recommendations on dose, precautions, and contraindications and determining the appropriate usage for the product. This is especially important in the case of drugs that are new or seldom used.

Chapter 1

Cardiology

1.1   Acute Coronary Syndromes

(Circ 2007;116:e148)

Cause: Atherosclerosis (85%) including spasm (NEJM 1983;309:220) with superimposed thrombus in 90% of those; emboli (15%) (Ann IM 1978;88:155); occasionally cocaine-induced spasm (NEJM 1989;321:1557).

In settings where pt is admitted for chest pain, after observation and evaluation, classify as one of the following.

- Acute coronary syndrome (ACS):
  - ST-elevation myocardial infarction (STEMI): si/sx of myocardial ischemia, ST elevation on EKG, elevated cardiac enzymes
  - Non-STEMI: si/sx of myocardial ischemia, possible EKG changes (but no ST elevation), elevated cardiac enzymes
  - Unstable angina (UA): si/sx of myocardial ischemia, EKG changes (except ST elevation), normal cardiac enzymes
    - Rest angina
    - New-onset severe angina
    - Crescendo angina (increasing in intensity, duration, or frequency)
- Non-ACS, cardiac cause:
  - Pericarditis
  - Myocarditis
  - Ischemia due to increased demand from aortic stenosis, hypertrophic cardiomyopathy

- Noncardiac cause, including the following:
  - GI: esophageal spasm, esophageal reflux, esophagitis, gastritis, peptic ulcer, biliary colic/cholecystitis
  - Musculoskeletal: costochondritis, muscle spasm, rib fracture, other trauma
  - Pulmonary: pleurisy (+/− lower respiratory tract infection, pneumonia), pulmonary embolism, pneumothorax
  - Vascular: aortic dissection
  - Psychiatric: panic disorder, acute stress, malingering
  - Neurologic: neuropathic pain due to zoster, nerve impingement
- Noncardiac cause, undefined (for billing purposes, though, always try to assign at least a possible cause)

Seventy-five percent of all ER chest pain pts are determined to have noncardiac cause (Ann IM 1998;129:845).

Epidem: Increased incidence with one or more of the following.

- Age: may be the most important risk factor (Am J Med 1997;102:350; Mayo Clin Proc 2002;77:515)
- Hypertension
- Elevated total and LDL cholesterol
- Diabetes mellitus
- Other vascular disease: carotid stenosis, peripheral vascular disease, aortic disease
- Family hx of premature MIs (males younger than 55 years or females younger than 65 years) (NEJM 1994;330:1041); sibling history sometimes stronger than parental (Circ 2004;110:2150)
- Obesity
- Smoking: increases risk by 3 times, but risk decreases to normal within 2 yr after stopping (NEJM 1985;313:1511); increases risk 5 times if greater than 1 ppd, or 2 times if 1–4 cigarettes qd in women (NEJM 1987;317:1303)
- Stress, day to day (JAMA 1997;277:1521), but not type A personality (NEJM 1988;318:65, NEJM 1988;318:110)

- Oral contraceptive use: increases risk twofold (NEJM 2001;345:1787)
- Carbon monoxide: acute exposures (e.g., firefighters); chronic carbon disulfide exposures (e.g., disulfiram [Antabuse] use, rayon manufacturing)
- Cocaine use or withdrawal (Ann IM 1989;111:876, NEJM 1986;315:1495); methamphetamine use
- Coffee, variable studies (NEJM 1990;323:1026, NEJM 1997;337:230, JAMA 1996;275:458)
- Exercise test showing ischemia (NEJM 1983;309:1085)
- Homocysteine levels greater than 15μmol/L, which correlate w/ worse prognosis (NEJM 1986;315:1438)
- Postmenopausal, if surgical and pts not placed on estrogen, but no sharp increase in natural menopause
- Sedentary work
- Sexual activity, which increases risk slightly, but not at all if regular exercise (e.g., 3x/wk) (JAMA 1996;275:1405)
- Viral URI in past 2 wk (Ann IM 1985;102:699), or chronic *Chlamydia pneumoniae* infections (Ann IM 1996;125:979, Ann IM 1992;116:273)

Decreased incidence with one or more of the following:

- Exercise, more than 6 METs, more than 2 hr/wk divided 3–4x/wk (NEJM 1994;330:1549)
- Fish intake 1–4/mo (JAMA 1995;274:1363, NEJM 1995;332:977, NEJM 1985;312:1205)
- 1–3 alcoholic drinks qd for men (NEJM 2003;348:109, Ann IM 1991;114:967); 2–3/wk for women (NEJM 1995;332:1245)
- Better control of hypertension, cholesterol, etc., in the United States (NEJM 1985;312:1005, NEJM 1985;312:1053)

Risk stratification is essential for decision-making regarding proper site of care (telemetry, CCU, transfer to other facility) as well as medical therapies and invasive approaches (timing and necessity of cardiac cath).

- TIMI Risk Score for UA/NSTEMI (JAMA 2000;284:835): increased risk with higher score; 1 point for each of the following.
  - Age older than 65
  - At least three risk factors for CAD
  - Prior coronary stenosis greater than 50%
  - ST segment deviation on EKG
  - At least two anginal events over past 24 hr
  - Use of ASA in past 7 d
  - Elevated serum cardiac markers
- Online model available at www.cardiology.org/tools
- GRACE risk model: score based on age, prior cardiac history, HR, blood pressure, ST-segment depression, serum creatinine, and cardiac enzymes; online calculator available at www.outcomes-umassmed.org/grace

Pathophys: Imbalance between myocardial oxygen supply and demand, mainly due to thrombus formation on an eroded plaque (or embolism from upstream source), but also vasospasm or arterial dissection; "secondary" ACS (aka demand myocardial ischemia) in which a noncardiac cause leads to increased myocardial stress (via fever, tachycardia), reduced coronary blood flow (systemic hypotension), or reduced oxygen delivery (severe anemia, hypoxemia).

Sx: Classic sx: chest pain/pressure (arm pain, jaw pain), dyspnea, nausea, diaphoresis; extreme fatigue a common presenting sign in elderly pts.

Sx that suggest noncardiac cause of pain: pleuritic pain, pain in mid to low abdomen or radiating to legs, pain reproduced with movement or palpation.

Responsiveness to NTG is not diagnostic of cardiac cause of chest pain: 35% of pts with chest pain and subsequently proven CAD had relief with NTG, vs 41% without evidence of CAD (Ann IM 2003;139:979); nor is response to "GI cocktail" (JAMA 2005;294:2623).

No recognizable sx ("silent") in approximately 25% of pts (Ann IM 2001;135:801; Ann IM 2001;134:1043), yet prognosis just as bad (Framingham, NEJM 1984;311:1144).

Si: S_4; mitral regurgitant murmur during pain.

Crs: ST depressions of greater than 1 mm especially those lasting more than 60 min at rest or asx are associated with an MI within 6 mo in 15% of the cases even when medically treated (NEJM 1986;314:1214).

Cmplc: Common and uncommon complications of MI include the following.

- Aneurysm of left ventricle: develops in first 48 hr; leads to emboli, CHF, and PVCs; 60% 1-yr mortality (NEJM 1984;311:100), though rate may be lower now with thrombolysis.
- Arrhythmias, especially PVCs and ventricular tachycardia, can occur.
- CHF (see Section 1.2).
- Dressler's syndrome: a delayed post-MI/CABG pericarditis (see Section 1.4).
- Heart block (MCCVD 1976;45:129) occurs in 5% of inferior MIs, 3% of anterior MIs, and 100% with anterior MI plus RBBB, causing a 75% mortality.
- Mural thrombi (with associated risk for embolism) can occur, especially with anterior MI (J Am Coll Cardiol 1993;22:1004).
- Papillary muscle rupture causes CHF with a normal-sized left atrium by echocardiogram; occurs most often with inferior MIs (NEJM 1969;281:1458).
- Pericardial tamponade from inflammation: r/o RV infarct, because both functionally constrict pericardial space acutely by fluid or dilated RV (NEJM 1983;309:551).
- Rupture of septal wall, usually on day 3 to 5, creates a ventricular septal defect (Circ 2000;101:27; NEJM 2002;347:1426)

that must be repaired asap; ruptures into pericardial sack, causing tamponade (NEJM 1996;334:319).

- Shock (7.5%) (NEJM 1991;325:1117): immediate revascularization improves survival (JAMA 2001;285:190).
- Stroke, especially if EF is less than 28% post-MI (NEJM 1997;336:251): prevent with warfarin anticoagulation.

Lab: Routine lab w/u: CBC with plt/diff; metabolic panel, +/− LFTs; cardiac enzymes (CPK, CK-MB, troponin); PT/PTT; fasting lipids, glucose within 24 hr.

Troponin (I or T, depending on your lab) has become the most utilized and important test; 30% of pts with ACS and neg CPK/CK-MB will be diagnosed with NSTEMI based on pos troponin assays (Circ 2006;114:790).

Non-ACS causes of elevated troponins include:

- Severe tachycardia: atrial fibrillation or other PSVT
- Left ventricular hypertrophy (LVH)
- Cardiac intervention: post-PCI, CABG
- Chest trauma
- Acute pericarditis, myocarditis
- CHF
- Acute intracranial hemorrhage or stroke
- Sepsis, acute respiratory failure, critical illness
- Burns
- Pulmonary embolism
- Severe pulmonary hypertension
- Chronic kidney failure

CK-MB still has utility because of shorter half-life than TnI, so may be useful in diagnosing recurrent infarcts (with persistently elevated TnI).

Myoglobin has fastest peak, but is rarely used in clinical practice (troponins are usually detected within 2 hr of injury).

Noninv: EKG: asap on arrival and with continued sx to look for progression or change over time.

- Normal EKG: Does normal EKG with chest pain rule out ACS? ER study of 387 pts with chest pain dx and normal EKG at time of analysis, analyzed by presence or absence of chest pain during the EKG analysis; 17% (67/387) subsequently ruled in for ACS by cardiac markers, stress testing, and/or greater than 70% stenosis on cath; no difference between pts with chest pain (16%) or without chest pain (20%) during normal EKG (Acad Emerg Med 2009;16:495).
- Nonspecific EKG changes: ST-segment deviation less than 0.5 mm or T wave abnormalities; look for Wellens' syndrome (deep anterior T wave inversions, severe left anterior descending or left main lesions on cath); but also can be seen in noncardiac conditions including stroke and other acute intracranial abnormalities, cholecystitis, drug effects (TCAs, phenothiazines).
- Q waves: Presence of significant Q's useful as sign of prior MI/CAD, but not diagnostic for ACS; differentiate from non-significant Q waves, by the following criteria:
  - Presence in two or more contiguous leads
  - Depth more than one-third the height of the corresponding R wave
  - Width more than 40 msec
- ST depressions: The most likely finding, with pain, in UA/NSTEMI.
  - Diff dx of ST depression: myocardial ischemia, LV strain in LVH (meets other criteria for LVH), reciprocal changes from STEMI, digoxin effect
- ST elevations: More than 2mm elevations in two or more contiguous leads, indication for thrombolysis or emergent PCI.
  - Inferior: II, III, aV_F
  - Anteroseptal: V_1–V_2; if ST elevation in V_1, consider RV infarct and get right-sided EKG to look for ST elevation in V_{3R}–V_{6R}

Test	Protocol	Positive Result	Comments	Estimated Sensitivity (%)	Estimated Specificity (%)
Standard treadmill or bicycle exercise	Patient able to perform adequate amount of physical activity Baseline ECG is normal or near normal (e.g., minimal ST-segment depression) Should not be used if patient has left-bundle-branch block or electronic pacemaker	New horizontal or down-sloping ST-segment depression ≥1 mm or ≥2 mm in presence of baseline repolarization abnormality	Blood-pressure response, exercise duration, ventricular arrhythmias, Duke treadmill score, and heart rate recovery should also be assessed Functional capacity and Duke treadmill score have significant prognostic value	65–70	70–75
Exercise stress echocardiography	Patient able to perform physical activity Two-dimensional echocardiogram immediately after exercise	One or more new segmental wall-motion abnormalities (hypokinesis, akinesis, or dyskinesis), left ventricular dilation, or both	Useful for abnormal baseline ECG (should not be used if patient has left-bundle-branch block or electronic pacemaker) Technically high-quality echocardiogram is essential	80–85	80–85
Dobutamine stress echocardiography	For patients unable to exercise adequately with or without abnormal ECG Incremental dobutamine infusion	Inducible segmental left ventricular wall-motion abnormalities, worsening of existing wall-motion abnormalities, or left ventricular dilation	Technically high-quality echocardiogram is essential	80–85	85–90

Exercise myocardial perfusion SPECT, with quantitative analysis	For patients able to perform physical activity Should be used when results of baseline ECG preclude assessment of ischemia (e.g., nonspecific ST-T changes) Can be used in patients with left-bundle-branch block or electronic pacemaker	Inducible single or multiple perfusion abnormalities; left ventricular dilation	Also can provide information on left ventricular function and wall motion	85–90	85–90
Pharmacologic myocardial perfusion SPECT, with quantitative analysis	For patients unable to exercise adequately Intravenous adenosine or dipyridamole Can be used in patients with left-bundle-branch block or electronically paced rhythm	Provides information similar to that provided by exercise SPECT		80–90	80–90
Electron-beam computed tomography	Calcium score closely correlates with extent of coronary atherosclerosis	If score is >100, consider follow-up stress test	Cannot predict coronary obstructions or detect vulnerable plaque or degree of stenosis Poor specificity	—	—

* Estimates of sensitivity and specificity are derived from multiple databases and from the chronic stable angina guidelines of the American College of Cardiology and the American Heart Association. The sensitivity, specificity, and predictive accuracy of all noninvasive stress-testing methods are influenced by age, sex, degree of coronary atherosclerosis, and, most important, the likelihood of coronary artery disease in the patient being tested. ECG denotes electrocardiogram, and SPECT single-photon-emission computed tomography.

Figure 1.1 Stress Testing Procedures

Reproduced with permission from Abrams J. Chronic stable angina. *NEJM.* 2005;352:2524. Copyright © 2005, Massachusetts Medical Society. All rights reserved.

- Anterior: V_3–V_4
- Anterolateral: V_5–V_6
- Posterior: R greater than S with ST depression in V_1 (diff dx of strong R-force in V_1: posterior MI, RBBB, RVH, WPW, lead misplacement, dextrocardia)
- Diff dx of ST elevation: acute myocardial injury, pericarditis (diffuse), myocarditis, early repolarization (especially in young males, look for old EKG to compare or follow serially to show no change), LV aneurysm (persistent ST elevation post-MI), WPW
- LBBB: Approach new LBBB in ACS similar to STEMI.
  - Look for old EKG asap to assess if new changes.
  - Difficult to assess for new MI in setting of chronic LBBB (Am Hrt J 1988;116:23).
    - Septal MI: new septal Q in aV_L or R in V_1; Q or late notching of S wave in two or more of V_3–V_5
    - Any area MI: new evolving ST segment or T wave changes
  - Pts with unchanged EKG have lower risk of MI and in-hospital mortality (NEJM 1985;312:1137).

CXR: R/o other causes of chest pain (pneumonia, pneumothorax, rib fx), but also r/o mediastinal widening (due to thoracic aneurysm) prior to giving thrombolytics or anticoagulants.

Echocardiogram: Evaluate LV function, look for mitral regurg, LV aneurysm, wall-motion abnormalities to suggest ischemia or mural thrombus.

Stress Testing: In cases of chest pain, uncertain cause, or unstable angina, can move to stress testing asap to help in diagnosis and decision-making re further invasive testing (cardiac cath); in pts with NSTEMI and STEMI, necessity and timing depend on multiple factors, determined after consultation with cardiology; see **Figure 1.1** for common tests used.

Rx: Therapies that follow focus primarily on rx of possible/probable ACS, UA, NSTEMI. Acute STEMI therapy, in most cases, involves early intervention with thrombolysis and/or PCI, more in the realm of ER and cardiology. See **Table 1.1** for overview of evaluation and therapies.

Anti-ischemic therapy

- Bed rest, reduced activity
- Supplemental oxygen therapy, especially if SaO_2 is less than 90%
- Nitrates
  - Reduce myocardial oxygen demand (afterload reduction, antihypertensive) and increase delivery (coronary artery dilation).
  - Give sublingual NTG 0.4 mg q 5 min up to three doses (or NTG spray).
  - If no relief, IV NTG; start at 10 mcg/min, titrate to pain relief, and keep SBP greater than 100–110 mmHg.
  - Transdermal NTG is helpful if mild persistent anginal sx, and for antihypertensive effect, but in urgent situations IV NTG will allow for better BP control and titration.
  - Avoid NTG in any form with recent use of sildenafil (Viagra) or similar meds within 24–48 hr, as it can precipitate life-threatening hypotension; study of IV NTG use in stable CAD pts showed average drop of SBP and DBP by 8–12 mmHg (Crit Care Med 2007;35:1863); other interventions are safe and suggest morphine or beta-blockers as appropriate anti-ischemic therapy; if nitrates are felt to be crucial, closely monitor BP response.
  - Give oral nitrates (isosorbide mononitrate and dinitrate) in chronic stable angina for sx and BP control.
  - Although helpful for sx control, there is no evidence of improved mortality with nitroglycerin in any form.

Table 1.1 Overview of ACS Evaluation and Acute and Chronic Therapy

	Low Risk	Moderate Risk	High Risk
Includes	• "Rule out MI" patients • Pain-free after initial presentation; no acute EKG changes; normal cardiac enzymes	• True ACS (mostly unstable angina) • Pain-free after rx; some EKG changes; normal or borderline elevated cardiac enzymes	• True ACS (unstable angina and NSTEMI) • Persistent or recurrent pain; EKG changes (ST depression, nonsignificant elevation, T-wave abnormalities); elevated cardiac enzymes)
Admission	• Consider outpatient evaluation in some patients • Observation admission for facilitated stress testing	• Inpatient admission	• Inpatient admission • In some settings, may require transfer to tertiary center for early invasive rx
Antiplatelet Rx	• ASA 325 mg on arrival and qd • Consider UFH/LMWH based on individual factors	• ASA 325 mg on arrival and qd • UFH or LMWH at therapeutic doses	• ASA 325 mg on arrival and qd • UFH/LMWH (UFH better choice if planning on early invasive strategy) • Clopidogrel 300 mg loading dose, then 75 mg qd (unless plan or at risk for early CABG) • Consider G IIb/IIIa inhibitors in pts with continued pain despite optimal therapies

Other Acute Rx	• NTG for pain and BP control (usually transdermal) • Beta-blockers in pts with HTN, tachycardia, but avoid in most, especially if planning on early treadmill testing	• NTG for pain and BP control (usually transdermal) • Beta-blockers in pts with HTN, tachycardia; individual factors will guide in others • Statin rx based on lipid testing	• NTG for pain and BP control (usually IV) • Beta-blockers in most, unless contraindications (bradycardia, hypotension, concern for early or frank cardiogenic shock)
Studies	• Serial cardiac enzymes and EKG • Noninvasive stress testing in most settings • Consider cardiac cath in pts with abnormal stress testing	• Serial cardiac enzymes and EKG • Noninvasive stress testing vs early cardiac cath • Consider echocardiogram • Consider cardiac cath in pts with abnormal stress testing	• Serial cardiac enzymes and EKG • Early invasive strategy with cardiac cath
Discharge Meds	• Depends on stress results; if nonischemic, may require no further therapies; if ischemic, treat as moderate-high risk patients • Risk factor modification • Consider statins for pts with CAD or strong family hx	• ASA 81–325 mg qd • Clopidogrel 75 mg qd, particularly if poststent or NSTEMI pts on medical mgt • Beta-blocker rx • ACEI for patients with LVEF <40% • Risk factor modification • Statins in most patients (goal LDL <70)	• ASA 81–325 mg qd • Clopidogrel 75 mg qd, particularly if poststent or NSTEMI pts on medical mgt • Beta-blocker rx • ACEI for patients with LVEF <40% • Risk factor modification • Statins in most patients (goal LDL <70)

- Morphine:
  - Give 1–5 mg IV initial and repeat doses.
  - Likely works by venodilation, reduced HR and BP, as well as direct analgesia.
  - Helpful for pain control unrelieved by NTG, and dyspnea in pts with pulmonary edema.
  - Watch for hypotensive effects; if BP drops, rx with IV fluid boluses and Trendelenburg positioning.
  - Can be a respiratory depressant; if severe, reverse with IV naloxone 0.4–2 mg.
  - As with NTG, no direct evidence of mortality benefit, but still clinically useful in many situations.
- Beta-blockers:
  - Reduce myocardial contractility, HR, BP.
  - In acute setting, consider for pts with continued pain, especially with tachycardia and hypertension.
  - Acute therapy: metoprolol 5 mg IV q 5 min for three doses; follow HR and BP between doses; then can start oral doses of 25–50 mg q 6–8 hr, depending on BP and HR response.
  - Although some still use acute beta-blockade in all ACS pts, utility and safety now under question with newer studies:
    - COMMIT study: Involved more than 45,000 pts in ER with acute MI, randomized to immediate IV and then PO metoprolol vs placebo until hospital discharge (or up to 4 wk); no difference between groups in primary outcomes of death or death/reinfarction; beta-blockade did reduce risk of reinfarction (2.0% vs 2.5%, NNT 200) and ventricular fibrillation (2.5% vs 3.0%, NNT 200), but increased the risk of cardiogenic shock (5.0% vs 3.9%, NNH 91) (Lancet 2005;366:1622).
    - Caution with use in ACS acutely, if presence of hypotension, CHF sx, conduction abnormalities.

- Early beta-blocker use (in ER) was prior CMS core measure for quality, but dropped after concerns for increased mortality with widespread use and studies.
- Major side effects include hypotension, bradycardia, worsening acute systolic heart failure, acute bronchospasm.
- Chronic therapy, though, especially in post-MI pts, has shown consistent, proven mortality benefit; all ACS pts should be discharged on beta-blocker therapy, unless clear contraindication (severe bradyarrhythmia, orthostasis, severe bronchospasm).
- In pts with low-risk ACS and plan for early stress testing, avoid beta-blockade if plan includes treadmill testing (attenuation of tachycardic response may lead to false negative test).
- Patient discharge on beta-blocker therapy after AMI (STEMI and NSTEMI) is a CMS core measure for quality; must document clear contraindication to use if pt is not discharged on beta-blocker.
- Calcium channel blockers:
  - Reduces myocardial contractility, HR, BP.
    - Nifedipine and amlodopine have antihypertensive effect, but no effect on AV/sinus node (and therefore, no direct effect on HR).
    - Verapamil and diltiazem have significant AV/sinus node effect, and some antihypertensive effect as well.
  - Helpful in pts with continued anginal sx, after primary therapies, especially with tachycardia and hypertension (similar indications to beta-blocker therapy, would use as alternative to beta-blockers in pts with prior intolerance or acute bronchospasm).
  - Avoid in pts with bradycardia, hypotension, acute systolic CHF, or severe LV dysfunction.
  - Avoid sublingual nifedipine in this setting, because of increased mortality due to significant hypotensive effects.

- Although some studies have shown reduced morbidity and mortality with acute CCB use (DAVIT, Eur Heart J 1984;5:516; DRS, NEJM 1986;315:423), meta-analysis has not shown benefit (Clin Cardiol 1998;21:633; BMJ 1989;299:1187).

Antiplatelet and anticoagulant therapies

- Aspirin:
  - Blocks cyclo-oxygenase to prevent plt activity.
  - Dose: 81–325 mg qd is acceptable.
  - VA Co-op study (NEJM 1983;309:396): 12 wk of 324 mg ASA vs placebo in unstable angina; reduced risk of death/nonfatal MI by 51% (NNT ~20).
  - Swedish study (J Am Coll Cardiol 1991;18:1587): 75 mg dose, 0.52 risk ratio at 1 yr.
  - Canadian study (NEJM 1985;313:1369): 325 mg qid; 51% RRR (NNT ~12) for death/nonfatal MI at 18–24 mo.
  - Avoid if active GI bleeding; but for high-risk pts consider GI protection with H2B or PPI.
  - ASA therapy within 24 hr of arrival for AMI is a CMS core measure for quality; must document clear contraindication to use if pt is not started on ASA in this setting.
- Clopidogrel (Plavix):
  - Reduces platelet activity by non-cyclo-oxygenase mechanism.
  - 75 mg qd; consider 300 mg one-time oral loading dose.
  - CAPRIE study: RCT of more than 19,000 pts, randomized to clopidogrel 75 mg qd vs ASA 325 mg qd; small but significant reduction in composite end point of stroke, MI, vascular death in clopidgrel pts (5.3% vs 5.8%, NNT 200) (Lancet 1996;348:1329).
  - CURE study (Circ 2004;110:1202): 3–12 mo of clopidogrel plus ASA reduced risk of composite end point of death/MI/stroke (9.3% vs 11.5%, NNT 45), but at the expense

of increased incidence of major bleeding (3.7% vs 2.7%, NNH 100); results similar for pts with medical therapy only vs PCI vs CABG.

- Consider avoiding if pt likely to need CABG during initial hospitalization because of perioperative bleeding; high risk for CABG would be diabetes, EKG or clinical sx suggestive of multivessel or left main disease.
- Clopidogrel is the primary alternative antiplatelet agent in pts allergic to ASA.
- Good additional med (with ASA) for up to 3–12 mo post-UA/NSTEMI in pts not deemed candidates for further interventions.
- Clear indication for use after PTCA with stent; bare metal stents for at least 1 month, preferably up to 1 year; drug-eluting stents for at least a year due to concerns for early stent thrombosis.

- Heparin, including unfractionated heparin (UFH) and low-molecular-weight heparin (LMWH):
  - Should be initiated asap in pts with ACS, either as IV UFH with loading bolus or SQ LMWH based on dosing guidelines for specific med; for example, enoxaparin (Lovenox), 1 mg/kg SQ q 12 hr.
  - Meta-analyses of smaller studies support use in ACS (Circ 2007;116:e148).
    - Combination of four smaller studies of UFH vs ASA alone in 999 pts reduced risk of death or recurrent MI by 53% (2.6% vs 5.5%, NNT 35).
    - Combination of six studies to include LMWH or UFH vs ASA in 2629 pts reduced risk of death or recurrent MI by 62% (2.0% vs 5.3%, NNT 30).
  - Which alternative (UFH or LMWH) is better?
    - Multiple studies have compared them, but due to different meds and protocols, it is difficult to assess completely; pooled studies of enoxaparin vs UFH showed

improved outcomes mainly driven by reduced risk of nonfatal MI with LMWHs.
- LMWH is often preferred because of ease of dosing and monitoring, especially in lower-risk settings ("r/o MI" pts awaiting stress testing).
- UFH may be better if the plan is for early invasive strategy (PTCA or CABG) because of ability to rapidly titrate off the anticoagulant effect.
- UFH initially dosed on weight-based protocols, then per frequent monitoring of PTT.
- LMWH does not require bolus, but use weight-based dosing; monitoring of anti-Factor Xa activity not required in ACS setting.
- Monitor for bleeding and thrombocytopenia (typically noted after 4 d of use, unless prior exposure to heparin with true HIT syndrome); can reverse UFH-associated bleeding with protamine, no specific reversal agent for LMWH.
- In pts with prior history of HIT or significant drop in plt on therapy, can use direct thrombin inhibitor, argatroban.
- Continued use for 48 hr to up to 5 d.
- Fondaparinux:
  - Direct Factor Xa inhibitor
  - Similar effect to LMWH (enoxaparin) in reducing short-term death and MI in ACS pts based on OASIS-5 trial (NEJM 2006;354:1464), with reduced risk of bleeding events (2.2% vs 4.1%, NNT 53).
  - Suitable alternative in ACS, but not used widely due to less substantial evidence.
  - No risk of thrombocytopenia (most appropriate choice in ACS pts with prior hx of HIT); no reversal agent for acute bleeding
- Warfarin:
  - Has no benefit in acute treatment of ACS because of delayed onset of action.

- Smaller studies have shown possible longer-term benefit in ACS pts, but most trials showed no benefit of adding warfarin to aspirin in ACS pts for long-term therapy.
- Warfarin should be used in setting of another clear indication (e.g., atrial fibrillation, mechanical heart valve), but few trials have looked at the safety or efficacy of "triple therapy" with ASA, clopidogrel, and warfarin in acute or chronic settings.
- Glycoprotein IIb/IIIa inhibitor:
  - Includes abciximab, eptifibatide, tirofiban; all IV infusions.
  - Most evidence surrounds use in peri-PCI time frame.
  - Meta-analysis of six large RCTs for glycoprotein IIb/IIIa inhibitors in ACS pts not taken for early revascularization shows reduced risk of death or MI at 30 d (10.8% vs 11.8%, NNT 100), but with equivalent increased risk of major bleeding over placebo (2.4% vs 1.4%, NNH 100) (Lancet 2002;359:189).
  - Would not use as routine strategy in ACS along with other agents, unless pt shows early recurrent ischemic symptoms, awaiting intervention.

Invasive vs conservative strategy regarding angiography and revascularization

- There is considerable hospital and regional variation in decisions re necessity or timing of PTCA in ACS (although widely utilized in STEMI as soon as possible); much of the decision-making here is likely dictated by local hospital practice.
- Invasive strategy usually denotes angiography within 4–24 hr (although some argue for immediate angiography, within 4 hr); conservative strategy delays angiography unless pts fail medical therapy, with persistent or recurrent anginal symptoms or ischemic changes on EKG or noninvasive testing.

- Many studies have significant rates of angiography in the conservative arms, and the main difference in the two populations is the time to angiogram and PTCA.
- Trials suggesting similar outcomes with either strategy include these:
  - TIMI IIIB: 1473 pts randomized to invasive vs conservative rx (also coincident study of thrombolytics in UA/NSTEMI, which showed no benefit); similar rates of composite end point of death/recurrent MI/abnormal stress test at 6 wk, but invasive approach did decrease LOS and readmission rates (Circ 1994;89:1545).
  - MAT trial: 201 pts randomized to invasive vs conservative rx; early invasive group did have reduced death and recurrent MI in-hospital (13% vs 34%, NNT 5), but outcomes did not sustain at long-term follow-up of up to 21 mo (J Am Coll Cardiol 1998;32:596).
  - VANQWISH study: 920 VA pts with ACS; no difference in death and/or recurrent MI between the two strategies (NEJM 1998;338:1785).
- Trials suggesting benefit of early invasive approach include these:
  - Meta-analysis of seven trials: More than 9200 pts with ACS; early invasive strategy reduced death/recurrent MI (12.2% vs 14.4%, NNT 45), but also suggested a higher in-hospital early mortality risk (1.8% vs 1.1%, NNH 142) (compare to MAT trial above with opposite results); pts at high risk with pos cardiac markers have more benefit from early invasive approach (JAMA 2005;293:2908).
  - Meta-analysis of seven trials: More than 8300 pts with NSTEMI; early invasive approach reduced 2-yr mortality (NNT 63) and recurrent MI (NNT 67), as well as recurrent hospitalization for unstable angina (J Am Coll Cardiol 2006;48:1319).

Secondary prevention and other considerations

- Medical therapy:
  - ASA for everyone, lifelong, 81–325 mg qd
    - This is a CMS core measure for quality for pts discharged with AMI.
  - Clopidogrel as above for poststenting pts and some pts with noninvasive strategy for NSTEMI
  - Beta-blockers for everyone, lifelong, as above
    - This is a CMS core measure for quality for pts discharged with AMI.
    - Use CCBs as alternative if beta-blockers not tolerated.
  - ACE inhibitors, lifelong, for post-AMI pts with LV dysfunction (EF less than 40%)
    - This is a CMS core measure for quality for pts discharged with AMI.
    - Also consider strongly in AMI pts with HTN or DM (even if preserved LV function).
  - Nitroglycerin preparations for sx (angina) control
- Lipid management:
  - Consider statin therapy in all post-MI pts regardless of baseline cholesterol.
    - A 2008 meta-analysis of statins in approximately 20,000 pts older than 65 showed significant reductions in all mortality (NNT 28), CHD mortality (NNT 34), nonfatal MI (NNT 38), and stroke (NNT 58) (J Am Coll Cardiol 2008;51:37).
    - A meta-analysis of 121,000 pts showed that statins reduced all-cause mortality by 12% (NNT 89) and CV mortality by 19% (Am J Med 2008;121:24).
  - Strive for goal of LDL less than 100 mg/dL (possibly less than 70 mg/dL).
  - Consider addition of niacin or fibrate if triglycerides are greater than 500 mg/dL.

- Consider addition of fish oil supplements: GISSI-HF trial for pts with CHF is described in Section 1.2 (Lancet 2008;372:1223); prevent future cardiovascular and sudden death in post-MI (Lancet 1999;354:447).
- BP control per JNC 7 guidelines: lower than 140/90 mmHg or lower than 130/80 mmHg if DM or CKD
- DM control with medical mgt to get HbA1c below 7%
- Smoking cessation:
  - Counseling for smoking cessation, in pts with any tobacco use within the past year, prior to discharge is a CMS core measure for quality in pts with AMI.
- Diet and exercise to maintain BMI of 18–25 kg/m^2
- Influenza vaccination if proper time frame
- Avoid NSAIDs, especially COX-2 inhibitors (celecoxib, rofecoxib), in acute setting and chronic long-term use due to concerns for increased risk of MI, death (Circ 2007;115:1634)
- Avoid postmenopausal hormone therapy

1.2 Congestive Heart Failure

(NEJM 2003;348:2007; J Am Coll Cardiol 2009;53:e1)

Cause: In the United States, most CHF is due to ASCVD, either as ongoing ischemia or due to prior MI; other causes include dilated cardiomyopathy from viral syndrome (see "Myocarditis" in Section 1.4 for other infectious causes), alcohol abuse, chemotherapeutic agents, postpartum, hemochromatosis; valvular disease (AS, MR), congenital heart disease; chronic hypertension, infiltrative diseases (amyloid, sarcoid), pericardial disease; rare "high-output" CHF from hyperthyroidism, large AV fistula, beriberi, severe anemia.

The American College of Cardiology (ACC) and the American Heart Association (AHA) have identified four stages of heart failure:

- Stage A: "At risk" for heart failure, including pts with CAD, HTN, or DM
- Stage B: Heart disease without si/sx of CHF, including prior MI, asymptomatic valvular disease, and cardiomyopathy
- Stage C: Heart disease with si/sx of CHF; most of the hospitalized population
- Stage D: Refractory or "end-stage" CHF

The New York Heart Association (NYHA) classification is helpful for prognosis and defining sx (but can change significantly over short periods with adjustment of therapies or complications):

- Class I: No dyspnea with moderate exertion
- Class II: Dyspnea with moderate exertion
- Class III: Dyspnea with mild exertion
- Class IV: Dyspnea at rest

Epidem: Incidence of 10 per 1000 persons older than 65 in the United States; factor in 20% of all hospital admissions of pts older than 65.

Increased mortality in the 1st month after hospitalization for CHF (Circ 2007;116:1482).

Pathophys: Complex interplay of structural heart disease and neurohormonal involvement of renin-angiotensin-aldosterone system, natriuretic peptides, and sympathetic nervous system leading to LV remodeling.

Important distinction is determination of type of CHF, as follows:

- Systolic dysfunction (NEJM 2010;362:228): Associated with "pump failure," LV dysfunction; imaging studies reveal reduced LV ejection fraction (less than 50%); accounts for most (up to 70%) of CHF and is the basis for much of the research and evidence on rx of CHF.
- Diastolic dysfunction (NEJM 2004;351:1097): "Stiff" LV from various causes (most common is chronic HTN, but also constrictive pericarditis, IHSS, restrictive cardiomyopathies, mitral

stenosis, atrial fibrillation with rapid ventricular response) prevents proper diastolic LV filling; preserved EF on imaging, but may be evidence on echo consistent w/ diastolic dysfunction; accounts for about 30% of CHF (higher in elderly), but may be more prevalent as increasingly recognized as important.

- Some pts have evidence of both types concomitantly.
- Determination of systolic vs diastolic dysfunction as well as acute vs chronic presentation is essential for proper billing and coding of hospital stay.

Sx: Common sx include dyspnea (at rest or with exertion), orthopnea, paroxysmal nocturnal dyspnea; nocturia; cough, productive of "frothy" sputum; chest pain/pressure (in setting of CAD); dizziness/presyncope (if low cardiac output).

Si: Common si include weight gain; peripheral edema; elevated JVP, hepatojugular reflex, displaced PMI; tachycardia is common especially in exacerbations.

Cardiac gallop also present: S_3 (usually with systolic) or S_4 (usually with diastolic); murmurs to suggest mitral regurgitation, aortic stenosis.

Crackles/rales detected on lung auscultation; employ percussion for effusion.

Hypoxemia determined by pulse oximetry or direct ABG assessment.

Crs: Symptomatic CHF has a 3-yr mortality of 41% in pts younger than 65, and 66% in pts older than 65, although may be improving with more widespread use of effective therapies (J Am Coll Cardiol 2000;36:2284).

Cmplc: Atrial fibrillation is common, probably due to LV remodeling, concomitant mitral regurgitation, and subsequent atrial enlargement; seen in both systolic (Circ 2003;107:2920) and diastolic CHF (J Am Coll Cardiol 2002;40:1636).

Higher risk for VTE, especially when hospitalized for exacerbations.

Sudden death is 6 to 9 times higher in CHF pts due to multiple causes, including ventricular arrhythmias, MI, PE.

Lab: Initial lab w/u in setting of pt with dyspnea: CBC with diff, electrolytes, BUN/Cr, serum glucose, cardiac enzymes with troponin, brain natriuretic peptide (BNP).

Consider D-dimer if concern for PE; consider ABGs in setting of respiratory failure; consider PT/PTT if bleeding risks or pt on chronic anticoagulation; consider digoxin level if pt on chronic therapy.

In cases of unexplained cardiomyopathy, consider iron studies to r/o hemochromatosis, as well as TSH, HIV, rheum panel, serum titers for *Treponema cruzi* (Chagas disease) based on history and risk factors.

For inpatients, consider daily assessment of electrolytes, BUN/Cr, which may fluctuate with therapies.

Are BNP levels helpful in the dx and rx of CHF? (NEJM 2008;358:2148)

- Evaluation of BNP in presumed or known CHF is an evolving field.
- BNP is a peptide (formed from the precursor NT-pro-BNP, which is also measured in some labs) released in response to hemodynamic stress related to ventricular dilatation; has natural effects of vasodilation, diuresis, and antagonism of the RAA system.
- Levels normally rise with age and are affected by any stressor that affects the ventricles, including elevated pulmonary artery pressures related to acute PE, COPD with cor pulmonale, pulmonary hypertension; cleared by the kidneys, so may be elevated in pts with acute and chronic renal failure.
- Most useful in the evaluation of pts with dyspnea to assess for possible CHF as the culprit.
  - Breathing Not Properly study: 1586 ER pts with dyspnea of uncertain etiology had BNP levels drawn and were then

independently evaluated for cause of sx; BNP had a negative predictive value of 96% at 50 ng/mL to rule out CHF as cause of sx (NEJM 2002;347:161).

- Assessment of BNP may also lead to faster diagnosis and institution of therapy in CHF pts, reducing hospital LOS and morbidity (Circ 2007;115:3103).

- Mixed results on the benefit of BNP-guided therapy for CHF (vs standard symptom-based); STARS-BNP trial showed decrease in CHF-related death and hospitalization (J Am Coll Cardiol 2007 49:1733); TIME-CHF trial did not show improved outcomes with similar strategy (JAMA 2009;301:383).

- Meta-analysis of 8 trials of BNP-guided CHF therapy for outpatients showed a reduction in mortality (RR 0.76) with BNP-guided rx, especially in pts younger than 75; however, no reductions in hospitalization rates; analysis of med use showed that BNP-guided therapy led to more use and titration of appropriate meds (ACEI, beta-blockers) (Arch IM 2010; 170:507).

- No studies have evaluated BNP-guided therapy for acute CHF exacerbations in the hospital, so unclear if it is helpful to measure BNP levels serially or near hospital discharge to assess for "baseline" levels; one study showed that a high BNP level (greater than 700 ng/L) was an independent predictor of death and readmission, but unclear if further adjustment to therapy could affect those outcomes or if it is just a predictor of severe disease.

Measurement of troponin levels in acute exacerbations of CHF:

- Mild elevations in cardiac troponins are common in pts with severe CHF and not necessarily indicative of active ischemia; 49% of pts with severe CHF awaiting cardiac transplant had elevated TnI in one study (Circ 2003;108:833).

- Poor prognosis is associated with pos levels: according to national registry data of pts with acute CHF and creatinine less than 2.0 mg/dL, 6% had (+) TnI or TnT, associated with lower blood pressure, lower EF, and higher in-pt mortality (NEJM 2008;358:2117).
- Determination of need for ischemic w/u depends on pts sx, EKG and serial enzyme measurement, and goals of therapy.

Noninv: CXR to look for pulmonary edema, effusions, cardiomegaly.

EKG to assess cardiac rhythm, presence of conduction abnormalities (LBBB), evidence of acute or prior CAD/ischemia.

Echocardiogram for multiple reasons.

- Assessment of LV function to diagnose CHF or determine type (systolic vs diastolic):
  - Assessment of LVEF is a CMS core measure for quality care of CHF; all pts with discharge dx of CHF need some prior assessment of LVEF (by echo, nuclear imaging, or cardiac cath), although not necessarily during that hospitalization.
  - Once dx of CHF is established, repeat echocardiograms do not need to be done regularly or with each exacerbation, unless concern for acute change in underlying disease (e.g., worsening valvular disease, new ischemic event).
- Evidence of CAD, prior MI by wall motion abnormalities
- Evidence of underlying valvular or congenital heart disease
- Rule out other causes of dyspnea: RV failure/strain associated with chronic lung disease or PE; pericardial effusion or thickening

Stress testing including nuclear imaging or cardiac catheterization can be considered in these cases:

- New dx of CHF/cardiomyopathy to r/o underlying ischemic disease that may require therapy
- New ischemic sx in setting of chronic heart failure
- Acute exacerbation of CHF with evidence of worsening EF, but repeat testing not required with each exacerbation per se

Rx: Largely depends on the type and presentation of heart failure; most studies of rx are focused on systolic CHF.

Rx of diastolic dysfunction focuses on the following:

- BP and HR control (especially if concomitant AF)
- Evaluation and rx of myocardial ischemia
- Rx of volume overload (similar to systolic dysfunction)

Main approach to inpatient rx of systolic CHF has four components:

1. Assessment of perfusion and rx of low CO
2. Assessment of volume status and rx of volume overload
3. Recognition and prevention of complications
4. Adjustment of chronic therapies to improve mortality and reduce hospitalizations

Assessment of perfusion and rx of low CO

- Probably the most critical assessment in the emergent setting.
- Most evaluation based on vital signs (BP and HR) and physical assessment of perfusion (pulses; skin assessment for mottling, cyanosis; capillary refill).
- Invasive monitoring can include the following:
  - Central line access and assessment of CVP: Often used, but very limited clinical efficacy in pts with CHF as CVP measurements are often high, even in setting of cardiogenic shock, and unreliable due to multiple causes.
  - In cases of CHF with cardiogenic shock, consider placement of PA catheter to measure PCWP (usually more than 18 mmHg in cardiogenic pulmonary edema; less than 18 suggests ARDS/noncardiogenic cause) and help to guide fluid and pressor management (NEJM 2005;353:2788).
- Do not confuse low blood pressure (common in many elderly pts with CHF and on chronic antihypertensive therapies) without si/sx of shock with true cardiogenic shock; base

assessment on evidence of end-organ involvement (low urine output, active cardiac ischemia, delirium/coma).

- Rx of cardiogenic shock includes the following:
  - Initial rapid treatment may require fluid boluses to boost BP, but may also require further ventilatory control (NPPV or intubation) if fluid resuscitation worsens pulmonary edema.
  - Vasopressor choices include dopamine or norepinephrine initially (both may exacerbate tachycardia), neosynephrine as pure vasoconstrictor if tachycardia is significant; all choices may exacerbate cardiac ischemia; although dobutamine infusions are used in rx of CHF, concern for initial use in cardiogenic shock arises because of variable effects on BP but may be used as 2nd-line agent with other pressors.
  - In some settings, consider intra-aortic balloon pump and quick assessment for emergent CABG.

Assessment of volume status and rx of volume overload

- Very important in the emergent setting, especially in pts presenting with dyspnea of unknown cause.
- Clinical si/sx as described above.
- In ER setting, many pts with significant dyspnea and adequate BP may safely receive emergent diuretic therapy while awaiting lab and imaging results.
- Diuretics are the mainstay of initial therapy, as follows:
  - Furosemide is the most common loop diuretic used; initial dose of 20–40 mg IV in "naïve" pts; in pts with known CHF on chronic therapy, give at least 1 to 1.5 times the usual dose in IV form, which is faster acting and 25–50% more effective; bumetanide 0.5-1 mg IV is an alternative.
  - Despite widespread use, actual clinical studies of diuretics in acute CHF are very limited.

- IV diuretics often continued for 24–72 hr, based on clinical response (close monitoring of vital signs, I/Os, daily weights), with conversion to oral therapy when stable.
- If inadequate response to diuretics, consider:
  - Increasing doses of loop diuretics, or starting continuous drip (furosemide 10–40 mg/hr, titrate based on urine output and sx).
  - Addition of second diuretic agent; metolazone is commonly used (2.5–5 mg PO qd), but thiazide diuretics or spironolactone can also be considered.
  - Hemofiltration/dialysis is used in select pts.
- Adverse effects can include hypokalemia from loop or thiazide diuretics, which should prompt oral or IV replacement; rapid fluid loss may lead to acute renal failure, hypotension.
- Vasodilator therapy is an important tool.
  - Strongly consider in the acute setting, especially if concomitant hypertension.
  - Nitroglycerin is often used, as strong venodilator, reducing RV/LV preload.
    - In emergent settings, continuous IV drip warranted with close monitoring (often in ICU).
    - Start drip at 5 mcg/min, titrate to clinical sx and BP response.
    - In nonemergent settings, transdermal nitroglycerin paste (0.5 to 2 in. q 6 hr) can be effective (or continuation of oral nitrates).
  - Nitroprusside is an alternative, especially if hypertensive crisis (see Section 1.5, covering hypertensive emergencies).
  - IV nesiritide (BNP) is also used, but studies are mixed; one study showed reduced PCWP and improvement in dyspnea when compared to placebo (NEJM 2000;343:246) but no difference in sx when compared to NTG (JAMA 2002;287:1531); there is a lack of large, primary outcome

studies, but more recent data suggest concern for increased mortality (JAMA 2005;293:1900) and renal failure (Circ 2005;111:1487).

- Fluid and salt restriction is also important.

Recognition and prevention of complications

- Acute respiratory failure:
  - Often seen in the acute/ER setting, due to the effects of pulmonary edema.
  - All pts should be initially treated with supplemental oxygen.
  - Assessment of oxygenation by pulse oximetry or ABG.
  - Role for acute noninvasive positive pressure ventilation (CPAP or BiPAP).
    - 3CPO trial: 1069 pts with acute pulm edema causing respiratory acidosis (pH less than 7.35), randomized to standard O_2 rx vs CPAP vs NIPPV; no difference in 7-day mortality or progression to intubation, but non-invasive ventilation did improve pt dyspnea, acidosis, hypercapnia, and tachycardia vs standard O_2 therapy (NEJM 2008;359:142).
  - In pts with severe respiratory symptoms or cardiogenic shock, need to consider intubation and mechanical ventilation.
- Comorbid disease:
  - Exacerbation of CHF often occurs with another presenting complaint (infection, trauma, PE, etc.), or as a complication in the post-op pt.
- Ventricular arrhythmias/sudden cardiac death:
  - ACC/AHA guidelines recommend consideration of implantable cardiodefibrillator (AICD) in the following settings:
    - CHF pts with reduced EF and prior hx of cardiac arrest, VF, or hemodynamically unstable VT

- CHF pts with ischemic heart disease (and at least 40 d post-MI) or nonischemic cardiomyopathy, EF less than 35%, NYHA Class II or III sx on optimal therapy, and reasonable expectation of survival
- Atrial fibrillation:
  - Is present in 10–30% of CHF pts, with higher incidence in pts with severe disease (NEJM 1999;341:910).
  - Is a risk factor for mortality in CHF.
  - Rapid ventricular response can worsen CHF by limiting ventricular filling (worsening diastolic dysfunction); goal is to control HR to 80–90 bpm at rest, 110–130 with activity.
  - In CHF, rx options include beta-blockers and digoxin for rate control; diltiazem can worsen CHF due to negative inotropic effects; see "Atrial Fibrillation" in Section 1.3 for more details.
- Venous thromboembolism:
  - Patients admitted with CHF exacerbation are at high risk for hospital-acquired DVT/PE.
  - Strongly consider medical VTE prophylaxis (or continuation of chronic anticoagulation in appropriate settings); see "VTE Prophylaxis in Hospitalized Patients" in Section 7.1 for details.
- Potassium metabolism:
  - Both hypokalemia and hyperkalemia can be present in pts with CHF.
  - Hypokalemia (also see "Hypokalemia" in Section 8.2):
    - Causes include kaliuresis from loop or thiazide diuretics; concomitant hypomagnesemia from diuretics.
    - Rx: In critical situations, can use IV potassium chloride (KCl), added to IVF; or if fluid-restriction, can give as IV piggyback, usually dosed at 10–40 mEq given 10 mEq per hr; but in most situations, oral

replacement is preferred as KCl given 20–40 mEq 1 to 3 times daily.

- Monitoring: Should check at least daily while inpatient, and then soon after hospital discharge if addition of KCl supplementation or change in other medications that could affect potassium levels.
- Hyperkalemia (also see "Hyperkalemia" in Section 8.2):
  - Causes include ACE inhibitor or ARB side effect (usually mild, less than 5.5 mEq/L); acute or chronic renal failure; potassium-sparing diuretic therapy; overly aggressive potassium supplementation.
  - Rx: In most cases, elevation is mild and not treated; may need to stop ACEI/ARB or K-sparing diuretic if severe; in setting of acute or chronic renal failure, can treat with oral Kayexalate.
  - Be particularly careful with hyperkalemia if concomitant use of digoxin or antiarrhythmic drugs.
  - Monitoring: As for hypokalemia; if significantly elevated, consider EKG to look for classic changes (peaked T waves, QRS prolongation).

Adjustment of chronic therapies to improve mortality and reduce hospitalizations

- In the inpatient setting, adjustment of chronic medications is usually reserved for later in the hospitalization when volume status and perfusion have returned to baseline.
- Continuation of chronic CHF meds on admission is usually advisable, except in certain circumstances:
  - Diuretics: Hold if evidence of volume depletion and acute renal failure, or significant metabolic disturbance (especially hyperkalemia with spironolactone in setting of acute renal failure).

- ACEI/ARB: Hold if significant acute renal failure or symptomatic hypotension/shock.
- Beta-blockers: Hold if acute bronchospasm, or if felt that recently added or titrated beta-blocker therapy may have contributed to current symptoms.
- Spironolactone: Hold if acute (or worsening chronic) renal failure, hyperkalemia.
- Digoxin: Hold if acute renal failure, bradycardia, or toxic levels.
- Medications to avoid in CHF (or that may have contributed to exacerbation):
  - NSAIDs: Cause sodium retention and edema, vasoconstriction, worsening renal function; should avoid all use in pts in Stage C or Stage D CHF.
  - Calcium channel blockers: Diltiazem and verapamil may exacerbate CHF sx; amlodipine and felodopine do not have same effect, but have no particular role in CHF except in BP control, especially for pts with chronic renal failure and CHF.
  - Antiarrhythmic drugs: If necessary based on comorbid arrhythmias, seek expert consultation for management.
  - Thiazolidinediones (e.g., pioglitazone): Should be avoided for routine DM therapy in pts with CHF, as can cause worsening edema and CHF sx.
- ACE inhibitors (ACEIs) are a mainstay of chronic CHF therapy.
  - Category includes lisinopril, enalapril, captopril, quinapril, and others.
  - Not only has chronic antihypertensive effect, but neurohormonal effects on RAA system also affect chronic LV remodeling.
  - Multiple studies have proven benefit in reducing CHF hospitalizations and mortality, especially in pts with EF less than 40%.

- 1995 meta-analysis of more than 30 trials of ACEI in pts with CHF and EF less than 40%; ACEI reduced mortality (OR 0.77) and reduced hospitalizations for CHF (JAMA 1995;273:1450).

- Contraindications include advanced chronic renal failure (serum Cr 2.5 mg/dL is a common cutoff in many clinical trials, although may still be used in some pts with stable CKD), bilateral renal artery stenosis, symptomatic hypotension, allergy/intolerance (cough is common, angioedema is rare).
- ACEI therapy is a CMS core measure for quality care of CHF: all pts discharged with a dx of systolic CHF should be on ACEI (or ARB) therapy unless a contraindication is present and documented.
- In most cases, should continue ACEI on admission; if no prior use, start at low doses and titrate to moderate dose (e.g., lisinopril 5 mg daily, titrated to up to 20 mg daily), following BP, renal function, and potassium levels closely.
- Usually reach limits of tolerance either because of renal dysfunction or hypotension; if pt has borderline low BP, probably better to add beta-blocker therapy as additional agent to ACEI rather than pushing ACEI to maximal dose.
- The role of angiotensin II receptor blockers (ARBs):
  - Category includes losartan, valsartan, and others.
  - Considered to be equivalent to ACEIs in setting of CHF therapy, but mostly used as 2nd-line drug if pt intolerant of ACEI (due to cough, which is not present with ARBs); evidence does not support the use of combination ACEI/ARB therapy in pts with CHF.
    - Valsartan in AMI trial: approximately 15,000 post-MI pts with CHF/LV dysfunction, randomized to valsartan, captopril, or both; no difference between the two primary drugs in 2-yr mortality; combo of ARB and

1.2   Congestive Heart Failure   **35**

ACEI increased side effects (hypotension, acute renal failure) without affecting mortality (NEJM 2003;349:1893).
- Other than cough, all other contraindications and side effects are similar to ACEI.
- Beta-blockers and CHF:
  - Blocks the effects of the sympathetic nervous system on cardiac function and LV remodeling; concern for negative inotropic effects is outweighed by positive effects in most pts.
  - Only two beta-blockers have proven efficacy in CHF rx and are FDA-approved for this indication: carvedilol and extended-release metoprolol (bisoprolol also has efficacy, but is not available in the United States).
    - Carvedilol study: 2289 pts with CHF, EF less than 25%; randomized to carvedilol titrated from 3.125 mg to 25 mg bid vs placebo; rx reduced mortality (11.2% vs 16.7%, NNT 18) and recurrent hospitalizations, with no increase in side effects (NEJM 2001;344:1651).
    - MERIT-HF study: Approximately 4000 pts with CHF, EF less than 40%; randomized to extended-release metoprolol, started at 12.5–25 mg daily and titrated to 200 mg daily; rx reduced mortality, symptoms, and hospitalizations (JAMA 2000;283:1295).
  - This class of drugs should be added early in the course of therapy for CHF pts, even if ACEIs have not reached maximal doses; concern with initiating therapy in pts with acute CHF exacerbation because of initial negative inotropic effects, which may temporarily worsen sx if started too early after exacerbation or at too-high doses.
  - Many pts do not reach the target doses seen in the studies because of limiting side effects, including bradycardia,

hypotension, bronchospasm, fatigue, weakness, depression.
- In pts already on beta-blockers, avoid abrupt withdrawal unless absolutely necessary because of rebound tachycardia and worsening symptoms.
- Aldosterone antagonists and CHF:
  - Spironolactone is most commonly used drug in this class; eplerenone is newer, more costly drug with limited clinical experience.
    - RALES trial: 1663 pts with CHF, EF less than 35%, already on ACEI and diuretic (more than 70% on digoxin as well); randomized to spironolactone 25 mg daily or placebo; rx reduced 2-yr mortality (35% vs 46%, NNT 9) as well as dyspnea and hospitalizations; had low rate of side effects and serious hyperkalemia in only 2% (NEJM 1999;341:709).
    - Based on this study, addition of spironolactone became very popular; but in clinical practice, higher rates of adverse events were seen, particularly hospitalizations for severe hyperkalemia (5 times higher than baseline rate prior to widespread use) (NEJM 2004;351:543).
  - Bottom line is that aldosterone antagonists are useful drugs in CHF pts with continued sx already on ACEIs, beta-blockers, and diuretics, but need to be monitored closely; should start at low doses (spironolactone 12.5 mg daily), avoid in pts with CrCl less than 30 or pre-rx potassium levels more than 5.0 mEq/L, discontinue potassium supplements initially, and monitor renal function and potassium levels very closely.
- Digoxin and CHF:
  - Positive inotropic effect through inhibition of the Na-K ATPase enzyme in cardiac muscle, but efficacy in CHF

may be due more to inhibition of sympathetic NS and RAA system.
- Although one of the more long-standing therapies for CHF, it has been replaced by ACEIs and beta-blockers as primary therapy; studies have shown reduced hospitalizations for CHF, but no effect on mortality.
  - Digitalis Investigation Group study: 6800 pts with CHF, EF less than 45%, already on diuretics and ACEIs; randomized to digoxin rx vs placebo; rx did not affect mortality but did reduce hospitalization for worsening CHF sx (27% vs 35%, NNT 12); 2% of pts needed admission for potential digoxin toxicity (NEJM 1997;336:525).
- Especially useful in pts with atrial fibrillation on rate control strategy (although beta-blockers should be 1st-line therapy because of improved efficacy of both rate control and CHF outcomes) and in pts not able to tolerate other drugs because of hypotension.
- Typically start at 0.125 mg daily; IV or PO loading is not necessary in treatment of chronic CHF (as opposed to atrial fibrillation); dose titration based on serum levels.
- Has multiple drug interactions and a narrow therapeutic window, especially in elderly pts with renal failure; toxicity usually related to serum dig levels more than 2 ng/mL and associated with nausea, dizziness, confusion, cardiac conduction abnormalities.
- Probably most effective in CHF pts at lower serum levels.
  - Analysis of digoxin levels in the DIG study group: pts with dig levels of 0.5–0.8 ng/mL had reduced mortality compared to placebo, but pts with intermediate levels (0.9–1.1 ng/mL) and high levels (1.2 ng/mL or more) had no difference and higher mortality, respectively (JAMA 2003;289:871). Note that the intermediate

and high-level groups are still within the therapeutic
window for most laboratories (up to 2 ng/mL).

- Using hydralazine/nitrates to treat CHF:
  - The combination of a venodilator (nitrates) and vasodila-
    tor (hydralazine) has dual effects and may inhibit the toler-
    ance that can develop from using nitrates alone.
  - Initial studies showed promising results:
    - V-HeFT I: VA study of 642 men with CHF already on
      digoxin and diuretic (no ACEI); randomized to hydrala-
      zine 300 mg daily and isosorbide dinitrate 160 mg daily
      vs placebo (3rd arm was given prazosin with no benefit);
      rx improved 2-yr mortality (26% vs 34%, NNT 13), but
      this study was conducted before widespread use of ACEI
      (NEJM 1986;314:1547).
    - V-HeFT II: 804 pts in same study population as V-HeFT
      I; randomized to hydralazine/isosorbide dinitrate (same
      doses) or enalapril 20 mg daily; ACEI rx reduced 2-yr
      mortality (18% vs 25%, NNT 14), but vasodilator
      therapy still had lower mortality than in prior placebo
      study (34%) (NEJM 1991;325:303).
  - As part of subgroup analyses of initial studies, African
    American pts tended to have better outcomes with the
    vasodilator therapy, which led to further study:
    - A-HeFT: 1050 African American pts with systolic CHF
      on standard therapies including ACEI, beta-blocker,
      digoxin, spironolactone; randomized to hydralazine and
      isosorbide dinitrate vs placebo; rx improved average
      10-mo mortality (6% vs 10%, NNT 25), and increased
      time to first hospitalization and QOL scores (NEJM
      2004;351:2049).
  - In addition to hypotension, most common side effects are
    headache and dizziness.
  - Consider as a 2nd-line therapy in pts unable to toler-
    ate ACEI/ARB, especially in chronic renal failure; or as

initial therapy in combination with ACEIs, beta-blockers, etc., in African American pts, if able to tolerate from BP standpoint.
- Consider ASCVD risk factors, and treat hyperlipidemia as appropriate (see Section 1.1, "Acute Coronary Syndromes," for details).
  - GISSI-HF trial: Approximately 7000 pts with CHF (regardless of EF); randomized to polyunsaturated fatty acids 1 gm daily (as found in fish oil supplements) vs placebo; rx was associated with reduction in 4-yr mortality (27% vs 29%, NNT 56) and hospital admission for cardiac reason (57% vs 59%, NNT 44) (Lancet 2008;372:1223).
- Other therapies for severe CHF:
  - Cardiac resynchronization therapy (CRT) (NEJM 2006; 355:288)
    - Consider for pts with severe systolic CHF and concomitant ventricular conduction deficits (QRS duration greater than 120 msec).
    - Dyssynchronous ventricular contraction may cause impaired ventricular filling and worsened mitral regurgitation; CRT is biventricular pacing to coordinate the AV contractions.
    - CRT (many times paired with an AICD) has been associated with improved mortality, CHF symptoms, and QOL (NEJM 2009;361:1329, NEJM 2002;346:1845, J Am Coll Cardiol 2004;44:810).
  - Inotrope therapy
    - Usually reserved for severe, end-stage CHF pts already on or having failed standard therapies, as an intermittent rescue medication.
    - Some research into chronic oral therapies, but no clear role for use yet.
    - Choices include dobutamine, dopamine, and milrinone.

- Usually requires ICU care and consideration of PA catheterization.
- Ventricular-assist devices (VADs) and cardiac transplants: considerations for younger pts with severe, end-stage disease

Discharge planning

- Crucial to improving patient care and reducing readmission rates.
- In addition to maximizing therapies to improve symptoms, pts should receive education on CHF and how to recognize and avoid exacerbations; discharge instructions should include the following:
  - Dietary advice re fluid and sodium restriction
  - Regular monitoring of weight, and advice for contacting primary care physician if weight gain
  - How to recognize worsening sx and who to contact if present
  - Activity recommendations and restrictions
  - Complete medication list (not just medications prescribed for CHF)
  - Avoidance of NSAIDs
  - Follow-up appointment with primary care physician.
- Meta-analysis of 18 studies of comprehensive discharge planning for CHF and postdischarge support showed reduced rates of readmission for CHF (35% vs 43%, NNT 12) (JAMA 2004;291:1358).
- Comprehensive discharge instructions for pts with CHF is a CMS "core measure" for quality; many hospitals have developed their own set of instructions given to pts; physicians need to make sure pts are given these (whether CHF is the primary or a secondary diagnosis) and that the medication list that the pt is given on discharge exactly matches that in the hospital discharge summary.

1.3   Arrhythmias

Ventricular Ectopy and Tachycardia

Cause: Definitions:

- Premature ventricular contraction (PVC): A spontaneous contraction of the heart arising from the ventricular conduction system, characterized by a wide (greater than 120 msec) and bizarrely shaped QRS complex without a preceding P wave and usually having a compensatory pause before the next normal beat.
- Ventricular bigeminy/trigeminy: Alternating PVCs and normal sinus beats (1:1 ratio for bigeminy, 1:2 ratio for trigeminy).
- Ventricular tachycardia (VT): Three or more successive PVCs with a rate greater than 100 bpm; if lasting more than 30 sec, defined as sustained ventricular tachycardia (less than 30 sec is nonsustained VT [NSVT]).
  - Monomorphic VT: all QRS complexes with similar appearance
  - Polymorphic VT: QRS complexes with varied appearance, axes
  - Torsades de pointes: QRS complexes with a rhythmic change in polarity and amplitude, seeming to twist on an axis

Diff dx of wide complex rhythms also includes SVT with aberrant conduction, use of class I antiarrhythmic agents, ventricular pacemakers, severe hyperkalemia, TCA overdose, acute STEMI (with "tombstone" ST-elevation fusing the QRS complex and T wave).

Cardiac causes include ischemic heart disease (ACS or chronic CAD), cardiomyopathy, valvular disease; idiopathic hypertrophic cardiomyopathy (HOCM), particularly in young athletes; prolonged QT interval.

Noncardiac precipitants include alcohol, tobacco, caffeine; metabolic abnormalities including hypokalemia, hyperkalemia, hypomagnesemia, acidosis, and hypoxia.

Antiarrhythmic drugs (flecainide, sotalol, quinidine), as well as antipsychotics (haloperidol, chlorpromazine, thioridazine), some antibiotics (quinolones, erythromycin), and TCAs, can precipitate VT (Torsades) by prolongation of the QT interval (J Am Coll Cardiol 2010;55;934).

Epidem: Incidence increases with age.

Pathophys: Possibly higher risk of sudden death in pts w/ early repolarization on EKG (NEJM 2008;358:2016).

Sx: Palpitations, dizziness, chest pain.

Si: Syncope, hypotension, shock, cardiac arrest.

Crs: PVC: not associated with increased mortality in pts without heart disease.

NSVT: 2-yr mortality increased by 30% in pts with LV dysfunction and NSVT on Holter monitoring (NEJM 1988;318:19).

Lab: In asymptomatic, hospitalized pts with frequent PVCs or NSVT, check electrolytes, magnesium, O_2 saturation.

Noninv: Conduct EKG to look for prolonged QT (greater than 470 msec in men, 480 msec in women, corrected for rate), evidence of CAD/prior MI. EKG can help determine VT vs SVT with aberrancy:

- QRS width greater than 160 msec is strongly associated with VT (Am J Cardiol 2008;101:1456).
- Presence of AV dissociation, fusion beats (formed by activation of myocardium by both a conducted atrial beat and ventricular activation), or capture beat (a normal-appearing QRS complex from a transmitted atrial beat, interspersed in VT) all suggest VT as origin of wide complex tachycardia (WCT).
- Brugada criteria to determine etiology of WCT had high sens (98.7%) and specif (96.5%) in initial study (Circ

1991;83:1649), but not as effective in f/u study (Eur Heart J 2007;28:589).

- Step 1: If no RS complex in any precordial (chest) lead, then VT; otherwise move to step 2.
- Step 2: If RS complex is greater than 100 msec, then VT; otherwise move to step 3.
- Step 3: If AV dissociation is present, then VT; otherwise move to step 4.
- Step 4: Conduct more detailed analysis of QRS morphology, which is likely not helpful in acute setting.

Perform echocardiogram to eval for LV and valvular dysfunction.

An electrophysiology study (EPS) can help determine the cause of heart rhythm disturbance and locate the site of abnormality.

Rx: PVCs and NSVT: No specific rx in most cases, except to correct underlying cause if able; continued monitoring and reassurance to pts and nursing.

Avoid routine antiarrhythmic rx in post-MI pts:

- CAST I: RCT of 1498 post-MI pts with asx or mild sx of ventricular arrhythmia randomized to class IC drug (encainide, flecainide); therapy increased mortality (5.7% vs 3.5%, NNH 45) and nonfatal cardiac arrests, even with proven initial suppression of events by Holter monitoring (NEJM 1991;324:781).
- CAST II: Similar to CAST I, but with class IC agent moricizine; also showed increased mortality with therapy (NEJM 1992;327:227).
- If pts complain of persistent disabling sx, consider rx with beta-blocker (JAMA 1993;270:1589).

Therapy for VT

- Acute therapy for VT includes the following approaches.

- For pt w/ pulseless arrest (VT/VF):
  - Start CPR per ACLS protocols.
  - Immediate unsynchronized DC cardioversion, start at 360 J (or standard for defibrillator).
  - Administer epinephrine 1 mg IV q 3–5 min (or vasopressin 40 U IV).
  - Consider amiodarone, lidocaine, or magnesium in specific settings.
- For unstable (hypotensive) pt:
  - Immediate synchronized DC cardioversion, start at 360 J.
  - Amiodarone 300 mg IV.
  - Alternative is lidocaine 1–1.5 mg/kg IV.
  - Magnesium 2 gm IV in torsades de pointes.
- For stable pt:
  - Amiodarone 150 mg IV over 10 min, then continuous infusion of 1 mg/min for 6 hr, then 0.5 mg/min
- Chronic therapy for VT includes the following approaches:
  - Drug therapy:
    - See previous discussion for class I drugs; studies have shown increased mortality with use of routine antiarrhythmic therapy.
    - Beta-blockers have mortality benefit for all CAD pts in reducing sudden death.
    - Consider amiodarone as well, but long-term adverse effects likely reduce the overall benefit in most pts.
      - While effective at reducing arrhythmia, side effects were seen in 86% of pts after 5 yr of therapy (which led to discontinuation of drug in 37%) (J Am Coll Cardiol 1989;13:442).
  - Automated implantable cardiodefibrillator (AICD):
    - Consider for pts in the following settings (Circ 1998 97:1325):

- Cardiac arrest from VT/VF not associated with a clearly reversible cause
- Spontaneous/sustained VT
- Syncope of unknown cause with electrophysiology studies showing inducible VT/VF
- NSVT in pts with CAD and LV dysfunction showing inducible VT/VF
- AICD has short-term improvements (3–12 mo) in QOL measures over medical rx, but no difference in physical functioning; no adverse QOL effects (NEJM 2008;359:999).
- 33% of pts received one or more ICD shocks; hazard ratio for death was approximately 11, highest within 24 hr; 1-yr survival rate after any shock is 82% (NEJM 2008;359:1009).

Supraventricular Tachycardia

(NEJM 2006;354:1039, Mayo Clin Proc 2008;83:1400)

Cause: Any tachycardia (HR greater than 100) originating from at or above the AV node:

- Sinus tachycardia, due to many causes
  - Underlying chronic illness: CHF, COPD, severe anemia, hyperthyroidism, deconditioning
  - Acute illness: ACS, sepsis, PE, other hypoxic respiratory failure
  - Volume depletion, acute blood loss
  - Fever
  - Drugs: caffeine, stimulants; abrupt withdrawal of antihypertensives, including clonidine and beta-blockers
  - Anxiety
  - Inappropriate sinus tachycardia, if no other cause apparent
- Atrial fibrillation and flutter (see "Atrial Fibrillation" later in Section 1.3)
- Multifocal atrial tachycardia

- Types of Paroxysmal SVT
  - AV nodal reentrant tachycardia (AVNRT) (60%) arises within the AV node.
  - AV reentrant tachycardia (AVRT) (30%) requires an accessory AV pathway.
  - Atrial tachycardia (10%), ectopic atrial focus overrides the sinus node.
  - Rarer forms include sinus-node reentrant tachycardia and junctional tachycardia.

Epidem: Incidence 35 per 100,000 people per year; increases with age and presence of cardiac disease.

Pathophys: Usually starts with a PAC or PVC; precipitants can include tobacco, alcohol, caffeine, drug use, ephedrine, hyperthyroidism, stress.

Sx: Palpitations (and sense of pounding in neck), anxiety, presyncope and syncope; chest pain/pressure is common and can be related to ischemia but not in most cases; sx usually start and end suddenly.

Si: HR greater than 100, and often difficult to assess by distal pulses.

Crs: Usually benign and not associated with ischemia or underlying heart disease, so does not affect long-term survival.

Cmplc: Long-term, unrecognized tachycardia can cause a cardiomyopathy (often reversible with rx).

Lab: No routine labs, but consider TSH to r/o underlying hyperthyroidism.

Noninv: EKG shows regular tachycardia (as opposed to irregular with AF), most PSVT with narrow QRS complex (dur less than 120 msec), but PSVT can have WCT in about 10% of cases due to one or more of the following:

- Preexisting conduction disease (BBB, IVCD); look for evidence on prior EKGs
- Rate-related conduction deficit (most common cause)

- Accessory pathway with preexcitation; look for signs of Wolff-Parkinson-White (WPW) syndrome on baseline EKG, including short PR interval, delta wave (slurred upstroke of the QRS), prolonged QRS interval, and tall R wave in V_1.

Get EKG during sx and at baseline to assess type and cause of PSVT; finding of underlying accessory pathway necessitates cardiology consult for electrophysiology study; look at baseline P waves (normally should be upright in the inferior leads) and P waves with tachycardia (if present and not lost in the QRS).

Can use the Brugada criteria to assess for VT vs PSVT with aberrancy (but may not be useful in the acute, emergent setting); see "Ventricular Ectopy and Tachycardia," earlier in Section 1.3.

Consider Holter monitoring as outpatient if dx is unclear.

Conduct echocardiogram to evaluate LV function and valvular disease, although structural heart disease is rare.

Rx: Emergent therapy is based on assessment of hemodynamics, as follows:

- For unstable pts (hypotensive, active coronary ischemia): Employ emergent synchronized DC cardioversion (start at 50–100 J).
- If regular, narrow complex PSVT in stable pt:
  - First consider vagal maneuvers (to stimulate vagus nerve and block sympathetics, slowing conduction through the AV node), including carotid sinus massage (only in pts without h/o carotid stenosis and no bruit on exam), Valsalva maneuver, or facial stimulation with cold water bath.
  - Adenosine IV: terminates PSVT in 60–80% of pts at 6 mg dose, and 90% of pts at 12 mg dose (Ann IM 1990;113:104); requires EKG monitoring and most have a transient AV block and post-rx sinus tachycardia; avoid in severe bronchospasm and in postcardiac transplant pts; also avoid in pts with wide complex tachycardia, unless absolutely certain PSVT with aberrant conduction is present,

because can precipitate ventricular fibrillation in VT pts; effects are reduced by concomitant theophylline use and potentiated by dipyridamole (component of Aggrenox); safe in pregnancy (most reports in 2nd and 3rd trimesters (Drug Saf 1999;20:85).

- If adenosine fails or is contraindicated, IV beta-blocker or calcium channel blocker is next, administered as follows:
  - Beta-blocker: Metoprolol 5 mg IV q 5 min up to three doses, monitor BP response; can use short-acting esmolol (0.5 mg/kg over 1 min) as well.
  - CCB: Verapamil 5 mg IV q 3 min up to three doses; monitor BP response and watch for AV blockade; or one dose of diltiazem 0.25 mg/kg IV bolus, repeating 0.35 mg/kg dose if no response.
  - If medical therapy fails, consider cardioversion.
- If regular, wide complex tachycardia, should treat as VT unless absolutely certain of PSVT with aberrancy; choices include IV procainamide, flecainide, propafenone, ibutilide, amiodarone, and cardioversion.

Long-term therapy for recurrent SVT episodes

- AV nodal dependent types (AVNRT, AVRT) should receive AV blockers, including beta-blockers, CCBs, or digoxin, with no 1st-line therapy shown to be superior to others in one RCT (Am J Cardiol 1984;54:1138).
- Class IC or III antiarrhythmics:
  - Flecainide: Oral flecainide in one placebo-controlled RCT reduced number (79% of pts free from PSVT events at 60 d vs 15% for placebo) and severity of tachycardic events, as well as time to first event after initiation (Circ 1991;83:119).
  - Propafenone: In one small RCT, oral propafenone reduced recurrence of symptomatic PSVT and paroxysmal atrial fibrillation vs placebo (Ann IM 1991;114:539).

- Amiodarone and sotalol are also alternatives.
- Despite these studies, long-term therapy is often avoided because of the risk of VT with class IC drugs and multiple long-term effects of amiodarone and sotalol.
- "Pill-in-pocket" approach: For pts with rare but prolonged recurrent episodes, can consider rx at home with single-dose therapy; choices include beta-blockers, CCBs, flecainide, propafenone.
  - 2001 study: 33 pts with infrequent PSVT (fewer than five episodes per yr) and inducible SVT with EPS were tested for effect of placebo, flecainide, and combo of diltiazem (120 mg) and propranol (80 mg); 61% responded to flecainide, 94% to diltiazem/propranol combo; pts sent home on most effective rx; during average 17-month follow-up, approximately 80% of episodes were terminated with either drug therapy with minimal side effects (J Am Coll Cardiol 2001;37:548).
- Consider electrophysiology study and catheter ablation based on sx and pt preference for therapy.

Atrial Fibrillation

(NEJM 2004;351:2408)

Cause: Linked to HTN, CAD; rheumatic heart disease, with either mitral stenosis or regurgitation; CHF, especially in setting of increased atrial size; hypertrophic cardiomyopathy; PE; COPD; pericarditis; hyperthyroidism; recent CABG or valve surgery; associations with alcohol ("holiday heart syndrome") and caffeine intake.

Epidem: Very common, increases with age, more prevalent in men.

Pathophys: Complex interplay of structural remodeling of cardiac myocytes, changes in the electrical currents via alteration of action potential conduction, and inflammatory reactions (Am Hrt J 2009:157:243).

Sx: Palpitations, dyspnea at rest or with exertion, dizziness; many, however, are asymptomatic (21% in Canadian Registry of new AF pts) (Eur Heart J 1996;17 Suppl C:48).

Si: Irregularly irregular tachycardia.

Crs: 2006 classification, per ACC/AHA/ESC guidelines (J Am Coll Cardiol 2006;48:854):

- Paroxysmal: spontaneous conversion to sinus rhythm within 7 d
- Persistent: no spontaneous conversion to sinus rhythm within 7 d (or terminated by cardioversion)
- Permanent: duration of more than 1 yr with failure or no attempt at cardioversion
- Lone: any atrial fibrillation in pts without structural heart disease (i.e., low risk for stroke complications)

    Per Framingham study, AF is a risk factor for increased mortality (Circ 1998;98:946).

Cmplc: Long-standing tachycardia can lead to cardiomyopathy (Am J Cardiol 1986;57:563).

Lab: Check TSH to look for hyperthyroidism; 1996 study of 726 pts with recent AF, low TSH in 5.4%, but only 1% had true clinical hyperthyroidism (sx and elevated T4) (Arch IM 1996;156:2221).

    Consider serial cardiac enzymes, but AF is not usually the only sign of an acute coronary syndrome (EKG should show signs of ST elevation or depression). Mild cardiac enzyme elevation ("troponin leak") not uncommon in elderly pts with known CAD and rapid AF, due to demand ischemia and subendocardial injury.

Noninv: Perform EKG to confirm irregular, narrow complex rhythm (with or without tachycardia); watch for mimics including the following:

- Sinus rhythm (or tachycardia) with sinus arrhythmia: may be irregular, but clear P waves present.

- Atrial flutter: Usually "regularly irregular" with variable conduction block; look for sawtooth P wave pattern in anterior chest leads, may be easier to see if slow ventricular conduction with vagal maneuver or meds; always consider in narrow complex tachycardia with steady rate of 150 bpm (2:1 conduction block, may not see sawtooth pattern due to tachycardia).
- Multifocal atrial tachycardia (rates greater than 100 bpm) or wandering pacemaker (rates less than 100 bpm): Irregularly irregular, but will have P waves with three or more morphologies; most common with underlying lung disease.
- Paroxysmal supraventricular tachycardia: May be difficult to distinguish at rates greater than 160 bpm; use calipers to determine irregularity to confirm AF (other PSVTs will be regular).

Order CXR to look for underlying lung disease, cardiac size/silhouette.

Perform echocardiogram: helpful to evaluate atrial sizes, LV and RV function, evidence of valvular disease; less likely to show LA thrombus; if true concern for cardiac embolic source of CVA, need to get TEE, but may not be necessary if planning on chronic anticoagulation (as will not change management).

Conduct treadmill testing, if there is concern for adequate rate control with exertion; stress testing with imaging only necessary if concern for underlying CAD.

Schedule Holter monitoring, if there is concern for paroxysmal episodes not noted while in hospital or to assess adequacy of rate or rhythm control as outpatient.

Rx: Major decisions for therapy include the following:

1. Hospitalization
2. Rate vs rhythm control
3. Anticoagulation for stroke prophylaxis

Hospitalization for new dx of AF

- Decision to hospitalize pts with new dx of atrial fibrillation depends on presenting sx, management strategies, pt compliance, and appropriate outpatient follow-up.
- If rate control strategy, may start oral meds if minimal symptoms and no hemodynamic instability.
- If rhythm control, and acute onset, can consider ER treatment with ibutilide or other drugs, but still should monitor for 6–12 hr for new arrhythmia; if onset unknown, need to admit for heparin and TEE if plan for cardioversion.
- If truly urgent need for DC cardioversion (active ischemia, hypotension/shock, pulmonary edema/CHF), do not need to wait for anticoagulation, because significant sx usually suggest abrupt onset (and lower risk of cardiac thrombus) and because risks of waiting outweigh potential benefits.
- Can start anticoagulation with warfarin (or ASA in low-risk) as inpatient or outpatient.

Rate control vs rhythm control strategies

- Rate control is use of medications to reduce ventricular response to rapid atrial stimulation.
- Rhythm control is use of medications or other interventions to convert AF to NSR.
- RACE trial: RCT of rhythm vs rate control in 522 pts with persistent AF post failed cardioversion; after 2 or more years, only 39% of rhythm control pts actually were in NSR (10% of rate control pts); no difference in primary end point of death from cardiovascular causes, heart failure, thromboembolic complications, bleeding, pacemaker insertion, or severe adverse drug event (NEJM 2002;347:1834).
- AFFIRM trial: RCT of rhythm vs rate control in 4060 pts with AF and high rates of CAD and HTN (i.e., high-risk stroke pts); no difference in mortality; more hospitalizations

and adverse drug events in rhythm control pts; similar risk of stoke in both groups.

- Atrial Fibrillation and Congestive Heart Failure Investigators trial: RCT of rhythm vs rate control in 1376 pts with systolic CHF (EF less than 35%); no difference in mortality, stroke, or worsening CHF (NEJM 2008;358:2667).
- So, based on these studies, rate control strategies seem to be indicated for most pts except in these settings: (1) severe symptoms accompany AF (hypotension, angina, worsening CHF), (2) inability to adequately control HR with medications, (3) pt preference for trial of rhythm control.

Rate control agents are presented in **Figure 1.2.**

- Primary choices are beta-blockers (metoprolol and atenolol, most commonly) and calcium channel blockers (diltiazem and verapamil).
- Acute therapy for rate control includes these meds:
  - Metoprolol 5 mg IV, q 5 min, up to 3 doses; monitor BP and HR response.
  - Diltiazem 0.25 mg/kg IV (20 mg for most adults, can use 10 mg in elderly); rebolus in 10–15 min if no improvement, and can start drip at 5 mg/hr and titrate up to 15 mg/hr.
  - Usually start with IV metoprolol, then change to diltiazem if no effect; watch for hypotension with either drug, and some risk of acute AV blockade leading to 3rd-degree heart block if used together.
  - Digoxin is 3rd-line agent; main benefit is lack of hypotensive response, so appropriate for use in pts unable to take beta-blockers or CCBs due to low BP; does not control rate well with exertion; has a longer time to take effect in acute settings; can load IV (0.5 mg IV, then 0.25 mg IV q 6 hr for 2 doses, then daily maintenance) or orally (same dosing); take care in pts with renal failure, same loading doses but may require less daily maintenance.
  - Amiodarone, possibly, in critically ill pts.

- Chronic therapy for rate control includes the following:
  - Beta-blockers: Can use oral metoprolol; usually start with short-acting 25–50 PO mg q 6 hr, then convert to longer-acting metoprolol SR (Toprol XL) or atenolol when stable.
  - Calcium channel blockers: Can use short-acting diltiazem starting at 30–60 mg PO q 6 hr and titrate to effect; convert to diltiazem LA once on stable dosing.
  - Digoxin: Dosing based on serum levels, use lowest dose possible to control rate and maintain serum levels less than 2 ng/mL.
- Rate control goals: resting, fewer than 80 bpm; fewer than 110 bpm with moderate activity; recent study showed that lenient rate control with goal of fewer than 110 bpm at rest was easier to achieve (fewer drugs and visits necessary) and no difference in composite outcome of adverse effects or AF-related risks as compared to standard guidelines for rate goals (NEJM 2010;362:1363).
- Special considerations in pts with acute need for rate control and hypotension:
  - If unstable, proceed to synchronized DC cardioversion, per ACLS protocols.
  - If mildly hypotensive but stable, can consider low test dose of IV metoprolol (controlling the rate may reduce diastolic dysfunction and improve cardiac stroke volume).
  - Also consider digoxin, but may not help acutely.

  Rhythm control agents are listed in **Figures 1.2 and 1.3.**

- DC cardioversion as 1st-line agent: Make sure to use synchronous mode to avoid "R-on-T" phenomenon, precipitating VF; overall success is 75–93% (J Am Coll Cardiol 2001;38:1498) but depends on duration of AF; multiple studies have shown that even with cardioversion, only 20–30% of pts remain in NSR for more than 1 yr.
- Drug therapy (see **Figure 1.3**): Amiodarone is probably most effective, but also has most potential long-term side effects; reserve for pts with CHF or hypertension with LVH.

Drug (Class)†	Purpose	Usual Maintenance Dose	Adverse Effects	Cautions and Contraindications
Metoprolol (II)	Rate control (rhythm in some cases)	50–200 mg daily, divided doses or sustained-release formulation	Hypotension, heart block, bradycardia, asthma, congestive heart failure	—
Propranolol (II)	Rate control (rhythm in some cases)	80–240 mg daily, divided doses or sustained-release formulation	Hypotension, heart block, bradycardia, asthma, congestive heart failure	—
Diltiazem (IV)	Rate control	120–360 mg daily, divided doses or sustained-release formulation	Hypotension, heart block, congestive heart failure	—
Verapamil (IV)	Rate control	120–360 mg daily, divided doses or sustained-release formulation	Hypotension, heart block, congestive heart failure, interaction with digoxin	—
Digoxin	Rate control	0.125–0.375 mg daily	Toxic effects of digitalis, heart block, bradycardia	—
Amiodarone (III)	Rhythm control (rate in some cases)	100–400 mg daily	Pulmonary toxic effects, skin discoloration, hypothyroidism, gastrointestinal upset, hepatic toxic effects, corneal deposits, optic neuropathy, interaction with warfarin, torsades de pointes (rare)	—
Quinidine (IA)	Rhythm control	600–1500 mg daily, divided doses	Torsades de pointes, gastrointestinal upset, enhanced atrioventricular nodal conduction	Prolongs QT interval; avoid with left ventricular wall thickness ≥1.4 cm
Procainamide (IA)	Rhythm control	1000–4000 mg daily, divided doses	Torsades de pointes, lupus-like syndrome, gastrointestinal symptoms	Prolongs QT interval; avoid with left ventricular wall thickness ≥1.4 cm

CARDIOLOGY

Disopyramide (IA)	Rhythm control	400–750 mg daily, divided doses	Torsades de pointes, congestive heart failure, glaucoma, urinary retention, dry mouth	Prolongs QT interval; avoid with left ventricular wall thickness ≥1.4 cm
Flecainide (IC)	Rhythm control	200–300 mg daily, divided doses	Ventricular tachycardia, congestive heart failure, enhanced atrioventricular nodal conduction (conversion to atrial flutter)	Contraindicated in patients with ischemic and structural heart disease
Propafenone (IC)	Rhythm control	450–900 mg daily, divided doses	Ventricular tachycardia, congestive heart failure, enhanced atrioventricular nodal conduction (conversion to atrial flutter)	Contraindicated in patients with ischemic and structural heart disease
Sotalol (III)	Rhythm control	240–320 mg daily, divided doses	Torsades de pointes, congestive heart failure, bradycardia, exacerbation of chronic obstructive or bronchospastic lung disease	Prolongs QT interval; avoid with left ventricular wall thickness ≥1.4 cm
Dofetilide (III)	Rhythm control	500–1000 μg daily, divided doses	Torsades de pointes	Prolongs QT interval; avoid with left ventricular wall thickness ≥1.4 cm

* The information in the table is adapted from Fuster et al. ACC/AHA/ESC guidelines for the management of patients with atrial fibrillation. *J Am Coll Cardiol.* 2001;38:1266.
† The Vaughn Williams class of antiarrhythmic drugs is given for those classified. Digoxin is not classified in this system.

Figure 1.2 Rate and Rhythm Control Agents for Atrial Fibrillation

Reproduced with permission from Page RL. Newly diagnosed atrial fibrillation. *NEJM.* 2004;351:2408. Copyright © 2004, Massachusetts Medical Society. All rights reserved.

1.3 Arrhythmias **57**

Underlying Disorder	Rate Control†	Rhythm Control		
		First Choice	Second Choice	Third Choice
Minimal or no heart disease	β-adrenergic blocker or calcium-channel blocker	Flecainide, propafenone, sotalol	Amiodarone, dofetilide	Disopyramide, procainamide, quinidine (or nonpharmacologic options)
Adrenergic atrial fibrillation with minimal or no heart disease	β-adrenergic blocker	β-adrenergic blocker or sotalol	Amiodarone, dofetilide	—
Heart failure	β-adrenergic blocker, if tolerated; digoxin	Amiodarone, dofetilide	—	—
Coronary artery disease	β-adrenergic blocker	Sotalol	Amiodarone, dofetilide	Disopyramide, procainamide, quinidine
Hypertension with LVH but wall thickness <1.4 cm	β-adrenergic blocker or calcium-channel blocker	Flecainide, propafenone	Amiodarone, dofetilide, sotalol	Disopyramide, procainamide, quinidine
Hypertension with LVH and wall thickness ≥1.4 cm	β-adrenergic blocker or calcium-channel blocker	Amiodarone	—	—

* LVH denotes left ventricular hypertrophy. The information in this table is adapted from Fuster et al. ACC/AHA/ ESC guidelines for the management of patients with atrial fibrillation. *J Am Coll Cardiol.* 2001;3 8:1266.
† β-adrenergic blockers include metoprolol and propranolol; calcium-channel blockers includes diltiazem and verapamil.

Figure 1.3   Antiarrhythmic Agents, by Cardiac Disorder
Reproduced with permission from Page RL. Newly diagnosed atrial fibrillation. *NEJM.* 2004;351:2408. Copyright © 2004, Massachusetts Medical Society. All rights reserved.

- Surgical options include surgical or radiofrequency catheter ablation techniques.
- If plan for rhythm control, need to assess for risk of cardiac thrombus and subsequent stroke, as follows:
  - If definite acute onset within 48 hr and no h/o cardiomyopathy or mitral valve disease, start IV heparin and plan for cardioversion.
  - If onset was more than 48 hr or unknown (most pts), can anticoagulate with warfarin for 3–4 wk (at goal INR), then plan for elective cardioversion; or alternatively, start IV heparin, get TEE to r/o cardiac thrombus, and perform cardioversion once TEE (–), but should still plan to start anticoagulation with warfarin after successful cardioversion.
  - ACUTE trial: RCT of 1222 pts with new AF more than 48 hr duration, randomized to TEE-guided strategy (heparin or 5 d of warfarin, TEE, cardioversion, warfarin for 4 wk postcardioversion) or conventional strategy (3 wk of warfarin, cardioversion, warfarin for 4 more wk); no difference between the groups in TIA, stroke, embolic events, but TEE-guided strategy had lower bleeding events (2.9% vs 5.5%, NNT 38) and obviously shorter time to cardioversion (NEJM 2001;344:1411).

Anticoagulation therapy for AF pts

- Embolic CVA occurs at similar frequency in pts with rate or rhythm control strategies, so need to consider anticoagulation for stroke prophylaxis in all pts with AF.
- Primary agent is warfarin, with goal INR of 2–3.
  - Strongly consider in all pts with risk of stroke, even in elderly and those at risk for falls.

- Risk of life-altering CVA may be much higher than that of significant bleeding events; cohort study showed warfarin for AF pts reduced risk of thromboembolism and mortality, with only moderate increase in intracranial hemorrhage and no increase in significant non-ICH bleeding events (JAMA 2003;290:2685).
- Anticoagulation with heparin advisable for hospitalized pts with AF *only* if acute onset (not just newly diagnosed) and if plan for early attempt at cardioversion; in all other cases, not indicated.
- Risk of stroke in pts with AF: Overall 3–5% per yr; risk increases with age and other comorbidities; use CHADS2 score to assess for risk of stroke: 1 point each for CHF, HTN, age older than 75, diabetes, and 2 points if prior CVA/TIA; for NNT with warfarin (vs ASA or no therapy) to prevent CVA, see **Table 1.2.**
- If CHADS2 score is zero, pt at very low risk for CVA; consider therapy with ASA only; all others should be considered for warfarin (JAMA 2003;290:2685, JAMA 2001;285:2864).

Table 1.2   CHADS2 Score and Warfarin Therapy in Atrial Fibrillation

CHADS2 Score	Risk of stroke w/ warfarin rx	Risk of stoke w/o warfarin rx	NNT to prevent one stroke
0	0.25%	0.49%	417*
1	0.70%	1.50%	125
2	1.30%	2.50%	83
3	2.20%	5.30%	32
4	2.40%	6.00%	27
5–6	4.60%	6.90%	44*

* Nonsignificant difference between stroke risks
Adapted from *JAMA*. 2003;290:2685.

- Addition of clopidogrel to ASA for CVA prophylaxis can be considered, but probably minimal benefit
  - ACTIVE trial: study of 7554 pts with AF, deemed unable to tolerate warfarin, randomized to ASA 75–100 mg qd only or ASA plus clopidogrel 75 mg qd; after 3.6 yr of follow-up, there was significant reduction in stroke (2.4% vs 3.3% per yr, NNT 111) but also an increase in major bleeding events (2.0% vs 1.3% per yr, NNH 142) in pts with clopidogrel added to ASA (NEJM 2009;360:2066).
- ACCP Consensus Conference recommends continuing low-dose ASA in CAD pts who receive warfarin for AF (Chest 2008;133:546S), but no real evidence either way and may slightly increase bleeding risks.
- Future options for CVA prophylaxis in pts with AF may include improved oral anticoagulants, such as dabigatran (NEJM 2009;361:1139), and surgical closure of the left atrial appendage (Lancet 2009;374:534).

1.4   Infectious and Inflammatory Cardiac Diseases

Infective Endocarditis

(NEJM 2001;345:1318; BMJ 2006;333:334; Lancet 2004;363:139)

Cause: Acute infection of native or prosthetic heart valve. *Staph. aureus*, streptococci, and enterococci are the most common causes (approximately 80% of cases); see **Figure 1.4.**

HACEK organisms may de difficult to incubate (and often a cause of "culture-negative" IE):

- *Haemophilus parainfluenzae, Haemophilus aphrophilus, Haemophilus paraphrophilus*
- *Actinobacillus actinomycetemcomitans*
- *Cardiobacterium hominis*
- *Eikenella corrodens*
- *Kingella kingae*

PATHOGEN	NATIVE-VALVE ENDOCARDITIS				PROSTHETIC-VALVE ENDOCARDITIS		
	NEONATES	2 MO–15 YR OF AGE	16–60 YR OF AGE	>60 YR OF AGE	EARLY (<60 DAYS AFTER PROCEDURE)	INTERMEDIATE (60 DAYS–12 MO AFTER PROCEDURE)	LATE (>12 MO AFTER PROCEDURE)
				approximate percentage of cases			
Streptococcus species	15–20	40–50	45–65	30–45	1	7–10	30–33
Staphylococcus aureus	40–50	22–27	30–40	25–30	20–24	10–15	15–20
Coagulase-negative staphylococci	8–12	4–7	4–8	3–5	30–35	30–35	10–12
Enterococcus species	<1	3–6	5–8	14–17	5–10	10–15	8–12
Gram-negative bacilli	8–12	4–6	4–10	5	10–15	2–4	4–7
Fungi	8–12	1–3	1–3	1–2	5–10	10–15	1
Culture-negative and HACEK organisms*	2–6	0–15	3–10	5	3–7	3–7	3–8
Diphtheroids	<1	<1	<1	<1	5–7	2–5	2–3
Polymicrobial	3–5	<1	1–2	1–3	2–4	4–7	3–7

*Patients whose blood cultures were rendered negative by prior antibiotic treatment are excluded. HACEK denotes haemophilus species (*Haemophilus parainfluenzae, H. aphrophilus,* and *H. paraphrophilus*), *Actinobacillus actinomycetemcomitans, Cardiobacterium hominis, Eikenella corrodens,* and *Kingella kingae.*

Figure 1.4 Bacterial Causes of Endocarditis

Reproduced with permission from Mylonakis E, Calderwood SB. Infective endocarditis in adults. *NEJM.* 2001;345:1318. Copyright © 2001, Massachusetts Medical Society. All rights reserved.

Epidem: Incidence of community-acquired native valve endocarditis 1.7–6.2 per 100,000 (Am J Cardiol 1995;76:933); up to 2,000 per 100,000 IV drug abusers (Clin Infect Dis 2000;30:374); males more than females by almost 2:1.

Risk factors include IV drug abuse (tricuspid valve most commonly involved), diabetes, hemodialysis, poor dental hygiene; valvular abnormalities including mitral valve prolapse and rheumatic heart disease.

Pathophys: Valvular vegetation composed of platelets, fibrin, microbes, and host cells.

Likely most cases preceded by transient bacteremia from nonsterile site (usually the mouth); can be stimulated by dental procedure but even just chewing or brushing teeth.

Sx: Fever in 90% of pts (BMJ 2006;333:334), anorexia, weight loss, night sweats.

Symptoms alone do not always necessitate w/u for IE with an echo: study of 500 pts referred for TTE to "rule out endocarditis"; only 8.6% had echo evidence of IE; if pt had none of the following five criteria, the risk of IE was zero: physical signs of embolism, pos blood culture, prosthetic valve, central venous catheter, h/o IV drug abuse (Heart 2003;89:273).

Si: Heart murmur, usually in cases of preexisting valvular disease rather than due to vegetation itself.

Classic physical findings of endocarditis include the following:

- Splinter hemorrhages under the nails of hands or feet
- Conjunctival petechiae
- Osler's nodes: tender subcutaneous nodules on the hands
- Janeway's lesions: nontender, erythematous lesions on the palms and soles
- Roth's spots: retinal hemorrhages

Crs: Mortality rates vary with causative organism (highest with *Staph. aureus*, Q fever, and hospital-acquired organisms) as well as complications (higher with neuro complications, as described below); overall mortality is 20–25% (mortality of right-sided IE in IV drug abusers is about 10%).

Strep. bovis endocarditis has high correlation with underlying colonic lesions, cancer; consider GI evaluation as appropriate.

Use the following guidelines to determine whether pts with Staph. aureus bacteremia (SAB) should be evaluated for IE:

- Study of 103 pts with SAB evaluated with both TTE and TEE; IE by Duke criteria dx in 25% of pts; although 41% had predisposing heart disease, only 7% had other clinical signs of IE; TEE identified vegetations in all 25% of the pts with IE (TTE only 7% of pts) (J Am Coll Cardiol 1997;30:1072).
- Risk factors for IE with SAB: Community-acquired SAB, absence of other obvious focus, metastatic sequelae, fever/bacteremia for more than 3 d after removal of indwelling catheter.
- TEE-guided strategy of managing SAB in pts with indwelling catheters, compared to either 2 or 4 wk of empiric rx, was considered more cost-effective (Ann IM 1999;130:810).
- Suggest TEE-guided strategy to r/o IE in all pts with proven SAB, unless clearly related to known source (including indwelling catheter or other site).

Cmplc: Valve destruction/regurgitation; CHF (more likely with aortic valve involvement).

Stroke syndrome:

- Etiology can be direct embolization of pieces of valvular vegetation; also mycotic aneurysms can form and lead to acute intracranial hemorrhage.
- CT +/− MRI can be used to evaluate neuro sx in setting of bacteremia/IE.
- Denmark study of 260 pts with native-valve IE with S. aureus; 35% of pts had neurologic complications, most common

was hemiparesis; more likely with mitral valve involvement; significantly increased mortality (74% vs 68% in pts without neuro complications) (Am J Med 1997;102:379).

- Finnish study of 218 pts with native-valve IE: 25% had neuro complications, more common with SAB, increased mortality with neuro disease (25% vs 20%) (Arch IM 2000;160:2781).

Additional complc include other septic embolic disease, including splenic, renal, and hepatic abscesses.

Lab: Blood cultures are the single most important diagnostic test; up to 93% of pts with true IE will have pos Cx, therefore very important to obtain multiple adequate Cx before starting antibiotic therapy; avoid drawing from an indwelling catheter because of concern about contamination; always consider IE risks in pts with pos blood Cx (especially *S. aureus* and viridans strep), even if minimally sx or asx.

Regarding "culture-negative" endocarditis:

- French study of 620 pts with IE : 14% of all pts had neg initial blood Cx, with causative organism eventually found in 17% of those pts; overall, initial negative Cx no effect on mortality, but more often had surgical intervention (Clin Infect Dis 1995;20:501).
- Most common associated factor was prior administration of antibiotics (48%).
- Consider serologic testing for *Chlamydia, Mycoplasma,* and Q fever (*Coxiella burnetii*).
- Other causes include HACEK organisms, fungal, *Legionella, Bartonella.*

Initial w/u besides blood Cx can include CBC with diff (often have leukocytosis and anemia of chronic disease), ESR, and CRP (although clinical utility is limited).

Repeat blood Cx on appropriate abx to confirm sterilization are recommended (Circ 2005;111:e394).

Noninv: EKG to look for evidence of conduction deficits.

Echocardiography: In most cases, can start with TTE, 98% specificity for vegetations but only 44% sensitivity; TEE has 100% specif and 64% sens (J Am Coll Cardiol 1991;18:391).

Consider TEE in following cases:

- Continued suspicion for IE with neg TTE (especially if SAB)
- Body habitus that may create difficult TTE windows (e.g., COPD with barrel chest, obesity, other chest wall deformities)
- Prosthetic valves

Duke criteria for dx of suspected IE (original article Am J Med 1994;96:200, modified Clin Infect Dis 2000;30:633): highly specific, 92% neg predictive value (J Am Coll Cardiol 1999;33:2023, Arch IM 2000;160:1185, Am J Cardiol 1996; 77:403):

- Definite cases: two major criteria, *or* one major and three minor criteria, *or* five minor criteria
- Possible cases: one major criterion and one minor criterion, *or* three minor criteria
- Major dx criteria are as follows:
  - Typical IE microbe on two blood cultures or pathologic specimen (or evidence of positive titer for *Coxiella burnetii*, difficult to grow in most settings)
  - Echocardiographic findings of new valve regurgitation or findings consistent with IE, including intracardiac mass/ vegetation, abscess, or new dehiscence of a prosthetic valve
- Minor dx criteria include the following:
  - Risk factors including predisposing heart condition (prosthetic valve, native valvular disease, congenital heart disease) or IV drug abuse
  - Fever higher than 100.4°F
  - Vascular findings (as above)

- Immunologic findings including positive rheumatoid factor, Osler's nodes, Roth's spots, glomerulonephritis
- Microbiologic findings including elevated CRP/ESR or pos blood Cx not meeting a major criterion

Rx: Mainstay of therapy is prolonged course of IV abx; generally 4–6 wk depending on organism, native vs prosthetic valve, abx choice—refer to AHA/IDSA guidelines (Circ 2005;111:e394); empiric therapy is not standardized, because in most clinical settings pt may be initially treated for another presumed source (until Cx and imaging results suggest IE); abx choice should be based on identification of sensitivities of specific microbe; in most cases of staph or strep endocarditis, penicillin (or derivative including nafcillin, oxacillin) can be used; vancomycin for MRSA; ceftriaxone is also a commonly used regimen because it allows once-daily IV dosing (JAMA 1992;267:264).

Consider surgical evaluation with the following conditions:

- Valve destruction w/ hemodynamic compromise
- Prosthetic valve involvement
- Persistent fever/bacteremia w/ appropriate abx therapy
- Large vegetations w/ embolic potential
- Perivalvular abscess formation

Anticoagulant therapy is not warranted (unless for another indication), despite risk of emboli and neuro complications; warfarin may actually increase the risk of intracranial hemorrhage and should be carefully monitored if used in IE pts.

Prophylaxis (Geriatrics 2008;63:12): includes single dose abx 30–40 min prior to procedure in pts with prosthetic valve, previous IE, unrepaired congenital heart disease, or cardiac transplant pts with valvular disorders (no longer recommended for mitral valve prolapse, rheumatic heart disease, or other valvular disease because of low overall risk); mostly concerns predental procedures, but also consider for hospitalized pts. In general, appropriate in these settings:

- Pts prior to oral/ENT surgery
- Pts with bronchoscopy (only with biopsies)
- Not necessary for GI/GU procedures

Antibiotic choices includes amoxicillin 2 gm PO; ampicillin 2 gm IM or ceftriaxone 1 gm IV if unable to take PO; clindamycin 600 mg PO or azithromycin 500 mg PO if penicillin-allergic.

Acute Pericarditis

(NEJM 2004;351:2195, Am Fam Phys 2007;76:1509)

Cause: 90% of cases are viral (and/or idiopathic); remaining 10% of cases derive from:

- Post-MI, or postcardiac surgery
  - Dressler's syndrome is delayed post-MI pericarditis due to autoimmune reaction; pericarditis associated with acute MI (2–4 d post-MI) is more common and fleeting.
- Bacterial or tuberculous infection, especially in pts with HIV/AIDS
- Dissecting aortic aneurysm (with hemopericardium)
- Chest wall trauma
- Neoplasm, especially primary lung, breast
- S/p radiation or chemotherapy
- Acute renal failure; uremia
- Autoimmune
- Rare adverse drug reaction

Epidem: 5% of ER pts (and 0.1% of hospitalized pts) with chest pain not due to AMI.

Pathophys: Normally, pericardium is a thin membrane surrounding the heart, containing 15–50 ml of serous fluid; pathologic disease can cause increase in fluid and thickening of the membrane.

Sx: Chest pain, usually substernal and pleuritic; worse when supine and improves when leaning forward.

Si: Pericardial friction rub in 85% of pts (Am J Cardiol 1995;75:378); best heard at lower left sternal border, with pt leaning forward and exhaling.

Crs: Almost 25% of all pts will have recurrence, usually within the first few weeks after acute therapy.

Cmplc: Watch for the following uncommon complications:

- Cardiac tamponade
  - Concern if hypotensive, tachycardic, elevated JVP, muffled heart sounds.
  - Pulsus paradoxus (PP): Drop in SBP of greater than 10 mmHg with inspiration; in emergent cases, PP is suggested with loss of radial pulse during inspiration.
  - More common in pts with cancer or infectious cause of pericarditis.
  - Accumulation of pericardial fluid increases intrapericardial pressure to greater than pressure in the right heart, leading to impaired RV filling, and RV failure.
  - Proceed urgently with pericardiocentesis for dx and rx; if not acutely available, consider aggressive fluid resuscitation to increase RV filling, especially in volume-depleted pts.
  - Recurrent effusions may require surgical intervention (i.e., "pericardial window" to drain to pleural space).
- Pericardial constriction (Circ 2006;113:1622)
  - Scarred pericardium impairs RV filling.
  - Sx include elevated JVP, signs of right heart failure (ascites, peripheral edema, without pulmonary edema).
  - Calcification may be seen on CXR, but echocardiogram is definitive test (may be difficult to distinguish from restrictive cardiomyopathy).

- Pleural effusion
  - May be associated with underlying disease (e.g., neoplastic, autoimmune).
  - If present, consider diagnostic thoracentesis instead of peri-cardiocentesis (unless required for therapeutic reasons).

Lab: CBC with diff to look for leukocytosis; ESR, CRP likely elevated but not clinically useful to determine cause or prognosis.

Consider ANA, RF if other sequelae of connective tissue disease.

Elevated troponin in 35–50% of pts, representing epicar-dial inflammation, not true transmural injury; usually returns to normal within 2 wk.

Noninv: EKG shows diffuse ST-segment elevation, possible T wave inversion, and PR-segment depression.

CXR to look for cardiomegaly (requires effusion of more than 250 mL) and to rule out other disease that may indicate cause (infection, aneurysm, mediastinal Ca).

Rx: General approach to pericarditis:
- Consider hospitalization in pts with severe pain to initiate pain control and watch for cmplc; pts at risk for cmplc or poor prognosis include those with temperature more than 100.4ºF, immunosuppressed, posttrauma, coagulopathic, or large effu-sion with evidence of tamponade.
- ASA or NSAIDs for anti-inflammatory effect and pain con-trol are mainstays of therapy.
  - ASA 2–4 gm qd; indomethacin 75–225 mg qd; ibuprofen 1600–3200 mg qd.
  - Consider addition of PPI to reduce GI side effects.
  - Concern for use in pts with known CAD/CHF and CKD, consider alternate therapies.
- Colchicine (0.6 mg bid):
  - CORE trial: 84 pts w/ 1st episode of recurrent pericardi-tis rx w/ ASA alone or ASA plus colchicine; addition of

colchicine reduced recurrence rate (NNT 4) and decreased symptoms at 72 hr (NNT 4) (Arch IM 2005;165:1987).

- COPE trial: Study population similar to CORE trial, but w/ 1st episode of pericarditis, rx w/ ASA plus colchicine 0.5–1 mg qd for 3 mo; showed similar results to CORE trial in regard to sx improvement and recurrence rates (Circ 2005;112:2012).
- Oral steroids (prednisone 1–1.5 mg/kg, then tapering dose) in recurrent or resistant cases, or in pts intolerant of, or contraindication to, ASA and NSAIDs.
- Rx of underlying disease is crucial, if possible.

Myocarditis

(NEJM 2009;360:1526, Circ 2006;113:876)

Cause: Multiple causes have been identified, including those listed below.

- Viral: Coxsackie B, adenovirus, parvovirus B19, hepatitis C (Circ Res 2005;96:144), EBV, CMV, HHV-6; HIV infection is a strong risk factor, may be some causative effect of virus, but also due to anti-HIV meds and opportunistic infections
- Bacterial: Mycobacterium, streptococcus, syphilis
- Other infectious: Lyme disease, ehrlichiosis, babesiosis, Chagas disease (*Trypanosoma cruzi*) (NEJM 2006;355:799)
- Medication/hypersensitivity: cocaine, antibiotics (including sulfa and cephalosporins), TCAs
- Infiltrative diseases: sarcoidosis, giant-cell myocarditis, amyloidosis, SLE, Wegener's granulomatosis

Epidem: Slightly more common in men (Am Heart J 2006;151:463); true incidence is very hard to determine as many pts do not have definitive diagnosis (and is an underdiagnosed cause of sudden death).

Pathophys: In most cases, the offending agent triggers a CD4+ T cell immune reaction causing direct damage to the myocytes.

Sx: Usually presents as dilated cardiomyopathy with typical CHF sx: dyspnea, chest pain, fatigue, edema.

May have viral prodrome in preceding weeks with fever, myalgias, cough, gastroenteritis.

Si: Similar to CHF.

Crs: Varies by type, as follows:

- Fulminant lymphocytic type: Viral prodrome, significant initial hemodynamic compromise, but has better long-term prognosis (NEJM 2000;342:690).
- Acute lymphocytic type: Onset is more insidious and less pronounced hemodynamic effects, but long-term prognosis is poor.

Cmplc: Sudden cardiac death due to ventricular tachycardia and fibrillation.

Bradyarrhythmias, including 3rd-degree AV block.

Lab: Many pts have elevated TnI but limited specif and sens for diagnostic purposes.

Definitive dx based on bx and pathologic diagnosis:

- Dallas criteria require presence of inflammatory cellular infiltrate with or without associated myocyte necrosis.
- However, there are significant limitations and low sensitivity because multiple samples are required to get diagnostic tissue; in postmortem study of pts with myocarditis, single sample yielded positive result in only 25% of cases, and more than five samples still failed to identify 33% of cases (J Am Coll Cardiol 1989;14:915, Mayo Clin Proc 1989;64:1235).
- Should consider biopsy in pts with acute onset of unexplained cardiomyopathy associated with hemodynamic compromise (and no evidence of ischemic cause) or progressive sx, especially with pronounced ventricular arrhythmias or heart block.

Noninv: EKG may show sinus tachycardia, nonspecific changes, or AMI-like patterns.

Echocardiogram can diagnose systolic dysfunction.

Cardiac catheterization (or noninvasive stress testing) can r/o ischemic disease as cause of cardiomyopathy.

Cardiac MRI can be used as an alternative to invasive diagnostics (Circ 2004;109:1250).

Rx: Primary treatment is similar to systolic CHF/LV dysfunction (acutely, hemodynamic support if needed, diuretics, vasodilators; chronically, ACE inhibitors, beta-blockers). See Section 1.2.

May require AICD in some cases (see recommendations for cardiomyopathy/CHF in Section 1.2).

Temporary or permanent pacemakers in setting of heart block.

Cardiac transplantation in severe cases.

Despite inflammatory causes, there is no clinically proven direct therapy for myocarditis, including steroids (NEJM 1989;321:1061), IVIG (Circ 2001;103:2254), immunosuppressants (NEJM 1995;333:269).

1.5 Hypertensive Crisis

(Chest 2007;131:1949, Lancet 2000;356:411)

Cause: Definitions:

- Hypertensive crisis: hypertension characterized by SBP greater than or equal to 180 mmHg, DBP greater than or equal to 110 mmHg; may be initial presentation of chronic hypertension (up to 28% had no prior hx of HTN) (HT 1996;27:144) or due to some other precipitating factor; will occur in 1–2% of chronic HTN pts; further defined as one of two types:
  - Hypertensive urgency (HU): BP more than 180/110, without evidence of symptoms or end-organ damage; typically requires therapy to improve BP within 24–48 hr, which may not require hospital admission.
  - Hypertensive emergency (HE): BP more than 180/110 with symptoms and evidence of end-organ damage;

typically requires hospital admission for immediate antihypertensive therapy and w/u; types of end-organ damage include the following:

- Neurologic: encephalopathy, stroke
- Cardiovascular: aortic dissection, ACS/AMI, acute diastolic heart failure
- Respiratory: acute pulmonary edema
- Renal: acute renal failure
- Obstetrical: preeclampsia, eclampsia, HELLP syndrome (hemolysis, elevated liver enzymes, thrombocytopenia)
- Hematologic: microangiopathic hemolytic anemia
- "Malignant" (or "accelerated") hypertension does not currently have agreed-upon definition and should not be used to describe hypertensive crisis.

Precipitating factors of hypertensive crisis (other than 1st presentation of chronic HTN) include the following:

- Illicit drugs, including cocaine, amphetamines, phencyclidine (PCP)
- MAO inhibitors with tyramine crisis
- Erythropoietin (EPO)
- OTC meds, including decongestants (oral and nasal preps)
- Medical emergencies including aortic dissection, ACS, and acute ischemic or hemorrhagic stroke
- Chronic alcohol abuse and acute alcohol withdrawal
- End-stage renal disease and hemodialysis
- Pregnancy-induced hypertension

Epidem: Higher incidence with age, males, African Americans, lower socioeconomic status (likely due to lack of primary care) (Am J Publ Hlth 1988;78:636, NEJM 1992;327:776).

Pathophys: Abrupt increase in SVR, leading to vascular endothelial injury and activation of coagulation cascade, leading to ischemic injury; activation of renin-angiotensin-aldosterone (RAA) system also creates further vasoconstriction.

Sx/Si: Most frequent initial sx/si: chest pain (27%), dyspnea (22%), headache (22%), neurologic complaints (21%), epistaxis (17%), presyncope (10%), agitation (10%) (HT 1996;27:144).

Also, back pain in setting of aortic dissection.

Crs: When first described, untreated HE had 1-yr mortality of 79%; likely much less now with increased outpatient BP screening and improved treatment strategies.

Cmplc: End-organ damage, as listed in the definition of *hypertensive emergency* at beginning of Section 1.5.

Lab: Initial w/u includes CBC, BMP; consider cardiac enzymes, BNP.

U/A can detect proteinuria.

Noninv: EKG to look for acute ischemic changes, LVH. EKG findings suggestive of LVH include the following:

- High voltages: depth of S wave in V_1 (or V_2) plus height of R wave in V_5 (or V_6) greater than 35 mm (false pos seen in young, athletic, thin adults); or height of R wave in aV_L greater than 11 mm.
- Strain pattern: characteristic voltage criteria plus pattern of ST depression and T wave inversions, especially in leads with tall R waves.
- Other nondiagnostic, but suggestive, signs: left axis deviation, IVCD or LBBB, left atrial enlargement (biphasic P wave in V_1 or large P waves [greater than 1 mm in size and 120 msec in duration] in limb leads).

CXR to look for pulmonary edema, mediastinal widening to suggest aortic dissection (if so, f/u with CT scan).

Consider echo once treatment has started to eval LV function, r/o LVH.

Rx: **Table 1.3** presents primary and secondary drug choices for hypertensive crisis, as well as strategies for inpatient management of chronic HTN.

Table 1.3   Drug Choices for Hypertensive Crisis and Inpatient Management of Chronic Hypertension

Drug	Route/Action	Dosing	Considerations
		Primary Agents	
Labetalol	IV; α-1 and nonselective β-blocker	20 mg IV loading dose, then can use repeated IV boluses or start drip at 1–2 mg/min and titrate to effect	• 1st-line drug for most hypertensive crises because despite effective drop in BP, maintains end-organ perfusion • Works within 2–5 min and lasts 2–4 hr • Safe in pregnant pts
Esmolol	IV; short-acting, cardio-selective β-blocker	0.5–1 mg/kg loading dose, then infusion starting at 50 mcg/kg/min and titrate to effect	• Works within 60 seconds and lasts 10–20 min • Helpful in acute postop HTN, because often only short-term therapy is needed • Will reduce HR and cardiac output • Very useful in cases of aortic dissection • Avoid in sympathetic crises (drug-induced, pheochromocytoma, MAOI with tyramine crisis), as unopposed α activity will lead to worsening of hypertension
Nitroprusside	IV; direct arterial and venous dilator	Start IV infusion at 0.3–0.5 mcg/kg/min, (but avoid doses >10 mcg/kg/min)	• Despite long hx of use, no longer considered a 1st-line agent due to side effects • Can actually have deleterious effect on end-organ perfusion, particularly to brain and heart

Nicardipine	IV; dihydropyridine CCB	Start IV infusion at 5 mg/hr, titrate to effect up to 15 mg/hr	• Works within seconds; lasts only a few minutes; very titratable • Prolonged use can lead to cyanide toxicity (metabolic acidosis, seizures, coma) • Contraindicated in pregnant pts • Strong vasodilator of cerebral and cardiac arteries • Useful in acute coronary syndromes and heart failure • Useful in sympathetic crises • Works within 5 min and lasts 4–6 hr
Fenoldopam	IV; direct vasodilator via dopamine-1 receptors	Start IV infusion at 0.1 mcg/kg/min, titrate to effect	• Works within 5 min and lasts 30–60 min
Secondary Agents			
Nitroglycerin	IV or transdermal; venodilator (arterial dilator at high doses)	Start IV infusion at 5 mcg/min and titrate to effect	• Limited use as primary agent due to primarily venodilatory effects • Helpful in ACS and acute pulmonary edema associated with HE
Phentolamine	IV; α-1 blocker	5–10 mg IV boluses to max of 20–30 mg	• Use only in setting of sympathetic hypertensive crises (drug-induced, pheochromocytoma, MAOI with tyramine crisis), as use of β-blocking agents can lead to worsening hypertension

(continued)

1.5 Hypertensive Crisis **77**

Table 1.3 Drug Choices for Hypertensive Crisis and Inpatient Management of Chronic Hypertension (*Continued*)

Drug	Route/Action	Dosing	Considerations
Hydralazine	IV; direct vasodilator	10–20 mg IV q 4–6 hr	• Limited use in HE because of variable BP effects • Most useful as antihypertensive rx in chronic HTN pts unable to take PO meds (postop, GI bleeds, etc.) • Safe in pregnant pts; often used as primary drug in preeclampsia pts
Enalaprilat	IV; ACE inhibitor	1.25 mg IV q 6 hr, up to 5 mg per dose	• Limited use in HE because of variable BP effects • Most useful as antihypertensive rx in chronic HTN pts unable to take PO meds (postop, GI bleeds, etc.) • Avoid in pregnant pts
Metoprolol	IV; cardioselective β-blocker	2.5–10 mg IV q 4–6 hr	• No use in HE due to variable effects (likely to reduce HR in excess of BP effect), unless associated ACS or tachyarrhythmia • Most useful as antihypertensive rx in chronic HTN pts unable to take PO meds (post-op, GI bleeds, etc.), especially in pts already on chronic β-blocker rx • IV forms of atenolol & propranolol also available

Clonidine	Transdermal; central-acting agent	0.1–0.3 mg/24 hr patch, change weekly	• No use in HE, but may be used in treating mild hypertensive urgencies in pts unable to take PO (especially in setting of alcohol withdrawal), or for patients on chronic clonidine to avoid rebound HTN

Avoid These Agents

Nifedipine	Sublingual	N/A	• Potent BP lowering effect has been associated with precipitation of acute stroke and ACS • Should not be used in any settings of hypertensive crisis
Diuretics (including furosemide)	IV or PO	N/A	• Because many cases of HE are associated with volume depletion (see Rx section), diuresis may lead to precipitous drop in BP and further end-organ damage • Consider only in cases of acute pulmonary edema (although NTG may be better 1st-line agent)

Adapted from *Chest.* 2007;131:1949.

CARDIOLOGY

Follow close monitoring in ICU; consider invasive arterial BP monitoring.

May require IV hydration, as high pressure can cause natriuresis and volume depletion (which may precipitate dangerous fall in BP with IV antihypertensive rx).

Goal BP reductions in HE: reduce DBP by 10–15% or to goal of less than 110 mmHg over 30–60 min (unless AMI or aortic dissection, which require more aggressive BP lowering).

For hypertension in setting of acute CVA, please refer to "Ischemic Stroke" in Section 6.1; avoid treatment except in cases of severe HTN (BP higher than 220/120) so as not to decrease cerebral perfusion pressures.

1.6 Syncope

(NEJM 2008;358:615, NEJM 2005;352:1004, J Am Coll Cardiol 2008;51:599)

Cause: Rapid and transient loss of consciousness, followed by complete recovery; presyncope is used to describe symptoms of faintness without loss of consciousness.

Even after evaluation, the cause of syncope may be unknown in up to 33% of pts (Am Fam Phys 2005;72:1492).

Causes fall into four main categories:

1. Reflex-mediated:
   - Vasovagal: parasympathetic stimulation leading to bradycardia, hypotension
   - Carotid sinus stimulation: either from direct carotid massage or due to head-turning, shaving, tight collar
   - Situational: for example, postmicturation, after a cough or sneeze
2. Cardiac:
   - Arrhythmia: bradycardia due to sick sinus syndrome or 2nd/3rd-degree heart block; ventricular tachycardia; pacemaker malfunction

- Structural heart disease (acute or chronic): aortic or mitral stenosis; ACS; pulmonary embolism; hypertrophic cardio-myopathy; pericardial tamponade
3. Neurologic:
   - Vascular: stroke/TIA, subclavian steal syndrome
   - Seizure, atypical migraines
   - Psychiatric: including conversion disorder, somatization, panic disorder
4. Orthostatic:
   - Dehydration
   - Medication-related (excessive antihypertensives, particularly in elderly); intoxication
   - Autonomic dysfunction with diabetes, Parkinson's, other degenerative neuro diseases

Epidem: 20–50% of adults will have a syncopal episode over their life-time (75% of pts older than 70) (Am Fam Phys 2005;72:1492).
Risk of orthostasis rises with age, and more prevalent in pts in NH settings (NEJM 2008;358:615).

Pathophys: Decrease in cerebral perfusion is the cause, regardless of underlying abnormality.

Sx: Vasovagal syncope in approximately 70% of cases has a prodrome of nausea, diaphoresis, weakness, dizziness; brief seizure activity may be seen with vasovagal syncope event.

Si: Check for orthostasis, defined as a drop in SBP of more than 20 mmHg or drop in DBP of more than 10 mmHg within 3 min of standing (with our without associated increase in pulse; increased HR or tachycardia suggest dehydration, bleeding).

Crs: Although recurrence is common, most cases of orthostatic or vasovagal syncope do not have long-term consequences.

Cmplc: No specific complications, unless associated trauma related to fall. Refer to sections on specific causes for more detailed complications.

Lab: Evaluation of syncope is controversial, and can be very expensive if tests ordered indiscriminately; best practice is a thorough history and physical examination with further evaluations based on clinical suspicion of underlying cause.

Initial w/u often includes CBC (r/o anemia), metabolic panel (r/o hypoglycemia, hypo- and hypernatremia, acute renal failure), cardiac enzymes, although lab studies rarely determine cause alone.

Noninv: EKG should be performed on all pts, unless clearly reflex-mediated cause, to evaluate rhythm, QT interval, evidence of conduction disease, or signs of acute or prior CAD/MI.

Testing depends on suspicion for underlying cause.

- Orthostatic and reflex-mediated may only require orthostatic BP and pulse, observation for further sx; can confirm reflex-mediated by inducing sx with carotid massage, situational circumstance, or tilt-table testing.
- Cardiac:
  - Inpatient telemetry monitoring vs outpatient monitor (24-hr Holter monitor if frequent sx; may require 7-d or longer event monitor if sx infrequent).
  - Echocardiogram to eval for valvular disease, r/o HOCM or underlying LV dysfunction.
  - Stress testing or angiography if concern for underlying ACS.
  - Electrophysiology study (EPS) if concern for underlying arrhythmia, especially if known CAD or cardiomyopathy.
- Neurologic: Probably the most over-ordered tests in the evaluation of syncope; most pts do not require w/u for neuro cause unless witnessed seizure activity or postsyncopal focal neurologic symptoms.
  - Head CT or MRI if concern for stroke, hemorrhage, or intracranial mass

- EEG if concern for seizure
- Carotid dopplers only if clearly due to TIA/stroke (syncope is not considered a symptom of cerebrovascular disease for the NASCET studies evaluating the role of carotid endarterectomy)

A study of diagnostic yield and cost-effectiveness of studies for evaluation of syncope (Arch IM 2009;169:1299) reported the following:

- Among the 1920 pts admitted for syncope evaluation, w/ mean age of 79 yr, many had comorbid HTN, CAD.
- Highest yield and most cost-effective test was postural BP measurement (affecting dx and mgt in up to 25% of pts, but only performed in 38% of all pts); see **Table 1.4.**

Rx: Hospitalize for evaluation in the following situations:

- Syncopal event associated with severe injury or driving

Table 1.4   Common Tests for Syncope

Test	Performed in (% of all patients)	Affected Management (% of tests obtained)	Cost per Affected Case
Electrocardiogram	99	7	$1,020
Telemetry	99	12	$710
Cardiac enzymes	95	1	$22,397
Head CT	63	2	$24,881
Echocardiogram	39	4	$6,272
Postural BP measurements	38	25	$17
Carotid ultrasound	13	2	$19,580
Electroencephalogram	8	1	$32,973
Head MRI	7	12	$8,678
Cardiac stress test	6	9	$8,415

Adapted from *Arch IM.* 2009;169:1299.

- Concern for cardiac cause: exercise-induced (to r/o HOCM or aortic stenosis); initial w/u indicating heart disease (abnormal EKG, cardiac enzymes); pts with pacemaker
- Focal neurologic symptoms to suggest TIA or postictal paralysis
- Severe orthostasis with reproducible symptoms and need for close monitoring of therapy or withdrawal of meds

For treatment of underlying neurologic or cardiac causes, refer to sections on treatment of those specific diseases.

Treatment of vasovagal syncope usually involves reassurance only; pts should lie down with prodromal sx; isometric exercises, increasing fluid and salt intake may help, especially in younger pts.

Medical therapies for recurrent episodes of syncope include the following:

- Beta-blockers: Have shown reduction in sudden cardiac death and VT in pts with known CAD, but little evidence to support routine use in syncope.
  - POST trial: 208 pts with vasovagal syncope randomized to metoprolol or placebo; no benefit in reducing further syncopal events (Circ 2006;113:1164).
- Fludrocortisone: Commonly used for orthostasis, but no RCTs have proven benefit; mineralocorticoid effect leads to fluid retention and increased BP, but watch for worsening HTN and CHF (and should definitely avoid concomitant use with antihypertensives); starting dose is 0.1 mg qd and can be titrated to a few doses per week based on effect; poorly tolerated in elderly due to hypokalemia, worsening HTN or CHF, depression, edema (Heart 1996;76:507).
- Midodrine: Alpha-agonist that causes peripheral vasoconstriction; proven effective in younger pts in multiple small studies (J Cardiovasc Electrophysiol 2001;12:935, Am J Cardiol 2001; 88:A7, JAMA 1997;277:1046, Neurol 1998;51:120); high

rate of intolerance in elderly pts because of HTN or angina exacerbation.

- SSRIs may help in some cases of recurrent syncope resistant to other therapies (J Am Coll Cardiol 1999;33:1227).

  Pacemakers in severe cases with recurrent syncopal events.
  Treatment of orthostatic hypotension involves the following:

- Volume repletion with isotonic fluid, if evidence of chronic dehydration; encourage fluid intake at home.
- Teach gradual movements; avoid rapid sitting/standing; isotonic exercises; avoid prolonged recumbency and raise head of bed when sleeping; consider custom-fit elastic stockings to reduce venous pooling.
- Consider adjustment to chronic antihypertensive therapy, especially medications directed mainly at HTN (vasodilators, CCBs) or symptoms (nitrates, diuretics); lowest tolerated doses of beta-blockers or ACE inhibitors in pts with known CAD, cardiomyopathy with LV dysfunction, DM with renal disease; many elderly pts with orthostasis have supine hypertension, so take care on making adjustments as inpatients (when most BPs are taken in bed), consider standing BP measurements once to twice daily to evaluate.
- Salt supplementation may be effective younger pts (Heart 1996;75:134), but avoid in elderly due to higher prevalence of HTN and CHF.
- Can consider medical therapies as with vasovagal above, but high rates of complications, intolerance.

Chapter 2

Endocrinology

2.1 Adrenal Disorders

Cushing's Syndrome

(NEJM 1995;332:791; Lancet 2006;367:1605)

Cause: Causes fall into four main categories:

- ACTH-dependent (80%): "Cushing's disease" from pituitary adenoma or ectopic ACTH or CRH production by small-cell lung cancer or other cancer (ovary, pancreas, pheochromocytoma); occasionally carcinoid tumors, especially of lung (Ann IM 1992;117:209)
- ACTH-independent (20%): cortisol overproduction from adenoma, carcinoma, or hyperplasia
- "Pseudo-Cushing's syndrome": hypercortisolism due to critical illness, severe depression (NEJM 1986;314:1329), or alcoholism (Lancet 1977;1:726)
- Factitious (less than 1%): excessive, intentional intake of oral glucocorticoids

Epidem: More common in women.

Pathophys: Hypothalamic-pituitary-adrenal axis: corticotropin-releasing hormone (CRH) produced in hypothalamus, converts precursor (pro-opiomelanocortin, POMC) to adrenocorticotropic hormone (ACTH) in pituitary gland, which stimulates cortisol production from adrenal gland; negative feedback loop of cortisol to hypothalamus and pituitary reduces production of CRH and ACTH.

Syndrome due to direct effects on tissue of excess glucocorticoids.

Sx: Muscle weakness, weight gain, easy bruising, decreased libido, amenorrhea.

Si: Truncal/central fat, edema, moon face, buffalo hump, abdominal striae, acne, ecchymoses, telangiectasias; virilization and hirsutism (more likely with adrenal carcinoma); muscle weakness.

Crs: Excellent prognosis unless underlying cancer (NEJM 1971;285:243).

Cmplc: Diabetes/glucose intolerance, hypertension (may be as high as 5% of pts with combined HTN and DM), ASCVD, "fatty liver," osteoporosis and fractures, increased number and severity of infections, peptic ulcers, depression and psychoses, nephrolithiasis.

Lab: (Ann IM 2003;138:980) Measure baseline serum cortisols; normal level is 5–25 mcg/dL in a.m., dropping to less than 10 mcg/dL in p.m.; random or morning serum cortisol levels have no value in evaluation.

- 1st step: Screen suspected pts (may require multiple tests).
  - Nighttime (11 p.m. to midnight) serum cortisol level: Less than 5 mcg/dL on repeated testing highly sensitive (99%) to r/o disease, but should be in a sleeping, non-stressed pt (may be hard to obtain in hospitalized pt).
  - Nighttime salivary cortisol: ELISA test, normal if less than 3–4 nmol/L; diagnostic for Cushing's if greater than 7 nmol/L; 93% sens, 100% specif (J Clin Endocrinol Metab 2002;87:4515).
  - 24-hr urine free cortisol (may be the best screen): Greater than 3 times normal levels strongly suggestive of Cushing's; baseline GFR less than 30 and incomplete urine collection

may confound results; false positives with digoxin and carbamazepine.

- Low-dose dexamethasone suppression test (DST): In normal pts, potent glucocorticoid will suppress ACTH production in pituitary, lowering cortisol levels (dexamethasone not detected on cortisol assays). Overnight test, dexamethasone 1 mg at 11 p.m. and check cortisol at 8 a.m.; less than 5 in normal; if greater than 10, r/o Cushing's (100% sens, 90% specif) (Ann IM 1990;112:738); false positives with phenytoin, carbamazepine, oral estrogens. If studies are indeterminate, then give 0.5 mg dexamethasone q 6 hr for 48 hr and measure serum cortisol. Both tests, however, have limited value (the three prior tests are easier and more helpful in screening).

- 2nd step: Determine whether ACTH-dependent or -independent; measure serum ACTH.
  - If low, investigate adrenal source.
  - If normal or high, suspect pituitary or ectopic source.
- 3rd step: Determine if ACTH-dependent Cushing's is due to pituitary or ectopic source; may be very difficult.
  - Perform imaging as described in the Noninv outline below.
  - High-dose dexamethasone suppression test no longer recommended (J Clin Endocrinol Metab 1997;82:1780).
  - CRH stimulation test: ACTH and cortisol increases after CRH is given indicate pituitary tumor, no increases indicate ectopic ACTH or adrenal tumor (Ann IM 1985;102:344). Perform petrosal venous sampling for ACTH levels (NEJM 1985;312:100).

Noninv: CT of adrenals if ACTH-independent, to look for solitary adrenal mass or bilateral hyperplasia; if (–) CT in setting of low ACTH levels, reconsider factitious syndrome.

If ACTH-dependent, MRI of brain with gadolinium enhancement, 71% sens, 87% specif; but 10% of the normal adult population have a lesion (Ann IM 1994;120:817); average size of adenoma is 6 mm, larger than 1 cm in only 6% of cases (J Clin Endocrinol Metab 2005;90:4963).

Rx: Combination of three modalities:

- Surgical transsphenoidal microadenomectomy, 90% successful (NEJM 1984;310:889) vs 76% (Ann IM 1988;109:487); bilateral adrenalectomy
- Irradiation of pituitary, 83% successful in pts who fail surgery (NEJM 1997;336:172)
- Medical therapies: aminoglutethimide, mitotane, metyrapone, and trilostane (Med Lett Drugs Ther 1985;27:87); bromocriptine; ketoconazole for its antisteroid synthesis effect (NEJM 1987;317:812)

Adrenal Insufficiency

(Endo Metab Clin N Am 2006;35:767;NEJM 2003;348:727)

Cause: Three main types:

1. Primary AI (destruction of more than 90% of adrenal glands) can be caused by any of the following:
   - Autoimmune disorder (classic Addison's)
   - Infectious or inflammatory destruction of gland, usually by hemorrhage or necrosis (Waterhouse-Friderichsen syndrome); classically associated with meningococcal infection, but has been related to multiple infectious types including bacterial (*Streptococcus, Pseudomonas*), mycobacterial (TB, MAI), viral (HIV up to 20% of cases, CMV), fungal (PCP, *Coccidiomycosis, Cryptococcus*) (South Med J 2003;96:888)
   - Cancer, including bilateral adrenal metastases
   - Drug-induced: etomidate (J Intensive Care Med 2007;22: 111, NEJM 2008;358:111), ketoconazole, progesterones

Rare: adrenoleukodystrophy, sarcoidosis, amyloidosis, Wilson's disease.

2. Secondary AI (loss of hypothalamic-pituitary axis) is caused by the following:
   - Chronic corticosteroid use (can occur in pts on as little as 7.5 mg prednisone qd, or 30 mg hydrocortisone, for 3 wk; risk may continue for months)
   - Pituitary irradiation or surgery (s/p rx for Cushing's)
   - Inflammatory infiltration of pituitary gland; sarcoidosis, tumor
   - Postpartum pituitary necrosis (Sheehan syndrome)

3. Functional or relative AI (inability to mount appropriate adrenal response in face of critical illness) is less well understood in terms of cause; most common in sepsis and systemic inflammatory response syndrome (SIRS).

Epidem: Primary and secondary AI are rare, less than 0.1% of population.

Pathophys: Hypothalamic-pituitary axis as described under "Cushing's Syndrome" at the beginning of Section 2.1; normal diurnal pattern to cortisol secretion (peak levels at 4 to 8 a.m.); cortisol circulates bound to corticosteroid-binding globulin (CBG).

Sx: Fatigue, anorexia, abdominal pain, myalgias.

Si: Hyperpigmentation, decreased/thinned body hair, postural hypotension.

In critically ill pts, may be difficult to evaluate; may just exhibit profound hypotension (refractory to IV fluid therapy) and fever.

Cmplc: Risks of chronic glucocorticoid rx include hyperglycemia, increased infection rates/immunosuppression, hypertension, delayed wound healing, acute psychosis, neuromuscular weakness (i.e., CCU myopathy).

ENDOCRINOLOGY

Lab: Electrolyte abnormalities: hyponatremia, hyperkalemia, hypercalcemia, hypoglycemia.

Eosinophilia in Addison's.

Early a.m. serum cortisol levels may be helpful as screening in nonacute pts.

Random cortisol level of less than 15 mcg/dL in critically ill pts suggests AI; level of greater than 34 mcg/dL suggests AI unlikely (NEJM 2003;348:727).

ACTH-stimulation tests (1 mcg and 250 mcg versions): give ACTH at specific dose im or IV and measure serum cortisol at baseline, 30 and 60 min after dose); any cortisol level greater than 19 mcg/dL (in noncritical pt) is normal response (i.e., not adrenally insufficient). In critical pts, initial study suggested that nonresponders to ACTH stimulation were those with cortisol rise of less than 9 mcg/dL and carried increased risk of death (JAMA 2002;288:862), but f/u study (NEJM 2008;358:111) did not corroborate findings and suggested no role for ACTH-stimulation tests in sepsis/SIRS.

Noninv: Consider CT or MRI imaging of the abdomen (adrenals) in some cases, especially if concern for primary adrenal cancer or metastases, but not required for diagnosis.

Rx: (JAMA 2002;287:236)

Classic AI: rx with oral glucocorticoid (hydrocortisone 20–30 mg qd, split doses) and mineralocorticoid (fludrocortisone 0.05–0.2 mg qd) replacement.

In setting of known AI, consider "stress dosing" in a variety of clinical scenarios; this may require only single doses or up to 48 hr of therapy for most surgeries or illnesses; no benefit to very high doses (hydrocortisone greater than 300 mg/d) or long courses of therapy; in critical pts, consider hydrocortisone 50 mg IV q 6 hr or 100 mg IV q 8 hr.

If plan for delayed stim testing, treat with dexamethasone (hydrocortisone will falsely elevate serum cortisol levels).

Steroid therapy for functional AI in sepsis/SIRS.

- 2002 French study (JAMA 2002;288:862): 300 pts with sepsis/SIRS, enrolled within 3 hr of arrival, randomized to hydrocortisone 50 mg IV q 6 hr and fludrocortisone 0.05 mg qd for 7 d; did ACTH-stim test on all pts and positive benefits were limited to pts with subnormal response to ACTH (increase of less than 9 mcg/dL); steroids reduced 28-d mortality (53% vs 63%, NNT 10) in the pts who were ACTH-nonresponders; reduced duration of vasopressor rx (7 d vs 9 d) in all pts who received steroids; no significant differences between groups in adverse events.
- CORTICUS study (NEJM 2008;358:111): 499 pts with sepsis/SIRS, enrolled within 72 hr of arrival, randomized to hydrocortisone 50 mg IV q 6 hr for 5 d (then tapered over 6 more days); did ACTH-stim test on all pts (nonresponders had increase of less than 9 mcg/dL); no significant difference in 28-d mortality between two groups (no difference in stim test responders or nonresponders); steroids improved duration of time to reverse shock (defined as SBP greater than 90 without pressors for 24 hr, 3.3 days vs 5.8 days) but no difference in percentage of pts with reversal of shock; adverse effects included higher rate of superinfection (OR 1.37 for new sepsis), hyperglycemia, hypernatremia.
- In summary, there is significant controversy regarding steroid use in sepsis/SIRS, as follows:
  - Steroids are likely to reduce duration of hypotension/shock and need for vasopressors, but may not reduce overall mortality.
  - ACTH-stim test can be performed, but conflicting results as to whether it helps determine who benefits.
  - Consider steroids in all cases of septic shock not quickly improved with IV fluid and pressor therapy, but be aware of potential adverse effects.

2.2 Thyroid Disorders

Myxedema (Severe Hypothyroidism)

(Endo Metab Clin N Am 2006;35:687; Am Fam Phys 2000;62: 2485; J Intensive Care Med 2007;22:224)

Cause: Usually pts with long-standing hypothyroidism, although may be new dx or noncompliance with meds.

Precipitating factors for myxedema include the following:

- Metabolic: hypoglycemia, hyponatremia, hypercalcemia (could be a cause or a result)
- Infection: pneumonia, UTI, sepsis
- Trauma, burns, surgery
- GI bleed
- Hypothermia
- Stroke
- Meds: amiodarone, beta-blockers, digoxin, lithium, diuretics, opiates, phenothiazines

Epidem: 4 times more common in women (80% of cases); exclusively in pts more than 60 years old; more frequent occurrence in winter months due to cold temperatures.

Pathophys: Hypothalamic-pituitary-thyroid axis: hypothalamic release of thyrotropin-releasing hormone (TRH), stimulates thyroid-stimulating hormone (TSH, aka thyrotropin) release from the pituitary gland; TSH stimulates thyroxine (T4) and tri-iodothyronine (T3) production in the thyroid gland; T4 is converted, mostly in target organs, to the active T3 by T4-deiodinase; T3 and T4 are synthesized and stored in larger protein thyroglobulin; negative feedback loop of T3 and T4, reduces synthesis of TRH and TSH.

Sx: Fatigue, constipation, weight gain.

Si: Coarse/brittle hair, dry skin, nonpitting edema (etiology of term myxedema), ptosis, macroglossia, decreased deep tendon reflex relaxation, altered mental status/delirium.

Hypothermia is the most concerning finding; may be less than 95.9°F.

Cardiovascular: hypotension, bradycardia.

Respiratory: hypoventilation, hypercarbic respiratory failure, sleep apnea.

Neurologic: progressive lethargy, delirium, psychosis, leading to coma.

In pts with limited hx, look for surgical scar on neck to suggest prior thyroidectomy.

Crs: Mortality of 30–60%, usually due to complications of the underlying illness; in one small study, mortality linked to lower GCS/consciousness and higher APACHE-II scores (J Endocrinol 2004;180:347).

Cmplc: Concern for concomitant adrenal insufficiency, may require ACTH-stim testing and stress dosing of hydrocortisone.

Lab: High TSH (usually critically elevated, but level does not correspond to severity of illness), low T3 and T4; TSH important to discriminate from euthyroid sick syndrome in ill pts (low T3 and T4 but normal/low TSH).

Hyponatremia due to SIADH-like syndrome with low serum osmolality, decreased clearance of free water.

Hypoglycemia, elevated CPK (when associated with hypotension and bradycardia, can mimic inferior wall MI, but rule out with lack of EKG changes and cardiac-specific troponin elevation), normocytic anemia, hyperlipidemia, elevated LDH, acute renal failure.

Noninv: EKG with bradycardia, low voltage in limb leads, nonspecific ST-T changes, prolonged QT interval.

Rx: Initial priority is supportive care.

- May require aggressive fluid replacement and rx of hypotension/shock.
- Recommend respiratory support with noninvasive and mechanical ventilation, especially for hypercarbia.

- Treat hyponatremia with fluid restriction like SIADH unless volume depleted. Hyponatremia for more details.
- Treat hypothermia with external warming, but take care not to cause peripheral vasodilation (and worsening hypotension) with warming blankets.
- Treatment of underlying illness, infection, etc., as appropriate.

Thyroid hormone replacement: some controversy surrounds type and dosing of thyroid replacement (expert opinion only), as follows:

- Initial dose of levothyroxine (T4): 250–500 mcg IV, then 50–100 mcg IV/PO qd; consider lower doses in elderly pts, with h/o CAD, active anginal symptoms; in small case series (Thyroid 1999;9:1167), excess mortality associated with high-dose replacement (greater than 500 mcg/d).
- Some suggest giving T3 because peripheral conversion of T4 to T3 in critical illness is reduced (Intensive Care Med 1985;11:259); start with 10 mcg IV for 1 dose, then continue q 8–12 hr until critical illness is resolved and pt is taking adequate oral intake.
- Once critical illness resolved, use chronic dosing of levothyroxine adjusted based on TSH levels.

Thyrotoxicosis (Hyperthyroidism, Thyroid Storm)

(Endo Metab Clin N Am 2006;35:663; BMJ 2006;332:1369)

Cause: Most common causes include the following:

- Grave's disease: autoimmune disease where antibody binds to and stimulates the TSH receptor on thyroid cells; leads to excess production of thyroid hormone
- Toxic adenoma or multinodular goiter: benign thyroid tumors, can be single or multiple
- Thyroiditis: postpartum, viral/bacterial, lymphocytic
- Thyroxine ingestion: excess treatment doses vs factitious disorder

- Drugs: lithium, alpha-interferon, amiodarone
- Nonthyroid gland causes: pituitary adenoma (secreting TSH), struma ovarii (ovarian teratoma), metastatic thyroid carcinoma

Thyroid storm precipitated by infection, surgery, trauma, acute MI/ACS, VTE, DKA, pregnancy, salicylate and pseudo-ephedrine use.

Epidem: More common in women (2%) than men (0.2%); increased risk with age; thyroid storm in less than 10% of pts with hyperthyroidism.

Pathophys: See "Myxedema (Severe Hypothyroidism)" earlier in Section 2.2 for the hypothalamic-pituitary-thyroid axis.

Sx: Heat intolerance, sweating, anxiety, palpitations, chest pain; fatigue, weight loss; menometrorraghia; diarrhea; hair loss; dyspnea.

Si: Tremor, tachycardia, diaphoresis; opthalmopathy in 30% of pts with Grave's (eye protrusion with periorbital swelling and inflammation); thyroid bruit in Grave's due to increased vascularity of gland; thyroid nodule or enlargement (toxic goiter); painful thyroid gland (thyroiditis).

Crs: Thyroid storm: marked fever, delirium, cardiovascular effects (sinus tachycardia, atrial fibrillation, high-output CHF); rating system for diagnosis (Endo Metab Clin N Am 1993;22:263).

Cmplc: Mortality rates of thyroid storm are 20–30%.

Lab: Suppressed TSH (unless very rare pituitary/central hyperthyroidism); elevated free T3 and T4; antithyroid antibodies present in Grave's.

Other lab abnormalities: hypercalcemia and elevated alkaline phosphatase (due to increased bone turnover), leukocytosis, hyperglycemia or hypoglycemia, elevated liver enzymes, elevated cortisol levels.

Noninv: Thyroid radioiodine uptake scan results:

- Increased uptake: Grave's disease

- Normal or increased uptake: toxic adenoma or multinodular goiter
- Reduced uptake: thyroiditis, factitious disorder

Thyroid ultrasound: diffuse enlargement/hypervascularity (Grave's); single or multiple nodules (goiter).

EKG: sinus tachycardia, atrial fibrillation (in 10–20% of cases, especially in elderly).

Echocardiogram in severe cases with CHF may show high-output failure (EF 70–75%).

Rx: Drug therapy (NEJM 2005;352:905):

- Inhibit hormone production: Thionamides; decrease T3/T4 synthesis, decrease antibody concentrations in Grave's; appropriate for excess production, does not work in thyroiditis; in severe thyroid storm, higher doses may be necessary.
  - Propylthiouracil (PTU) 200–400 mg PO q 6–8 hr
  - Methimazole 20–25 mg PO q 6 hr
  - Adverse effects: itching, fever, arthralgias, hives; uncommonly, agranulocytosis, elevated transaminases, vasculitis
- Inhibit thyroid hormone release: Iodine preparations, use only after initiating thionamides (30–60 min), as can initially stimulate increased hormone production.
  - SSKI 5 drops PO q 6 hr
  - Lugol's solution 4–8 drops PO q 6 hr
- Beta-blockade: Control peripheral response, mostly cardiovascular, to thyroid hormone.
  - Propranolol 60–80 mg PO q 4–6 hr; can be given IV 0.5–1 mg doses.
  - Esmolol drip when cannot use PO dosing; very short-acting.
  - Atenolol 50–200 mg qd (may need to be split bid) or metoprolol (100–200 mg qd in split doses); cardioselective preferred in pts with active bronchospasm.

- Use with care in acute heart failure; but even in these set-tings, control of diastolic dysfunction due to tachycardia is important; close ICU monitoring may be necessary.
- Other considerations:
  - Glucocorticoids: Hydrocortisone 50 mg IV q 6 hr or 100 mg IV q 8 hr if hypotensive and concern for relative AI, also reduces peripheral T4 to T3 conversion.
  - Anticoagulation for AF as CVA prophylaxis; controversial if short-term, reversible; see "Atrial Fibrillation," Section 1.3, for more details.
  - APAP for fever (avoid ASA, as it can increase hormone levels).
  - Dextrose-containing IVF if depleted glycogen stores, caus-ing hypoglycemia.

  Definitive therapies: Long-term antithyroid meds may be enough in some cases, but most get radioactive iodine (I-131) therapy and/or thyroidectomy.

2.3   Diabetic and Glucose Disorders

Hyperglycemia, Inpatient (Including Diabetes Mellitus)

(NEJM 2006;355:1903)

Cause: Most cases due to preexisting or new diagnosis of Type 1 or Type 2 DM, but also may be due to stress hyperglycemia from acute illness in up to 33% of cases; stress hyperglycemia defined as elevated blood sugar in the setting of acute illness, but no agreed-upon diagnostic criteria.

Epidem: More than 2000 consecutive pts in Atlanta hospital: 38% had hyperglycemia on admission, 33% of those had no prior hx of DM (new diagnosis vs stress hyperglycemia) (J Clin Endocrinol Metab 2002;87:978).

Pathophys: Possible mechanisms of stress hyperglycemia include increased circulating counterregulatory hormones (cortisol, epinephrine, glucagon), increased lactate levels, and increased insulin resistance, leading to increased gluconeogenesis and decreased glycogen synthesis.

Sx/Si: Most pts asx (aside from concomitant illness); severe hyperglycemia causing typical sx of fatigue, polyuria, polydipsia.

Crs: Hyperglycemia is linked to poor outcomes including increased mortality, LOS, and complications, across multiple illnesses, as follows:

- Post-op wound infections, including cardiac surgery (Ann Thorac Surg 1997;63:356; Diab Care 1999;22:1408).
- Acute MI: increased mortality, shock, and CHF (Lancet 2000;355:773, Diab Med 1996;13:80).
- Stroke: increased mortality (Arch Neurol 1985;42:661, Arch Neurol 1990;47:1174).
- Trauma, burns: increased mortality, infection rates, graft compromise (J Trauma 2001;51:540).
- Pneumonia: increased mortality and complications (Diab Care 2007;30:2251, Diab Care 2005;28:810).
- COPD exacerbation: increased mortality, LOS, multiple respiratory pathogens (Thorax 2006;61:284).
- All-cause mortality: of 2030 consecutive pts admitted to Atlanta hospital (see Epidem discussion above), new dx of hyperglycemia was associated with increased mortality (16% vs 1.7% for normoglycemic pts), longer LOS, higher rates of discharge to nursing facility (vs home); known diabetics were more similar to normoglycemic pts, suggesting increased severity of illness in pts with newly diagnosed or, more likely, stress hyperglycemia (J Clin Endocrinol Metab 2002;87:978); in separate study of more than 900 consecutive inpatients in Australian hospital, only independent predictors of mortality were age older than 75 and admission BS more than

100 mg/dL, and in pts without prior hx of DM there was a 33% increase in mortality with each 18-point increase in admission BS (Med J Aust 2008;188:340).

Cmplc: Main complication of therapy is hypoglycemia (see "Hypoglycemia" later in Section 2.3).

Lab: For most pts (even if normoglycemic on initial labs), consider BS checks with each meal and at bedtime for first 24–48 hr; if abnormal, continue through hospital stay; in well-controlled Type 2 DM, could cut back to qd or bid in stable pts with prolonged stay; consider early a.m. checks in some pts with morning hyperglycemia to rule out Somogyi phenomenon (early a.m. hypoglycemia stimulates stress hormones causing later a.m. hyperglycemia); in critical illness with insulin infusions, q 1-hr checks are standard.

HbA1c may reliably diagnose DM in pts admitted with random hyperglycemia: small 2003 study (50 pts) showed A1c more than 6.0% as 100% specific for dx of DM in setting of random admission hyperglycemia; less than 5.2% was 100% sensitive to r/o chronic DM (Diab Care 2003;26:1064).

Consider diabetes screening in some Type 2 pts with inadequate outpatient f/u: lipid panel, spot urine for microalbumin/creatinine ratio.

Rx: Type of care depends on severity of illness and previous level of glucose control; most data regarding outcomes of rx come from critical care pts, and then extrapolated to the less severe illnesses.

ICU studies of "tight glucose control" with continuous insulin infusion:

- Leuven 1 (aka Van den Berghe SICU study): Largest and most prominent positive outcome study to date re insulin infusion therapy; more than 1500 pts in surgical ICU (62% post-op cardiac surgery) randomized to intensive insulin rx (IV insulin infusion if BS more than 110 mg/dL, with goal of 80–110) vs conventional care (IV insulin infusion if BS more than

215 mg/dL, with goal of 180–200); achieved average glucose levels of 103 in intensive arm, 153 in conventional; intensive therapy led to significant reductions in ICU mortality (4.6% vs 8.0%, NNT 30) and all mortality (NNT 27), with highest mortality benefit in pts in ICU more than 5 d (NNT 11); also reduced morbidity with fewer ICU days, fewer ventilator days, less renal failure and need for dialysis, less sepsis and antibiotic use; main harm was hypoglycemia (BS less than 40 mg/dL), which occurred in 5% of intensive control pts (NNH 23) (NEJM 2001;345:1359).

- Leuven 2 (aka Van den Berghe MICU study): Follow-up to first study, 1200 medical ICU pts, across a variety of illnesses (43% respiratory illness) and baseline APACHE II score of 23; same design for intensive and conventional control as for Leuven 1 study; no difference in this study in ICU mortality, except in pts who remained in ICU more than 3 days (but unable to predetermine which pts met this criterion) (31% mortality in intensive rx vs 38% in conventional, NNT 15); 90-day mortality also reduced in this population (NNT 14); despite controversy about mortality benefit, intensive rx did improve morbidity with faster weaning from ventilator, fewer ICU days, and shorter overall LOS (even more prominent in pts in ICU more than 3 days); higher rates of hypoglycemia in this study than in surgical pts (18.7% in intensive rx, NNH 6) (NEJM 2006;354:449).

- DIGAMI 1 study: 620 pts with DM and acute MI, randomized to conventional rx vs intensive inpatient and outpatient (3 mo posthospital) rx; reduced 1-yr mortality in intensive rx group (26.1% vs 18.6%, NNT 13), which persisted up to 3.5 yr later; reduced inpatient mortality in a prespecified group of hyperglycemic patients without prior insulin therapy and thought to have low cardiovascular risk (possibly stress hyperglycemics) (BMJ 1997;314:1512).

- DIGAMI 2 study: Follow-up to first study, which removed potential confounder of outpatient rx by creating three arms including one only for intensive inpatient control; 1253 pts with DM and acute MI; failed to show any mortality benefit between the groups, but underpowered to prove this (Eur Heart J 2005;26:650).
- Krinsley study: Patients in a mixed med-surg ICU ("real-life"), with less intensive goals (started if BS more than 200 mg/dL, with goal less than 140), reduced in-hospital mortality (14.8% vs 20.9%, NNT 16) (Mayo Clin Proc 2004;79:992).
- VISEP study: 537 pts with sepsis, paired with separate intervention of pentastarch therapy for resuscitation; despite lower average BS values (112 mg/dL vs 151 in conventional group), there was no difference in mortality; however, study was stopped early due to more hypoglycemia events (BS less than 40 mg/dL) in intensive rx group (17% vs 4.1%, NNH 8).
- Despite variable outcomes in large studies, most hospitals have moved toward intensive insulin therapy in the ICU (and many have pushed for more aggressive care in floor settings as well).

Recommendations for target blood glucose levels: ADA recommends close to 110 mg/dL for ICU pts; fasting less than 126 mg/dL and random less than 180 mg/dL for ward pts (same as outpatient) (Diab Care 2008;31 Suppl 1:S12); controversy exists among experts as to whether the goals should be less strict (consider less than 140 in critical illness, less than 180 in ward pts).

In critically ill pts, choose intensive insulin therapy; deciding on a specific protocol is more problematic, as there are little head-to-head data comparing efficacy; a 2007 review of 12 protocols showed the extensive variability in the different types (Diab Care 2007;30:1005); many facilities use a modification of the traditional Yale protocol (Diab Care 2004;27:461).

In non-ICU inpatients, insulin infusions are generally not warranted or practical; however, glucose control measures are still likely to have a benefit (although unproven in this population); traditional practice was "sliding scale" insulin therapy with glucose measurements q 4–6 hr and escalating doses of short-acting insulin; this practice has not proven effective and, in fact, seems to be associated with higher rates of severe hyperglycemia, due to a "roller coaster" effect (good review of history of sliding scale: Am J Med 2007;120:563).

Generally, avoid use of oral hypoglycemics in the inpatient setting; in select pts, without critical or concomitant illnesses, and with good oral intake, can use safely; see **Table 2.1.**

Table 2.1   Oral Hypoglycemic Medications

Drug Class	Examples	Contraindications in Inpatients
Sulfonylureas	glyburide, glipizide, glimeperide	Hypoglycemia (can be severe and prolonged), especially if poor oral intake, acute renal failure, or in elderly patients; rarer cases of hyponatremia, hepatitis, hematologic abnormalities
Metformin	—	Avoid in renal and hepatic failure; lactic acidosis, especially in cases of severe illness; avoid if exposed to iodinated contrast dye
Thiazolidinediones ("glitazones")	pioglitazone, rosiglitazone	Avoid in fluid overload states, particularly CHF, as can cause worsening heart failure; dose adjustments necessary in liver failure; fluid overload may exacerbate anemia
Meglitinides	nateglinide, repaglinide	Hypoglycemia if poor oral intake; needs dose adjustments in renal and hepatic failure
Alphaglucosidase inhibitors	acarbose, miglitol	Ineffective in setting of poor oral intake; needs dosage adjustment in renal failure; may cause liver dysfunction in rare cases

Consider using a regimen of subcutaneous insulin based on three components (NEJM 2006;355:1903):

- Basal insulin: Long-acting insulin (NPH q 12 hr, insulin glargine q 24 hr, insulin detemir q 12–24 hr) to control fasting and premeal glucose levels; can be used even if pt has minimal or no oral intake; in pts not previously on insulin, start dosing at 0.2–0.3 units/kg/day (divided into 1–2 doses as per type of insulin) and adjust based on a.m. fasting sugars.
- Prandial (mealtime) insulin: Short-acting insulin (regular, aspart, or lispro) to control glucose excursions at mealtime; give 0–15 min prior to meal (can be given postmeal in some situations, if missed); in pts not previously on insulin, start dosing at 0.05–0.1 U/kg/meal; can be held in pts who do not eat, but should be given before meal even if prandial BS is normal.
- Correctional insulin (similar to "sliding scale"): Short-acting insulin (choose same type as for prandial insulin so can be given as single injection) to control unexpected premeal hyperglycemia; consider 1–4 U for each increment of 50 mg/dL over 150 mg/dL (based on assessment of pt's own insulin sensitivity); if using high doses of correctional insulin daily, consider increasing doses of basal and prandial insulin to improve overall control.

See **Figure 2.1.**

Diabetic Ketoacidosis (DKA)

(Endo Metab Clin N Am 2006;35:725, Am Fam Phys 2005;71:1705)

Cause: New onset/dx of Type 1 (or rarely Type 2) DM; infections (pneumonia, gastroenteritis, UTI); acute coronary syndromes/MI; pancreatitis; CVA; trauma; alcohol, drugs (especially cocaine), meds (lithium, atypical antipsychotics).

Epidem: Incidence rising, but mortality falling over past 15 yr; accounts for 25% of all Type 1 DM health costs.

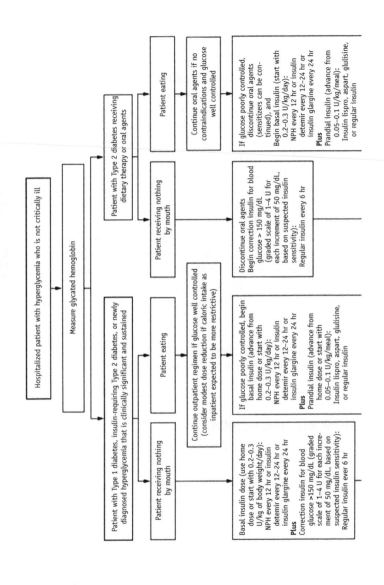

Hospitalized patient with hyperglycemia who is not critically ill

Measure glycated hemoglobin

Patient with Type 1 diabetes, insulin-requiring Type 2 diabetes, or newly diagnosed hyperglycemia that is clinically significant and sustained

Patient receiving nothing by mouth

Basal insulin dose (use home dose or start with 0.2–0.3 U/kg of body weight/day):
NPH every 12 hr or insulin detemir every 12–24 hr or insulin glargine every 24 hr
Plus
Correction insulin for blood glucose >150 mg/dL (graded scale of 1–4 U for each increment of 50 mg/dL, based on suspected insulin sensitivity): Regular insulin ever 6 hr

Patient eating

Continue outpatient regimen if glucose well controlled (consider modest dose reduction if caloric intake as inpatient expected to be more restrictive)

If glucose poorly controlled, begin basal insulin (advance from home dose or start with 0.2–0.3 U/kg/day):
NPH every 12 hr or insulin detemir every 12–24 hr or insulin glargine every 24 hr
Plus
Prandial insulin (advance from home dose or start with 0.05–0.1 U/kg/meal):
Insulin lispro, aspart, glulisine, or regular insulin

Patient with Type 2 diabetes receiving dietary therapy or oral agents

Patient receiving nothing by mouth

Discontinue oral agents
Begin correction insulin for blood glucose > 150 mg/dL (graded scale of 1–4 U for each increment of 50 mg/dL, based on suspected insulin sensitivity):
Regular insulin every 6 hr

Patient eating

Continue oral agents if no contraindications and glucose well controlled

If glucose poorly controlled, discontinue oral agents (sensitizers can be continued), and
Begin basal insulin (start with 0.2–0.3 U/kg/day):
NPH every 12 hr or insulin detemir every 12–24 hr or insulin glargine every 24 hr
Plus
Prandial insulin (advance from 0.05–0.1 U/kg/meal):
Insulin lispro, aspart, glulisine, or regular insulin

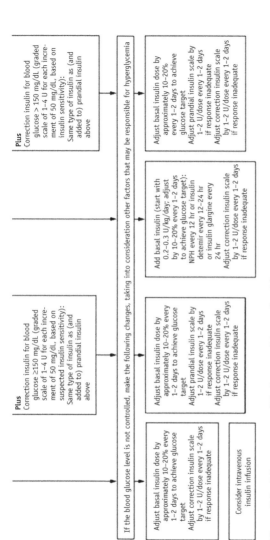

Plus
Correction insulin for blood glucose ≥150 mg/dL (graded scale of 1–4 U for each increment of 50 mg/dL, based on suspected insulin sensitivity): Same type of insulin as (and added to) prandial insulin above

Plus
Correction insulin for blood glucose > 150 mg/dL (graded scale of 1–4 U for each increment of 50 mg/dL, based on insulin sensitivity): Same type of insulin as (and added to) prandial insulin above

If the blood glucose level is not controlled, make the following changes, taking into consideration other factors that may be responsible for hyperglycemia

Adjust basal insulin dose by approximately 10–20% every 1–2 days to achieve glucose target
Adjust correction insulin scale by 1–2 U/dose every 1–2 days if response inadequate

Consider intravenous insulin infusion

Adjust basal insulin dose by approximately 10–20% every 1–2 days to achieve glucose target
Adjust prandial insulin scale by 1–2 U/dose every 1–2 days if response inadequate
Adjust correction insulin scale by 1–2 U/dose every 1–2 days if response inadequate

Add basal insulin (start with 0.2–0.3 U/kg/day; adjust by 10–20% every 1–2 days to achieve glucose target): NPH every 12 hr or insulin detemir every 12–24 hr or insulin glargine every 24 hr
Adjust correction insulin scale by 1–2 U/dose every 1–2 days if response inadequate

Adjust basal insulin dose by approximately 10–20% every 1–2 days to achieve glucose target
Adjust prandial insulin scale by 1–2 U/dose every 1–2 days if response inadequate
Adjust correction insulin scale by 1–2 U/dose every 1–2 days if response inadequate

Figure 2.1 Management of Diabetes in Hospitalized Patients
Reproduced with permission from Inzucchi SE. Management of hyperglycemia in hospital setting. *NEJM.* 2006;355:1903. Copyright © 2006, Massachusetts Medical Society. All rights reserved.

ENDOCRINOLOGY

Pathophys: Triad of hyperglycemia, ketosis, acidosis:

- Hyperglycemia due to lack of insulin causing decrease in muscle uptake of glucose and increase in liver production of glucose.
- Ketosis due to lipolysis leading to increase in FFA and their conversion to ketones in liver.
- Acidosis due accumulation of ketones (acetoacetate [AA] and beta-hydroxybutyrate [BHB] are the active ketones; acetone present but does not contribute to acidosis).

Sx: Initially due to hyperglycemia: polyuria, polydipsia, weight loss.

Neurologic sx if associated hyperosmolarity.

Abdominal pain, N/V in up to 50%, related to degree of acidosis.

Si: Dehydration: tachycardia, hypotension, delayed capillary refill, skin tenting.

Obtundation, altered mental status

Acetone breath: "fruity" odor

Kussmaul respirations: tachypneic with deep breathing due to metabolic acidosis

Rarely fever, usually blunted by peripheral vasoconstriction, even with underlying infection

Crs: Sx usually develop more rapidly (over 2–3 d) than HHS due to acidosis.

DKA is resolved when (1) anion gap is normal, (2) neurologic status is at baseline, (3) pt able to take PO.

Cmplc: Most mortality related to underlying illness, rather than metabolic disturbances; prognosis worse with age, neurologic sx, hemodynamic instability.

Cerebral edema: worsening mental status 12–24 hr after acute presentation; more common in children, may be due to rapid correction of hyperosmolarity; prevent by initial use of isotonic saline (0.9% NS), addition of dextrose once BS is less than 200.

Lab: Routine labs in management of DKA.

- Glucose: Usually 500–800 mg/dL at time of diagnosis; "euglycemic" DKA described in pregnancy and poor nutritional states; usually follow q 1 hr while on insulin infusion.
- Electrolytes: Should check BMP q 2–4 hr during acute phase.
  - Sodium: Variable, directly reduced by hyperglycemia, but then loss of free H_2O from osmotic diuresis can lead to hypernatremia; "pseudohyponatremia" due to hyperlipidemia. See Hyponatremia section for details.
  - Potassium: Most have overall potassium deficit due to renal and GI losses, but initial levels may be normal or high due to hyperosm, acidosis, and insulin deficiency.
  - Anion gap metabolic acidosis: Anion gap = Na − (HCO_3 + Cl), less than 12 is normal; more than 15 indicates DKA (or other metabolic acidosis, see "Metabolic Acidosis" section for more details); better marker of improvement than ketones, less painful/invasive than serial ABGs.
- Ketones: Nitroprusside reaction converts acetoacetate to acetone; may not be helpful in recovery phase as acetone takes longer to clear through the lungs, but acidosis from AA and BHB resolved (acetone does not contribute to anion gap acidosis); helpful in initial diagnosis, but probably not necessary to follow (anion gap is a better indicator of progress and resolution of DKA).
- Phosphate: Similar to K, usually body-depleted, but initial hyperphos due to renal dysfunction.
- Others: Leukocytosis (even in the absence of infection); increased amylase/lipase (even in absence of pancreatitis).

    Consider EKG, CXR, blood/urine Cx on admit to look for underlying causes.

Rx: Mainstays of therapy: (1) close monitoring, (2) fluid repletion, (3) insulin therapy, (4) electrolyte replacement.

Most ICU status with hourly glucose, BMP q 2–4 hr, and venous pH.

- Fluids:
  - Most important initial therapy is isotonic saline (up to 1000 mL/hr), will boost intravascular volume and renal blood flow (which may drop initial BS up to 70 mg/dL without insulin rx).
  - Switch to 0.45% NS in subacute phase or if 40 mEq KCl/L needed (therapeutically equivalent to 0.75% NS).
  - Add dextrose to fluids (e.g., D5 NS) once BS is less than 200 to allow resolution of ketoacidosis without precipitating hypoglycemia.
- Insulin:
  - Hold until potassium measured; ensure initial K at least 3.3 mEq/L so as not to precipitate severe hypokalemia.
  - IV bolus of regular insulin 0.1 U/kg, then 0.1 U/kg/hr IV infusion.
  - Consider hourly SQ insulin instead of infusion in mild to moderate cases (Int J Clin Pract 2006;60:429; Am J Med 2004;117:291).
  - Goal is to decrease BS by 50–70 mg/dL per hour; if no improvement in first hour, rebolus and increase drip rate.
  - Resume long-acting SQ insulin with 1–2 hr overlap with IV drip once DKA resolved (see Crs description above).
- Potassium:
  - If initially critically high and EKG changes, rx with insulin bolus (alternative is sodium bicarb [1 mEq/kg over 5 min], but insulin probably more effective).
  - Begin K repletion once K is less than 5.3 mEq/L; add to IVF or piggyback depending on rate (do not exceed 20 mEq/hr unless severe, life-threatening; rates greater than 10 mEq/hr may require central access).

- Bicarbonate:
  - Controversial; 1 small RCT (Ann IM 1986;105:836) did not show improved outcomes with use.
  - Consider using if pH is less than 7.0 with cardiac dysfunction or life-threatening hyperkalemia.
- Phosphate:
  - Can drop in subacute phase as renal function improves.
  - Usually does not require replacement unless less than 1.0 mg/dL with sx (respiratory, cardiac, hemolysis).
  - If needed, 20–30 mEq K-phos per liter can replace KCl in IVF.

Hyperosmolar Hyperglycemic State (HHS; Hyperosmolar Nonketotic Coma)

(Endo Metab Clin N Am 2006;35:725; Am Fam Phys 2005; 71:1705)

Cause: New onset/dx of Type 2 DM; infections (pneumonia, gastroenteritis, UTI); acute coronary syndromes/MI; pancreatitis; CVA; trauma; alcohol, drugs, multiple meds.

Epidem: Much less common than DKA.

Pathophys: See "Diabetic Ketoacidosis (DKA)" earlier in Section 2.3; do not develop ketoacidosis, possibly because of enough insulin sensitivity to avoid lipolysis, ketogenesis; massive hyperglycemia causes osmotic diuresis and hyperosmolarity.

Sx: Initially due to hyperglycemia: polyuria, polydipsia, weight loss; neurologic sx predominate (confusion, coma).

Si: Dehydration: tachycardia, hypotension, delayed capillary refill, skin tenting; obtundation, altered mental status.

Crs: Sx more insidious than DKA because lack of acidosis blunts initial sx (N/V, abd pain, neuro sx) and allows for more profound dehydration.

Cmplc: Most mortality related to underlying illness, rather than metabolic disturbances; prognosis worst with age, neurologic sx, hemodynamic instability.

More concern for cerebral edema because of hyperosmolarity; prevent by initial use of isotonic saline to avoid rapid drops in serum osmolality and adding dextrose once BS in less than 300.

Lab: Routine labs in the management of HHS.

- Glucose usually 500 mg/dL, and may exceed 1000 mg/dL; poor GFR leads to significant hyperglycemia (as opposed to younger Type 1 diabetics with better renal function).
- No anion gap acidosis or ketosis (although pts with shock may have anion gap due to lactic acidosis).
- Sodium: Variable, directly reduced by hyperglycemia, but then loss of free H_2O from osmotic diuresis can lead to hypernatremia.
- Potassium: Most have overall K deficit due to renal and GI losses, but initial levels may be normal or high due to hyperosmolality, acidosis, and insulin deficiency.
- Phosphate: Similar to K, usually body-depleted, but initial hyperphos due to renal dysfunction.

Consider EKG, CXR, blood/urine Cx on admit to look for underlying causes (even more likely than in DKA).

Rx: Mainstays of therapy: (1) close monitoring, (2) fluid repletion, (3) insulin therapy, (4) electrolyte replacement.

Most significant treatment issues may be related to underlying cause.

Most ICU status with hourly glucose, BMP q 2–4 hr , venous pH.

- Fluid therapy: See "Diabetic Ketoacidosis (DKA)" earlier in Section 2.3.

- Insulin: See "Diabetic Ketoacidosis (DKA)" earlier in Section 2.3.
  - Due to insulin resistance, likely will require higher insulin doses.
  - Add dextrose to fluids once BS is less than 300 (different threshold than DKA).
- Potassium: See "Diabetic Ketoacidosis (DKA)" earlier in Section 2.3.
- Bicarbonate not necessary given lack of acidosis, except for severe hyperkalemia.
- Phosphate: See "Diabetic Ketoacidosis (DKA)" earlier in Section 2.3.

Hypoglycemia

(NEJM 1986;315:1245,NEJM 1995;332:1144)

Cause: In most inpatient situations, due to effects of insulin or oral hypoglycemics; especially extended sulfonylurea action in acute renal failure and pts receiving hypoglycemic meds in setting of reduced or no oral intake (J Hosp Med 2007;2:234); occasionally, due to med error; more rarely, postprandial hypoglycemia, factitious syndromes, insulinoma.

Epidem: Higher rates with intensive insulin regimens, especially continuous infusions.

- Leuven 2 (MICU study) had hypoglycemia rates of 18%; see "Hyperglycemia, Inpatient" earlier in Section 2.3 (NEJM 2006;354:449).
- Risk factors for hypoglycemia in nondiabetics include renal failure, hypoalbuminemia, sepsis, malignancy, CHF (J Am Ger Soc 1998;46:978).

Pathophys: Whipple's triad: neuro symptoms, BS less than 40 mg/dL, relief of sx with glucose administration.

In the pancreatic beta-cells, proinsulin is cleaved to insulin, with release of C-peptide as by-product.

Sx: Patients report sx with only 15% of episodes (J Intern Med 1990;228:641); sympathetic activation causes sweating, anxiety, nausea, palpitations; neuro sx include fatigue, dizziness, headache, difficulty concentrating.

Si: Sympathetic activation causes tremor, tachycardia; neurologic symptoms include confusion, delirium, rarely seizures and coma.

Crs: Despite higher rates of hypoglycemia in intensive insulin regimens, one ICU study found no association between hypoglycemic events and in-hospital mortality (Crit Care Med 2006;34:2714); in nondiabetic, elderly pts, hypoglycemia was a predictor of increased inpatient mortality (OR 3.7) (J Am Ger Soc 1998;46:978); in a different study of diabetic and nondiabetic elderly, hypoglycemia was common and associated with increased mortality, but not an independent predictor in multivariate analysis (Arch IM 2003;163:1825).

Lab: STAT fingerstick for glucose; confirm if needed with serum glucose; rx for symptoms and/or BS less than 60 mg/dL (some pts with long-standing hyperglycemia/poor control will have sx at higher glucose levels).

In nondiabetic pts, if persistent hypoglycemia, get plasma insulin, pro-insulin, C-peptide levels, and sulfonylurea assay:

- Insulinoma: elevated levels of insulin, pro-insulin, and C-peptide
- Factitious syndrome due to insulin: elevated insulin, but low levels of C-peptide and pro-insulin
- Factitious syndrome due to sulfonylureas: elevated levels of insulin, pro-insulin, and C-peptide; positive assay for sulfonylureas

Noninv: In select pts with difficulty determining cause and extent of events, consider monitored 72-hr fast.

Rx: First step is to avoid (69% of hypoglycemic events in small study were considered preventable) (Am J Health Syst Pharm 2005;62:714).

- Frequent glucose monitoring (especially with infusions).
- Avoid "U" for "units" in written orders, as may be seen as an extra "0", e.g., 10U may be misread as 100.
- Avoid NPO status; add IV dextrose solutions if NPO; discontinue prandial insulin if NPO (but can still use basal insulin in most cases).
- Avoid oral hypoglycemics in inpatients, unless stable renal and hepatic function and taking good PO.
- Avoid sliding scale insulin and insulin stacking (repeated, frequent doses of short-acting insulin) as primary inpatient mgt.
- Coordinate preprandial insulin dosing with meals (avoid timed dosing, rather, order to be given with meal).
- Watch for pts with extreme insulin sensitivity: low-weight pts, cystic fibrosis, postpancreatectomy.

In pts who can swallow, give 15 gm of carbohydrate (0.5–1 cup of fruit juice or soda) and recheck BS in 15–30 min.

In pts who cannot swallow, 12.5 gm dextrose IV (25 mL of D50 solution) and repeat BS in 15–30 min.

In settings of prolonged effect of oral hypoglycemics, will need to closely follow BS (usually q 1–2 hr to start) and rx with continuous IV solution with dextrose; intermittent D50 doses may not be sufficient to maintain normoglycemia.

Reevaluate inpatient diabetic regimen:

- Consider stopping oral meds.
- Evaluate for change in renal function.
- Consider decreasing prandial (if occurring premeal) or basal (if occurring in a.m.) insulin doses.
- Evaluate oral intake with nursing/dietary, consider calorie counts.

2.4 Mineral Disorders (Calcium/Magnesium/Phosphorus)

Hypocalcemia

Cause: Most likely causes in a hospitalized pt are the following:

- Low serum albumin (hypoalbuminemia):
  - 40% of circulating calcium is bound to albumin.
  - Correct using this formula: (Serum calcium + 0.8 [4 − Serum albumin]); but may underestimate true hypocalcemia especially in elderly pts (Arch Gerontol Geriatr 1992;15:59) and critically ill (Crit Care Med 2003;31:1389).
- Critical illness: Greater than 80% of ICU pts (ionized Ca less than 1.16 mmol/L), correlates with both mortality and APACHE-II scores (Am J Kidney Dis 2001;37:689).
- Hypoparathyroidism (low PTH): Due to surgical removal of glands (associated with thyroidectomy), autoimmune, infiltrative diseases, HIV.
- Vitamin D deficiency.
- Hypomagnesemia: Causes both decreased PTH secretion and PTH resistance, usually associated with Mg levels less than 1 mg/dL.
- Excess calcium deposited in bone/tissues: hyperphosphatemia, acute pancreatitis, metastatic cancer.
- Increased calcium binding intravascularly: respiratory alkalosis (increases binding to albumin).
- Calcium loss in urine: Chronically hypoparathyroid pts treated with loop diuretic (Ann IM 1977;86:579).
- Meds: bisphosphonates, cinacalcet, cisplatin, 5-fluorouracil and leucovorin, foscarnet.

Pathophys: Calcium and phosphate metabolism due to interplay and feedback mechanisms of parathyroid hormone (PTH) and vit D (from dietary intake and converted to active form by enzymatic activity in the kidney, liver, and skin); drop in serum PTH slows bone turnover, decrease in renal resorption of calcium, and decrease in gut absorption, all causing a drop in serum calcium; vit D (active form, calcitriol) has similar actions as PTH.

Sx: Neuro: fatigue, anxiety, tetany and seizures in severe hypocalcemia.
> Skin: hyperpigmentation, dermatitis
> GI: steatorrhea

Si: Trousseau's sign: carpal spasm with BP cuff inflation for 3 min; Chvostek's sign: facial twitching from tapping on facial nerve anterior to ear; hyperactive reflexes
> Cardiovascular: hypotension, bradycardia

Crs: See description of critical illness under Cause, above; linked to poor outcomes in critically ill pts.

Cmplc: Reduced sensitivity to digoxin.

Lab: Confirm low calcium, especially in elderly and critically ill, with ionized calcium (i.e., free, unbound calcium); if true hypocalcemia, check renal function, Mg, phos; consider PTH and vit D levels (calcidiol and calcitriol) in lone hypocalcemia not associated with other critical illness.

Noninv: EKG may show prolonged QT interval.

Rx: For most pts with chronic hypocalcemia, oral repletion of calcium at 1500–2000 mg calcium (carbonate or citrate usually) per day is adequate; however, hospitalized pts usually have acute hypocalcemia and rx is more problematic; little evidence to help guide therapy, especially in cases due to severe illness; some animal studies even suggest potential harm to calcium therapy (Cochrane 2008;CD006163).

- Mild, asymptomatic hypocalcemia does not require therapy (usually ionized Ca greater than 3.2 mg/dL).
- Consider rx in pts with resistant hypotension/shock, si/sx of neuromuscular irritability and tetany, prolonged QT intervals.

- IV therapy: IV bolus over 5–10 min, usually as 1 gm of calcium chloride (272 mg of elemental Ca; very painful, should give through central line) or calcium gluconate (90 mg of elemental Ca; usually preferred); bolus effects usually only short-acting and so consider repeat Ca levels and start continuous infusion of 0.5–1.5 mg/kg elemental Ca per hr (may be able to titrate down further and even off as repleted).
- Adverse effects: Watch for vein irritation, necrosis if extravasated; will precipitate in solution with phosphate or bicarbonate; can cause bradycardia and heart block with rapid administration, especially in pts on digoxin.

   If Mg-depleted, Ca will not correct until Mg repleted. See "Hypomagnesemia" later in Section 2.4.

Hypercalcemia

(NEJM 1992;326:1196)

Cause: Most likely causes in a hospitalized pt are the following:

- Hyperparathyroidism via renal calcitriol (activated vit D) production (90% of all pts with hypercalcemia, although lesser percentage in pts requiring hospitalization)
- Soft tissue cancers, especially lung, breast, and hepatoma; leukemia/lymphoma (Ann IM 1994;121:633, Ann IM 1994;121:709); multiple myeloma (see Section 4.4) by:
  - PTH-like protein secretions (NEJM 1990;322:1106; Ann IM 1989;111:484)
  - Secretion of other bone-resorbing substances
  - Tumor conversion of 25-OH vit D to 1,25-OH vit D (calcitriol)
  - Local osteolytic mets
- Inflammatory/infectious
  - Sarcoidosis
  - Tuberculosis, via extrarenal calcitriol production in granulomas

- Cat-scratch disease (JAMA 1998;279:532)
- Disseminated coccidiomycosis (NEJM 1977;297:431)
- Vitamin D intoxication (NEJM 1992;326:1173) including the milk-alkali syndrome (Mayo Clin Proc 2009;84:261)
- Endocrine: thyrotoxicosis (Ann IM 1976;84:668), adrenal insufficiency (Calcif Tissue Int 1982;34:523)
- Prolonged immobilization, especially with underlying Paget's disease
- Meds: thiazides (NEJM 1971;284:828); vit A (Ann IM 1974; 80:44) and vit D; lithium; theophylline (J Clin Endocrinol Metab 2005;90:6316)
- Benign familial hypocalciuric hypercalcemia (autosomal dominant) (Ann IM 1985;102:511)

Pathophys: Calcium and phosphate metabolism due to interplay and feedback mechanisms of PTH and vit D (from dietary intake and converted to active form by enzymatic activity in the kidney, liver, and skin); rise in serum PTH stimulates bone turnover, renal resorption of calcium, and increased gut absorption, all causing increases in serum calcium; vit D (active form, calcitriol) has similar actions as PTH.

Sx: Fatigue, weakness, sleepiness, nausea/anorexia, constipation, polyuria, polydypsia, and volume depletion.

Si: Confusion, delirium, drowsiness, coma.

Cmplc: Pancreatitis; increased risk of digoxin toxicity.

Lab: Calcium elevated (after correction for low albumin, see Cause section in "Hypocalcemia"), 10.5 mg/dL or more; sx usually between 11 and 12 mg/dL; severe toxicity if more than 14 mg/dL; consider ionized calcium to confirm.

Low serum chloride suggests malignancy-related (Am J Med 1997;103:134).

PTH to evaluate for hyperparathyroidism; if PTH negative, consider PTHrp levels and vit D levels; in certain clinical settings, SPEP/UPEP to r/o myeloma, TSH to r/o hyperthyroidism.

Noninv: EKG shows short QT interval with normal T wave, but short-ened ST segment.

Specific imaging not warranted; hypercalcemia due to malignancy is usually present with a clinically apparent tumor, but if none known, can consider CXR, mammogram, CT abdomen, etc.

Rx: Acute rx for Ca more than 13 mg/dL, to decrease within hours.

- Normal saline to assure intravascular volume adequately replaced:
  - In hypotensive pts, IV boluses until stable, and then 200–300 mL/hr (as tolerated) and titrate to urine output of 100–150 mL/hr initially.
  - In critically ill, hypotensive, consider CVP or PA catheter monitoring.
  - Previous practices suggested addition of loop diuretic for more calciuresis, but more recent study suggests to avoid furosemide initially (Ann IM 2008;149:259), as may contribute to dehydration; may be needed after volume replaced to prevent volume overload and accelerate renal calcium clearance.
- Bisphosphonate therapy:
  - Inhibits osteoclast-induced bone resorption.
  - Zoledronic acid (Zometa) 4 mg IV, one dose given over 15 min (need to adjust dose in pts with renal disease); normalized serum calcium within 4 days in 50% of pts in one study, 88% within 10 days (J Clin Oncol 2001; 19:558).
  - Pamidronate (Aredia) 60–90 mg IV, one dose given over 2 hr (J Clin Oncol 1992;10:134,Am J Med 1993;95:297).
  - Can repeat as soon as 7 d later, but many pts require therapy less often.
- Calcitonin:
  - Inhibits osteoclasts and increases calciuresis.

- SQ or im injection: Initially 4 U/kg q 8–12 hr, but can increase up to 8 U/kg; nasal calcitonin is not useful (small study) (Calcif Tissue Int 1992;51:18).
- Good for acute therapy because it works faster than bisphosphonates, but no real role in long-term rx because of tachyphylaxis.
- Gallium nitrate IV infusion over 5 days; although effective, role limited due to side effects and need for prolonged infusion; consider in pts resistant to bisphosphonate therapy (Cancer 2006;12:47, Ann IM 1988;108:669).

Chronic rx; consider with myeloma and metastatic cancer, as diminishes sx and allows hospital discharge (Ann IM 1990;112:499).

- Biphosphonates: Can give further IV dosing q 4 wk; Cochrane review in myeloma pts suggested reduction in vertebral fractures (NNT 10), pain (NNT 11) (Cochrane 2002;CD003188).
- Steroids, primarily for sarcoid pts (e.g., prednisone 20 mg PO tid) (Ann IM 1980;93:269, Ann IM 1980;93:449).
- Avoid thiazide diuretics, supplemental calcium, and vit D.

Hypomagnesemia

(Lancet 1998;352:391)

Cause: Most likely causes in a hospitalized pt are the following:

- GI fluid loss: NG suction, diarrhea/malabsorption, malnutrition, fistulae, pancreatitis
- Renal fluid loss: loop and thiazide diuretics, chronic IV therapy and volume expansion
- Other: hypercalcemia, hypophosphatemia, osmotic diuresis (DM with glucosuria or drugs), alcoholism

Epidem: 12% of inpatients; 65% of ICU pts (Am J Clin Path 1983;79:348); 30% of inpatients with alcoholism.

Pathophys: Normal serum Mg (1.7–2.2 mg/dL), accounts for only 1% of total body Mg.

Low Mg inhibits PTH secretion, which in turn causes hypocalcemia (NEJM 1970;282:61); alcohol inhibits PTH secretion, thus also contributing (NEJM 1991;324:721).

Sx: Cramps, dizziness, weakness.

Si: Most due to concomitant hypocalcemia: carpopedal spasm, Chvostek's sign, Trousseau's sign, delirium, muscle tremor and bizarre movements, seizures.

Crs: Ataxias take months to clear.

Cmplc: Hypocalcemia; hypokalemia (present in 40–60% of cases) does not respond to K replacement until Mg corrected (Arch IM 1992;152:40); ventricular arrhythmias; long term can contribute to osteoporosis, ASCVD, DM.

Lab: Chem: Mg less than 1.6 mEq/L.

Noninv: EKG shows prolonged PR, widening of QRS, inverted T's.

Rx: Oral replacement preferred if possible (high dose IV infusion can acutely decrease renal reabsorption, leading to higher urinary losses of Mg).

Mg chloride or Mg lactate tablets provide about 3 mmol (~60 mg) of magnesium; six to eight pills/day in split doses.

IV administration for NPO or critically ill pts, severe sx, tetany, or arrhythmia; 1–2 gm Mg sulfate over 5–10 min, followed by infusion of 0.5–1 gm/hr; watch for possible hypotension with rapid infusion.

Hypermagnesemia

(Lancet 1998;352:391)

Cause: Renal failure, often parallels hyperkalemia; IV infusions (particularly in preeclampsia pts); chronic Mg-containing antacid and laxative use; enemas, especially in megacolon, with Mg-containing soaps.

Epidem: Less common than hypomagnesemia (10–15% of inpatients).

Pathophys: Avg daily intake = 20–40 mEq; total body stores = 2000 mEq, half in bones, the rest intracellular, approximately 1% extracellular (serum).

Sx: Constipation, urinary retention; nausea; drowsiness.

Si: Depressed DTRs, hypotension, bradycardia (Ann IM 1975;83:657).

Cmplc: Heart block, respiratory paralysis.

Lab: Chem: Mg more than 2.2 mEq/L. Make sure to check renal function.

Noninv: EKG shows heart block.

Rx: In most clinical settings, mild to moderate hypermagnesemia requires no therapy other than monitoring and treatment of underlying disease.

Discontinue oral Mg; hemodialysis in ESRD pts; life-threatening sx: calcium gluconate 5–10 mEq (10–20 cc of 10% solution).

Hypophosphatemia

(Lancet 1998;352:391)

Cause: Causes include the following:

- Redistribution: respiratory alkalosis (can be severe, but usually asx); postmalnutrition "refeeding" syndrome; DKA; sepsis
- Urinary loss: Hyperparathyroidism, vit D deficiency, volume overload, alcoholism, acidosis
- Intestinal malabsorption: dietary restriction, antacids, vit D deficiency, chronic diarrhea

Epidem: Found in about 1% of all inpatients, but much higher in alcoholics, critical illness.

Pathophys: Total body phos approximately 700 gm: 85% in bone, 15% in fluid/soft tissues.

Sx: Most asymptomatic; higher risk of severe depletion and sx in alcoholics, DKA pts, malnourished pts with refeeding.

Weakness, dyspnea, confusion.

Si: Myopathy, dysphagia, ileus; hypotension (consider as confounding issue in cases of "resistant" shock).

Cmplc: Rhabdomyolysis; hemolysis, thrombocytopenia; impaired immunity; encephalopathy; respiratory failure.

Lab: Phos less than 2.5 mg/dL (usually asx unless less than 2.0 mg/dL; severe sx at less than 1.0).

Rx: Mild, asx cases do not require rx; if levels are less than 1.0 or sx, replete.

Oral therapy preferred if pt able to tolerate; sodium or potassium phosphate up to 2–3 gm qd (oral preps contain 250 mg phosphorus per dose, variable amounts of Na and K); give with meals to aid absorption.

IV rx can precipitate hypocalcemia (correct severe hypocalcemia first), renal failure, and arrhythmias, close monitoring essential; potassium phosphate: 3 mmol (93 mg) of PO_4, 4.4 mEq of $K+$ (doses of 10–30 mmol KPhos over 6 hr depending on pt weight and severity of depletion).

Vit D supplementation if deficient.

Hyperphosphatemia

(Lancet 1998;352:391)

Cause: Caused by the following:

- Increased load: oversupplementation, vit D intoxication, phosphate enemas; rapid cell breakdown due to rhabdomyolysis, tumor lysis syndrome, malignant hyperthermia, hemolysis, severe acidosis
- Reduced excretion: renal failure (most common), hypoparathyroidism, bisphosphonates, Mg deficiency
- "Pseudo"-hyperphos with multiple myeloma: circulating proteins bind phos and raise measured serum levels

Pathophys: Rapid increases can lead to hypocalcemia; soft tissue deposition of Ca in setting when calcium phosphate product (serum Ca multiplied by serum phos) is greater than 70.

Sx: See "Hypocalcemia" earlier in Section 2.4.

Si: See "Hypocalcemia" earlier in Section 2.4.

Crs: Long-term deposition in ESRD, particularly if vit D supplementation.

Lab: Serum phos more than 2.5 mg/dL.

Rx: Acute, severe hyperphos (in pts with normal renal function): responds to IV saline infusion, but watch for worsening hypocalcemia (if present, consider dialysis).

Chronic: phosphate binders given orally (containing aluminum, Mg, or Ca) to reduce intestinal absorption; low protein diet.

Chapter 3

Gastroenterology

3.1 Abdominal Pain in Adults

Cause: Differential dx of abdominal pain by system:

- Gastrointestinal:
  - Upper GI: GERD/esophagitis, peptic/duodenal ulcers, gastric outlet obstruction
  - Small bowel: appendicitis, gastroenteritis, Crohn's disease, mesenteric ischemia, bowel obstruction, neoplasm, bowel perforation with peritonitis
  - Lower GI: infectious colitis, ulcerative colitis, ischemic colitis, diverticulitis
- Pancreaticobiliary:
  - Pancreas: acute/chronic pancreatitis, pancreatic cancer
  - Biliary: biliary colic, cholecystitis, choledocholithiasis, ascending cholangitis
- Hepatic:
  - Hepatitis: viral, alcoholic, toxic
  - Liver abscess, primary or metastatic cancer, passive congestion from CHF
- Pulmonary
  - Lower lobe pneumonia, pleurisy, pneumothorax, pulmonary embolism, subphrenic abscess
- Cardiac and vascular
  - Acute coronary syndrome, MI, pericarditis
  - AAA, aortic dissection

- Renal and urologic
  - Pyelonephritis, cystitis, prostatitis
  - Nephrolithiasis/urolithiasis, bladder outlet obstruction with urinary retention
- Gynecologic
  - Female: ovarian cancer, ovarian torsion, ectopic pregnancy, pelvic inflammatory disease and tubo-ovarian abscess, mittelschmirtz (ovarian pain with ovulation), ovarian cysts, dysmenorrhea
  - Male: testicular cancer or torsion (with undescended testicle)
- Abdominal wall and other
  - Muscle strain, herpes zoster, umbilical or ventral hernia
  - Acute intermittent porphyria, DKA, sickle cell crisis, narcotic withdrawal, familial Mediterranean fever

Epidem: Chief complaint for 6.5% of all ED visits (Med Clin N Am 2006;90:481).

Crs: Study of 380 ER pts older than 65 yr presenting with abdominal pain (Acad Emerg Med 1998;5:1163) reported the following:

- About 50% require admission, about 20% require surgical intervention, about 5% mortality
- Final dx: infection 19%, obstruction 15%, ulcers 7%, urinary tract disease 7%, malignancy 7%
- Risk factors for poor outcome: hypotension, leukocytosis, fever, abnormal bowel sounds

Lab: Initial labs include CBC, metabolic panel, renal function, liver function, amylase, lipase.

Others to consider: PT/PTT in pts on anticoagulants; cardiac enzymes in pts at risk for CAD; lactate level and ABG if concern for mesenteric ischemia; U/A with micro and Cx; blood cultures if fever, leukocytosis; urine pregnancy test in premenopausal women.

Noninv: CT scan of abdomen is primary imaging in most cases; oral and IV contrast preferred unless acute/chronic renal failure, or high likelihood of kidney stones (noncontrast CT preferred).

Abdominal US for evaluation of RUQ pain, pelvic pain in young women.

Plain Xrays for evaluation of N/V to look for obstruction.

3.2 Gastrointestinal Bleeding (Including Upper and Lower GI Sources)

(Med Clin N Am 2000;84:1183; NEJM 2008;359:928)

Cause: Terminology:

- Upper GI bleeding (UGIB): Any GI source above the ampulla of Vater (pancreatic duct).
- Mid GI bleeding: Small bowel source from ampulla of Vater to terminal ileum.
- Lower GI bleeding (LGIB): Source is in the colon, sigmoid, rectum, or anus.
- Occult GI bleeding: Bleeding not associated with frank symptoms, usually initially unrecognized by patient and physician; diagnosed by fecal occult blood test (FOBT) or anemia (usually iron deficiency).
  - Incidental finding of iron deficiency anemia in elderly pts requires GI w/u, especially to rule out colon cancer (although most can have it done after hospital discharge).
- Obscure GI bleeding: Bleeding (may be frank or occult) without an apparent source after standard w/u of common upper and lower sources.

Causes of GI bleeding by site (most common causes listed first):

- Upper GI source:
  - ENT: epistaxis (with ingestion of blood)

- Esophagus: esophageal varices, Mallory-Weiss tears (due to repeated vomiting or rarely instrumentation), esophagitis (related to GERD, medications including bisphosphonates, fungal and viral infections), esophageal cancer
- Gastric: peptic ulcer disease, gastritis (due to NSAIDs, viral infections, alcohol, critical illness), gastric varices and portal gastropathy, gastric cancer (commonly adenocarcinoma, but also lymphoma, metastases), arteriovenous malformations (AVMs), Dieulafoy's lesions (large submucosal vessels that can bleed without associated ulcer), Cameron lesions (gastric ulcers within a hiatal hernia), iatrogenic (NG tube erosions, postbiopsy), aortoenteric fistula, gastric antral vascular ectasia (GAVE, "watermelon stomach")
- Duodenal: duodenal ulcer disease, duodenitis, pancreatic hemosuccus and hemobilia, small bowel or pancreatic cancer, AVMs, iatrogenic (postbiopsy, post-ERCP), aortoenteric fistula
- Mid GI source:
  - Small intestine: angiodysplasia, small bowel cancer, aortoenteric fistula, Crohn's disease, Meckel's diverticulum (congenital small bowel pouch, remnant of the connection from the umbilical cord to the gut, containing gastric and pancreatic tissue; present in about 2% of population, but most are asx), mesenteric ischemia
- Lower GI source:
  - Colon and sigmoid: diverticulosis, AVMs, colon cancer, Crohn's and ulcerative colitis, infectious colitis (including *C. difficile*, *Salmonella*, *Shigella*, *E. coli*, *Giardia*), ischemic colitis, aortoenteric fistula, postprocedural (polypectomy)
  - Rectal/anal: hemorrhoids, anal fissure, cancer, radiation proctitis

Epidem: Upper GI bleeds account for about 100 to 150 cases per 100,000 pts per yr in the United States (PUD/DUD about 50%) (NEJM 1999;341:1738); lower GI accounts for less, about 20 to 50 per 100,000, but many more lower GI bleeds go unaccounted for because of lack of seeking care.

Pathophys: More than 90% of peptic ulcers can be attributed to *Helicobacter pylori* infection (48%), NSAID or aspirin use (24%), and smoking (21%) (J Clin Gastroenterol 1997;24:2); also consider "stress ulcer" (more accurately, the sloughing of gastric mucosa) in critical illness; steroids; bisphosphonate use.

NSAIDs cause ulcers by blocking cyclo-oxygenase and inhibiting prostaglandin formation (which stimulate gastric mucous and bicarbonate secretion, increase gastric blood flow).

Varices (esophageal and gastric) represent collateral blood flow that forms due to elevated blood pressure in the portal system from increased resistance; possibly related to levels of endothelin-1 and nitric oxide (NEJM 2001;345:669).

Sx: Upper GI source usually presents with hematemesis or "coffee ground" emesis as well as melena; may have hematochezia if brisk bleeding, but can usually distinguish from lower source by significant hemodynamic instability.

Mid and lower GI source present with melena and/or hematochezia.

Sx of blood loss can include weakness, fatigue, delirium (especially in elderly), syncope.

Most acute bleeding episodes are not associated with abdominal pain, unless sx from associated ulcer (postprandial or nocturnal epigastric pain), esophagitis (postprandial or nocturnal burning, substernal chest pain), inflammatory bowel disease (IBD) (diffuse crampy pain, associated with frequent stools), or ischemic bowel disease (diffuse pain, usually severity of pain out of sync with abdominal exam findings).

GASTROENTEROLOGY

Dark stools confused for melena can be from iron or bismuth subsalicyclate (Pepto-Bismol) ingestion; red stools can be associated with ingestion of beets or red dye-containing liquids.

Si: Signs include orthostatic hypotension to frank hypovolemic shock, tachycardia; pallor associated with severe anemia.

Look for signs of liver disease to suggest risk for varices: jaundice, spider angiomas and telangiectasias, palmar erythema, ascites, "caput medusa" (prominent subcutaneous abdominal veins, suggesting portal hypertension), gynecomastia, hepatosplenomegaly.

Bowel sounds are typically hyperactive due to the cathartic action of blood in the gut.

Crs: Most sources stop bleeding spontaneously (80% in PUD) (JAMA 1989;262:1369), unless concomitant coagulopathy.

See rebleeding rates in discussion of endoscopy under Noninv below.

Mortality higher for upper GI bleeding (about 7–10% vs less than 5% for LGIB); despite advances in therapy with endoscopy, PPIs, rx of varices, mortality has remained unchanged due to aging population; risk factors for death include severity of initial bleed with hemodynamic compromise, rebleeding, pt age, and other comorbidities (BMJ 1995;311:222; Gut 1996;38:316).

Variceal bleeding occurs in 40% of pts with cirrhosis (Semin Gastrointest Dis 1997;8:179); initial episode mortality is about 20–30%, with 1-yr mortality better than 50% (GE 1981;80:800); rates of rebleeding after first event approach 70%.

Cmplc: Blood loss anemia is a primary complication.

Another risk is myocardial infarction (usually NSTEMI): 12% in one series (Chest 1998;114:1137), but probably even higher with the advent of more sensitive troponin assays; most pts do not have angina, but may have dyspnea, syncope, or no symptoms; represents a demand ischemia/infarct related to anemia and hypotension; supportive therapy (oxygen, beta-blockers), but unable to anticoagulate (ASA, heparin, etc.) in most pts because of active bleeding.

Lab: Initial labs include CBC with platelets, electrolytes, renal and liver function tests, PT/PTT; serial testing of H&H suggested (q 4–8 hr for 24–48 hr depending on severity of symptoms and initial degree of anemia).

Consider cardiac enzymes in at-risk pts.

Elevated BUN often seen with upper GI source, thought to be due to breakdown and digestion of high-protein blood, but may be more related to renal failure from hypovolemia (Am J Gastroenterol 1980;73:486); may have limited value as a discriminatory test in pts without hematochezia; pts with BUN/Cr ratio less than 33 had specif only 17% for LGIB (Am J Gastroenterol 1997;92:1796).

Elevated INR, thrombocytopenia, low albumin, elevated liver function tests may help distinguish cirrhotic pts at risk for variceal bleeding.

After initial evaluation, consider utility of serum *H. pylori* testing (ELISA antibody test for prior infection); unhelpful if previously diagnosed and treated; unnecessary if direct biopsy performed on endoscopy; also consider urease breath test.

Noninv: Most imaging tests (plain films, CT, MRI) are not specifically useful in GI bleeds, unless trying to r/o another comorbid condition (aspiration pneumonitis, metastatic cancer, bowel obstruction or perforation).

Early endoscopic evaluation and therapy for UGIB

(Ann IM 2003;139:843)

- It allows for quick assessment of cause and possible therapeutic intervention.
- When performed within 24 hr of admission, early endoscopy is associated with reduced risk of rebleeding and reduced LOS (Gastrointest Endosc 1999;49:145).

GASTROENTEROLOGY

- In pts with PUD, appearance of ulcer has prognostic value (Med Clin N Am 2000;84:1183).
  - Highest risk: Active bleeding or oozing vessel has 60–80% rebleed rate.
  - High risk: Visible, but nonbleeding vessel has about 40% rebleed rate; with adherent clot has 14–36% rebleed rate.
  - Low risk: Flat, pigmented spots and "clean" ulcers have low rate of rebleeding, 5–10%.
- Endoscopic treatment options for high-risk lesions include epinephrine injection or other sclerotherapy, mechanical clips, thermal ablation, argon plasma coagulation; consensus recommendations for epinephrine injection plus a second therapy instead of epinephrine alone (GE 2004;126:441).
- Highest risk of failure of endoscopic therapy is in pts with recurrent PUD history, shock on arrival, active bleeding on initial endoscopy, large ulcers (2 cm or larger) (NEJM 2008;359:928).
- Routine "second-look" endoscopy after 24–48 hr is controversial; some say useful to reduce rebleeding rates after interventional rx (Gastrointest Endosc 1994;40:34), but guidelines say unnecessary and not cost-effective (Ann IM 2003;139:843).

Evaluation of mid GI bleeding (small bowel)

(GE 2007;133:1694).

- The mid GI tract is the source of most cases of obscure bleeding (another common cause is missed lesions on upper and lower endoscopy).
- Capsule endoscopy has changed management over past 10 yrs and is now the primary test for evaluation.
  - Patient swallows a wireless video camera in pill shape, which captures sequential pictures of the gut as it is moved through by peristalsis.

- In animal model, capsule endoscopy showed significantly greater sens for small bowel lesions than push enteroscopy (64% vs 37%) (GE 2000;119:1431).
- Other options for diagnosis include push enteroscopy (longer EGD scope) and intraoperative enteroscopy.
- Tagged RBC scans and angiography may help in cases of rapid bleeding, but otherwise fail to diagnose or effectively localize lesions.
- If concerned for Meckel's diverticulum, Meckel's scan uses nuclear imaging to detect gastric tissue in the small bowel.

Evaluation of lower GI bleeding

- Colonoscopy is primary diagnostic test, should be performed if possible within 24–48 hr of bleeding episode.
  - While can be done urgently, many times test is difficult due to blood and stool obscuring view; given that most episodes of LGIB resolve without therapy, watchful waiting and supportive care may be best for the first few days.
  - Should attempt bowel cleansing (most use polyethylene glycol, GoLytely) to improve diagnostic yield, which can be as high as 90% (Gastrointest Endosc 1998;48:606).
  - Usually colonoscopy is preferred over sigmoidoscopy because of higher yield, except in young pts with likely hemorrhoids or lower GI infection as probable cause and lower risk of colon cancer.
- Tagged RBC scans can be used to localize bleeding, but have significant limitations; must be done at the time of active bleeding (requires bleeding rate of at least 0.1 mL/min) and many centers do not have 24-hr nuclear imaging capabilities; positive findings show a "blush" over the bleeding area, which may not be accurate enough to proceed with surgical intervention.

- Angiography has better yield than nuclear imaging, but requires active bleeding as well, and is not available in many centers.

Rx:

Treatment considerations for all GI bleeds

- Initially, stabilize pt, ABCs.
- Obtain IV access with at least two large-bore (18 gauge or larger) IVs; CVC may be necessary if lack of good IV access, but large-bore peripheral IVs preferred for initial resuscitation.
- Provide supplemental oxygen; NPO status; telemetry monitoring.
- In settings of massive hematemesis, especially associated with altered mental status, consider intubation and mechanical ventilation to protect airway and prevent aspiration.
- Assess the degree of hemodynamic compromise:
  - Orthostasis and resting tachycardia suggest 10–15% volume loss, frank hypotension more than 30%.
  - Initiate fluid repletion with IV crystalloid (NS or LR); can usually give rapid boluses (1–2 L/hr or faster) unless concern for CHF/pulmonary edema.
- If source unclear, consider placement of NG tube for aspiration of stomach contents; presence of blood in NG aspirate is highly specific for UGIB source (specif for high-risk ulcer bleeding ~75%, NPV 78%) (Gastrointest Endosc 2004;59: 172), but not sensitive; up to 15% of high-risk lesions may have negative NG aspirate (i.e., cannot r/o upper source if negative aspirate, as may have already stopped bleeding); relative contraindication to blind NG tube placement in pts at high risk for varices, as may cause trauma and worsening bleeding.
- Consider the following in rx of blood-loss anemia:
  - Transfusion practices are often dictated by hospital policies; many consider transfusion with Hgb less than 9–10 gm/dL (Hct less than 30%) with active bleeding, as

likely Hgb will drop further, but if bleeding is more remote in pt without comorbid disease, could use a lower trigger (as low as 7 gm/dL) (Crit Care Med 2009;37:3124); see Section 4.1, "Anemia (Including Transfusion Practices)."

- Evaluate for coagulopathy and treat as appropriate:
  - Get medication history including ASA, NSAIDs, clopidogrel, heparins (UFH and LMWH), warfarin.
  - Administer fresh frozen plasma if comorbid coagulopathy from meds; protamine in pts on heparin; no specific reversal agents for other meds.
  - Vitamin K can be given in IV form for warfarin reversal, but may also require FFP until vit K effect can occur (within 24 hr).
    - Although pts with cirrhosis have elevated INR and coagulopathy, there are no studies to guide vit K administration for variceal bleeding in cirrhotic pts (Cochrane 2008;CD004792).
  - Transfuse platelets if plt count is less than 50K with active bleeding.
- Institute PPI therapy for UGIB unless clearly not related to ulcer (see below).
- Assess risk for varices based on patient history, exam, risk factors; if high risk, consider octreotide therapy (as described below under "Specific therapy for variceal bleeding").
- Prepare for early endoscopy.

Gastric acid suppression in UGIB

- In vitro elevation in gastric pH (greater than 6) is associated with improved clotting (Gut 1989;30:1704).
- Mainly, PPI therapy is proven in the setting of UGIB from PUD/DUD, although often used in all pts initially (as ulcer cause is most common) until endoscopy is performed.
  - Initial 1997 study of 220 pts with ulcer bleeding; randomized to omeprazole 40 mg PO q 12 hr for 5 d vs placebo;

rx reduced rebleeding rates (11% vs 36%, NNT 4) and need for surgery (7% vs 23%, NNT 6), but not powered for mortality benefit (NEJM 1997;336:1054).

- 2005 meta-analysis of 21 trials showed similar reduced rebleeding rates (NNT 12) and need for surgery (NNT 20), but no mortality benefit (BMJ 2005;330:568).
- Despite initial studies with PO PPIs, most now use IV PPIs in the initial setting due to NPO status; can use intermittent therapy (e.g., pantoprazole 40–80 mg IV q 12 hr) or bolus-infusion (e.g., pantoprazole 80 mg IV bolus, then 8 mg/hr drip for 72 hr).
  - 2002 meta-analysis of 4000 pts suggested reduced rebleeding rates with continuous infusion therapy rather than intermittent bolus (Crit Care Med 2002;30:S369).
- No role for H2B therapy in acute setting, with the widespread availability of PPIs.
- In pts with low-risk findings on early EGD, no need to continue IV PPI therapy; can transition to PO in anticipation of discharge.
- After initial therapy, longer term gastric suppression is warranted to allow for ulcer healing.
  - 1997 meta-analysis of PPIs and H2Bs showed better healing rates with PPIs at 4 wk of therapy (85% vs 75%, NNT 10) (Eur J Gastroenterol Hepatol 1995;7:661).
  - Most pts don't require therapy for longer than 6–8 wk, unless recurrent or severe disease, continued risk factors, *H. pylori* (–).

Other treatment considerations in pts with PUD

(Am Fam Phys 2007;76:1005)

- Some pts may be eligible for early discharge to home after endoscopy, reducing LOS from 6 to 7 days down to 2 to 3 days:
  - Young, otherwise healthy pts (younger than 60 yr), hemodynamically stable, Hgb more than 8–10 gm/dL

without need for transfusion, no coagulopathy, low risk findings on EGD, and good f/u plans (JAMA 1997;278: 2151; Am J Med 1998;105:176; Gastrointest Endosc 1999; 50:755)

- Eradication of *H. pylori* greatly reduces risk of recurrence.
  - 67% risk reduced to 6% risk of recurrence in gastric ulcers; 59% reduced to 4% in duodenal ulcers (GE 1996;110:1244).
  - Various combinations of acid suppression (PPI or H2B) plus antibiotics (penicillins, tetracycline, fluoroquinolones, macrolides) for 7 to 14 days can be used.
  - American College of Gastroenterology suggests the following regimens (Am J Gastroenterol 2007;102:1808):
    - Clarithromycin PLUS amoxicillin (or metronidazole) PLUS any PPI for 14 days
    - Metronidazole PLUS tetracycline PLUS bismuth subsalicylate PLUS any PPI or H2B for 10 to 14 days
- Avoid NSAID use, if possible; if requires long-term ASA or NSAIDs, consider long-term PPI therapy or misoprostol (oral prostaglandin) (Cochrane 2002;CD002296).
- Avoid alcohol, smoking, drug use.
- Surgical options for treatment still exist, but are used much less frequently in the current era of frequent, prolonged PPI use.

Specific therapy for variceal bleeding

(NEJM 2001;345:669)

- Acute medical therapy:
  - No benefit has been shown to acid suppression (H2B or PPI), but often used initially until bleeding source identified.
  - Octreotide: A somatostatin analog that reduces liver and gut blood flow, portal hypertension; when added to endoscopic therapy, reduces rebleeding rates (NNT 6) and transfusion needs (NEJM 1995;333:555; Lancet 1995;

GASTROENTEROLOGY

346:1666); vasopressin has similar results, but more side effects (coronary and distal ischemia); terlipressin also effective but not available in the United States.

- Preventive therapy:
  - Beta-blockers: Reduce gut blood flow and portal pressures; nonselective beta-blockers preferred (propranolol and nadolol); proven efficacy in prevention of first and recurrent bleeding episodes; dosage unclear (difficult to measure portal pressure), but suggest titrating to maximal dose that keeps resting HR more than 55–60 bpm.
    - Prevention of first bleeding: Meta-analysis of four trials (~600 pts) showed reduced bleeding events and severity-adjusted mortality in cirrhotic pts rx with propranolol or nadolol vs placebo (NEJM 1991;324:1532).
    - Prevention of recurrent bleeding: Meta-analysis of 12 trials showed reduced recurrent bleeding (NNT 5) and mortality (NNT 14) with addition of beta-blockers (Hepatol 1997;25:63).
  - Nitrates: Reduce portal pressures and cause gut vasoconstriction due to compensation for primary vasodilatory effects; one study, however, of monotherapy with isosorbide mononitrate showed no effect on bleeding episodes and increased mortality associated with treatment (GE 1997;113:1632); combination therapy with beta-blockers showed improved portal pressures, but no clinical outcomes (Ann IM 1991;114:869); many pts will not tolerate combo therapy because of hypotensive side effects.
- Emergent endoscopy for sclerotherapy or band ligation; both have similar results in stopping initial bleeding (~80%), but sclerotherapy associated with more complications (NEJM 1992;326:1527).
- If uncontrolled bleeding, consider gastroesophageal balloon to tamponade vessels (i.e., Minnesota tube, Sengstaken-Blakemore tube); up to 80% effective in resistant bleeding

(GE 1978;75:566), but risks include perforation, pressure-induced ulcers.

- If further uncontrolled bleeding, consider urgent transjugular intrahepatic portosystemic shunt (TIPS) procedure; intravascular placement of a metal shunt from hepatic vein to the portal vein through the liver tissue to reduce portal hypertension; reduces rebleeding rates, but at the expense of increased hepatic encephalopathy (Ann IM 1997;126:858).
- Antibiotics: In cirrhotic pts with ascites and acute variceal bleeding, addition of prophylactic abx (usually a 3rd generation cephalosporin or fluoroquinolone) reduces infection rates (particularly spontaneous bacterial peritonitis, SBP) and improves short-term mortality (Hepatol 1999;29:1655).

Treatment considerations for mid and lower GI bleeding

- Most episodes of small bowel bleeding are self-limited and do not require acute therapy, other than supportive care.
- Most diverticular bleeds resolve spontaneously (75%), but have a high rate of recurrence (38%) (Ann Surg 1994;220:653).
- LGIB lesions can be treated endoscopically similar to EGD therapies; polypectomy as needed.
- Surgical intervention is required for severe, uncontrolled bleeding or recurrent episodes.

Stress ulcer prophylaxis

(Gastro Clin N Am 2009;38:245)

- In critical illness, local gut ischemia and inflammatory factors can cause gastric mucosal damage, leading to GI bleeding.
- Mucosal damage occurs in 75–100% of critically ill pts, leading to occult bleeding (guaiac positive stool or drop in Hgb) in up to 50% and clinically significant bleeding in about 5%; significant GI bleeding in this critically ill population is associated with high mortality (~50%) (Gastro Clin N Am 2009;38:245).

- The two main risk factors for stress ulcers are respiratory failure and coagulopathy (NEJM 1994;330:377), as well as hypotension, sepsis, chronic kidney and liver disease, alcohol abuse (Crit Care Med 1996;24:1974).
- Choices for prophylaxis include the following:
  - There is good evidence of reduction in GI bleeding with H2 blockers (famotidine is the most potent) (Ann IM 1985;103:173) and sucralfate; limited evidence for PPIs (Dig Dis Sci 1997;42:1255; Am J Crit Care 2008;17:142) but presumed effective due to more reduction in gastric acidity than H2Bs.
  - Choice depends on institutional norms, individual patient factors, costs; little evidence to suggest one choice is superior.
- Who should get prophylaxis?
  - American Society of Health System Pharmacists suggests stress ulcer prophylaxis for pts in the ICU with any of the following additional risks (Am J Health Syst Pharm 1999;56:347):
    - Mechanical ventilation for more than 48 hr
    - Coagulopathy with plt less than 50K, INR more than 1.5, PTT more than 2 times normal
    - Severe trauma, burns, spinal cord injury, s/p transplant or liver resection
    - Hx of GI bleeding or ulcer within the past yr
    - Liver failure
    - GCS 10 or less
    - Also consider for sepsis: ICU LOS more than 1 wk, occult GI bleeding, high-dose steroids
  - There is no clinical evidence to suggest need for stress ulcer prophylaxis in non-ICU pts, but individual decisions can be made based on pts' risk factors (Am J Health Syst Pharm 2007;64:1396).

- Risks of prophylaxis include these:
  - Infections: Increased risk for pneumonia (JAMA 2004;292:1955; NEJM 1998;338:791), possibly C. *diff* colitis (JAMA 2005;294:2989; Clin Infect Dis 2006;43:1272).
  - Cost: Not only direct inpatient costs, but evidence of prolonged use as inpatient (56–76%) (Ital J Gastroenterol Hepatol 1997;29:325; Am J Gastroenterol 2000;95:3118) and on discharge (25% of ICU pts started on stress ulcer prophylaxis were discharged on the med without an appropriate indication) (Ann Pharmacother 2007;41:1611).
  - Drug interactions: PPI use may reduce the antiplatelet efficacy of clopidogrel (Cardiol Rev 2009;17:198; Lancet 2009;374:989).
- Bottom line is to consider stress ulcer prophylaxis in ICU pts, especially with coagulopathy or requiring mechanical ventilation; reassess regularly, and in most pts can discontinue prophylaxis when critical illness resolved; make sure not to continue prophylaxis on discharge unless a clear indication for continued use.

3.3 Pancreaticobiliary Diseases

Biliary Tract Disease (Including Cholecystitis, Bile Duct Obstruction, Cholangitis)

(NEJM 2008;358:2804; Med Clin N Am 2008;92:925)

Cause: Definitions:

- Cholelithiasis: Presence of gallstones in the gall bladder (GB), may be sx or asx.
- Biliary colic: Intermittent episodes of pain associated with gallstone impaction in the cystic duct of the GB.

- Cholecystitis: Infection of the gall bladder associated with an impacted gallstone (90% of cases) or critical illness ("acalculous cholecystitis").
  - Risk factors for acalculous cholecystitis (other than critical illness) include diabetes, HIV and other forms of immunosuppression, TPN administration, acute renal failure (Med Clin N Am 2006;90:481).
- Choledocholithiasis: Obstruction of the common bile duct (CBD) by a gallstone. CBD obstruction can come from other causes (~15% of cases) including pancreatic, GB, or duodenal tumor; GB "sludge" or microlithiasis (controversial); stricture; foreign body/blocked stent; Mirizzi's syndrome (impacted cystic duct stone causes indirect compression of the CBD without stone passage to CBD); primary sclerosing cholangitis (PSC).
- Ascending cholangitis: Infection associated with obstruction of the CBD.

Epidem: 60% of pts with acute cholecystitis are women, but actually higher rate in men with known gallstones (men have about half the risk of women for stone formation) (GE 1999;117:632); higher risk in diabetics and more severe course (Arch Surg 1988;123:409).

Pathophys: Gallstones: Most (80–90%) are cholesterol stones; remaining are black or brown pigmented stones related to other chronic or underlying illnesses.

Cholecystitis: Impaction of stone in cystic duct leads to inflammation, GB wall edema, and pericholecystic fluid; bacteria can then grow in the static fluid leading to infection; in severe cases, gangrene and gas can form.

Sx: Most gallstones are asx, diagnosed on imaging for another indication.

Biliary colic is usually postprandial or nocturnal RUQ or epigastric, lasting from a few minutes up to 6 hr; associated N/V;

with cholecystitis and cholangitis, pain is prolonged, with fever, tenderness on exam, and may have associated sepsis.

Cholangitis classically has Charcot's triad (fever, jaundice, RUQ pain) in up to 70% (J Hepatobiliary Pancreat 2007;14:52) and Reynolds' pentad (Charcot's triad plus hypotension and delirium) in about 5% (but poor prognosis) (Arch Surg 1982;117:437).

Si: Murphy's sign: Patient stops inspiration during palpation of the gall bladder when asked to breath deeply; also performed at the time of US imaging ("ultrasonographic Murphy's sign").

Crs: Annual risk associated with gallstones: colic in 1–4%; acute cholecystitis in 0.3% (~10–30% of pts with prior colic); symptomatic choledocholithiasis in 0.2%; pancreatitis in 0.04–1.5% (Med Clin N Am 2008;92:925).

Cmplc: Necrotic or gangrenous cholecystitis; emphysematous cholecystitis (due to anaerobic organisms); GB perforation (in 8–12% with 20% mortality) (Med Clin N Am 2006;90:481); gallstone ileus (large passed gallstone causes bowel obstruction, usually at the ileocecal valve); local effects can include abscess formation and pleural effusion.

Lab: Initial labs as described for abdominal pain in Section 3.1; blood cultures in all pts with concern for cholangitis.

Typical findings:

- Colic: Labs are usually normal.
- Cholecystitis: Leukocytosis; usually LFTs are normal (exception is Mirizzi's syndrome, see Cause above).
- Choledocholithiasis: Elevated liver enzymes, including AST/ALT, alkaline phosphatase (and GGTP, although rarely adds anything further to alk phos evaluation), and bilirubin (conjugated hyperbilirubinemia).
- Cholangitis: Same as for choledocholithiasis, with leukocytosis. Presence of associated sepsis may lead to acute renal failure and metabolic abnormalities.

CRP and ESR likely elevated in infection, but rarely add to the clinical picture.

Elevated amylase/lipase suggest concomitant pancreatitis.

Noninv: Ultrasound is the initial imaging choice for these reasons:

- US is more than 95% specific and sensitive for cholelithiasis and cholecystitis.
- Findings in cholecystitis include thickened GB wall, pericholecystic fluid, and ultrasonographic Murphy's sign.
- Ultrasonographic Murphy's plus stones in the GB has 92% PPV and 95% NPV for acute cholecystitis (Radiol 1985;155:767).
- Also can identify CBD dilation indicating choledocholithiasis, but poor sens (25–60%); study showed that sens of both US (63%) and CT (71%) for choledocholithiasis was much less than endoscopic US and ERCP (Gastrointest Endosc 1997;45:143), as they miss small stones that obstruct the duct but cause minimal dilation.

CT imaging is indicated if concern for other causes of abdominal pain, and may be better for identification in pts with evaluation suggesting cholangitis or pancreatitis to eval CBD and pancreas.

HIDA (hepatobiliary iminodiacetic acid) scan is nuclear imaging for GB filling; lack of filling within 60 min suggests cystic duct obstruction (up to 90% sensitive); although it may have better accuracy than US (Surg 2000;127:609), the ease and availability of US make it the first choice; HIDA scans usually reserved for second evaluation of pts with recurrent or persistent RUQ sx despite negative US (but true value may be limited) (J Emerg Med 2007;33:47).

MRI (MRCP) reserved for eval of RUQ sx associated with pancreatitis; 90% sens and 95% specif for choledocholithiasis (Abdom Imaging 2008;33:6); direct visualization with ERCP usually preferred if concern for CBD obstruction, as can provide direct therapy at the same time (i.e. removal of stone, stenting, etc).

Rx: Most with colic alone do not require admission; all others likely require admission for further monitoring and therapy.

General measures for treatment of pts with biliary tract disease

- Pain control with opiates and/or NSAIDs (e.g., IV ketorolac)
- NPO status and bowel rest; IV fluids for dehydration and maintenance
- Detection and treatment of coagulopathies, if present
- Antibiotics for pts with cholecystitis and cholangitis
  - Abx typically cover Gram-negatives and anaerobes; consider broader-spectrum coverage in pts with prior episodes requiring instrumentation of the biliary tract or immunodeficiency.
  - Common abx regimens include ampicillin-sulbactam, ceftriaxone, combo of fluoroquinolone and metronidazole.
  - If concern for MDR organisms, use piperacillin-tazobactam, cefepime, carbapenems.
  - Typically treat until clinically improved and for 7 to 14 days total, although shorter course may be used if early cholecystectomy (Aust N Z J Surg 1990;60:539).
- GI and surgical consults as needed
  - ERCP for common bile duct (CBD) obstruction (see below)
  - Early vs delayed surgery for cholecystitis

Surgical options for cholecystitis

- Laparoscopic surgery has replaced laparotomy as primary rx choice, even in pts with acute cholecystitis, due to decreased risks, recovery time, and LOS.
- Debate as to timing of surgery: "early" (within a few days to week of acute infection) vs "delayed" (weeks to months after).
  - Cochrane review of five trials (451 pts) showed no difference between early or delayed surgery in CBD injury at

GASTROENTEROLOGY

surgery or need for conversion to open cholecystectomy; no mortality in any of the trials; in pts with plan for delayed surgery, 17% required emergency surgery due to recurrent or nonresolving disease; pts with early surgery had reduced LOS (Cochrane 2006;CD005440).

- In pts deemed not appropriate for surgery due to critical illness (including most with acalculous cholecystitis), consider placement of percutaneous cholecystostomy to allow for GB drainage; usually can be done with radiographic guidance and local anesthesia (Radiol 1989;173:481).

ERCP for CBD obstruction

(NEJM 1999;341:1808)

- ERCP is best test to initially diagnose and treat choledocholithiasis; RCT of ERCP vs surgery for acute cholangitis showed reduced mortality in pts with ERCP (10% vs 32%, NNT 5) (NEJM 1992;326:1582).
- When stone found, ERCP allows for removal by direct retrieval with sphincterotomy (~80–90% effective).
- ERCP has minimal adverse effects: pancreatitis in about 5%, bleeding in about 2%, cholangitis in about 1% (NEJM 1996;335:909).
- Stones that cannot be removed by ERCP can be managed with placement of stent (to allow for gradual fragmentation and dissolution), lithotripsy, or surgical removal.

Pancreatitis, Acute and Chronic

(Med Clin N Am 2008;92:889; NEJM 2006;354:2142)

Cause: Determination of cause is crucial to determining therapy and risk of recurrence. Causes include:

- Gallstones and other mechanical obstruction represent the most frequent (40%) cause. Other ductal obstruction occurs much less commonly; includes pancreatic and duodenal cancer, parasitic obstruction from *Ascaris*, blood clots, pancreas divisum (congenital malformation of the pancreatic ducts), sphincter of Oddi stenosis.

- Alcohol (35%) is another common cause, but usually only in severe alcohol use (more than 8 drinks per day for 5 yr or more) (Am J Gastroenterol 2001;96:2622), and in only 5–10% of all alcoholics. Smoking may be associated with increased risk (OR 4.9) and coffee intake with decreased risk (OR 0.85) (Am J Gastroenterol 2004;99:731); more common in males (2.5:1), younger pts (younger than 35 yr), and African Americans.
- Hypertriglyceridemia (2%) can contribute to pancreatitis, usually with trig levels more than 2000 mg/dL.
- Post-ERCP accounts for a small proportion (2%) of cases.
- Drug-induced causes are also infrequent (2%). Many drugs have been suggested; commonly used offenders include estrogens (including tamoxifen), diuretics (thiazides and loop), antibiotics (metronidazole and tetracyclines), valproic acid, azathioprine, sulfasalazine, mesalamine, statins (GE 2007;132:2022).
- Rarer causes include hypercalcemia, posttraumatic, autoimmune (SLE, vasculitis), infectious (usually viral; mumps most common prior to widespread immunization, also HIV, CMV, EBV), complication of cystic fibrosis; up to 15% are determined "idiopathic" as no cause is evident.

Chronic pancreatitis in the United States is primarily a result of alcoholic pancreatitis.

Epidem: Accounts for 200,000 to 300,000 U.S. hospitalizations per year and 20,000 deaths.

Pathophys: Activation of trypsinogen to trypsin without elimination from the gland causes autodigestion of the pancreatic tissue; inflammatory cascade worsens the course.

Chronic disease forms due to destruction of the endocrine and exocrine pancreatic glands from repeated bouts of inflammation (GE 2007;132:1557).

Sx: Abdominal pain, typically epigastric, but may be RUQ, LUQ, boring through to back; associated N/V; typically worse with eating or drinking (particularly fatty meals and alcohol).

Fever is seen in some cases, usually with associated SIRS in severe cases.

Chronic disease characterized by chronic abdominal pain (can be intermittent or persistent); loss of digestive enzymes leads to steatorrhea, weight loss.

Si: Abdominal tenderness; guarding is more common than rebound tenderness; hypoactive bowel sounds.

Due to poor PO intake and 3rd spacing of fluids, many will show signs of severe dehydration, including tachycardia, hypotension, syncope, oliguria, dry mucous membranes.

Grey Turner's sign: extension of pancreatic enzymes and inflammation causing retroperitoneal hemorrhage with flank ecchymosis; Cullen's sign: extension of pancreatic enzymes and inflammation causing abdominal wall hemorrhage with periumbilical ecchymosis (Gastrointest Radiol 1989;14:31).

Crs: Determination of severity is important in determining prognosis and therapy (particularly nutrition, antibiotics, and surgery/intervention); about 20% of all cases are classified as severe (with mortality of severe cases up to 30% vs less than 1% for mild cases) (JAMA 2004;291:2865); see **Figure 3.1** for overview.

Ranson's criteria (see **Figure 3.1**) are the most well-known, requiring determination of 12 clinical and lab values over the

Criterion and Marker	Threshold Value	Severe Pancreatitis
Atlanta criteria*		Indicated by any positive factor listed
Ranson's score†	≥3	
APACHE II score‡	≥8	
Organ failure		
Shock	Blood pressure of <90 mm Hg	
Pulmonary insufficiency	Partial pressure of arterial oxygen of ≤60 mm Hg§	
Renal failure	Creatinine level of >177 μmol/liter (2 mg/dL) after hydration	
Systemic complications		
Disseminated intravascular coagulation	Platelet count of ≤100,000/mm³ Fibrinogen level of <1 gm/liter Fibrin-split products level of >80 μg/mL	
Metabolic disturbance	Calcium level of ≤7.5 mg/dL	
Local complications		
Pancreatic necrosis	Present	
Pancreatic abscess	Present	
Pancreatic pseudocyst	Present	
Ranson's score†		Indicated by a total score ≥3, with 1 point for each positive factor
At presentation		
Age	>55 yr	
Blood glucose level	>200 mg/dL (10 mmol/liter)	
White-cell count	>16,000/mm³	
Lactate dehydrogenase level	>350 IU/liter	
Alanine aminotransferase level	>250 IU/liter	
Within 48 hr after presentation		
Hematocrit	>10% decrease	
Serum calcium	<8 mg/dL (2 mmol/liter)	
Base deficit	>4 mEq/liter	
Blood urea nitrogen	>5 mg/dL (1.8 mmol/liter) increase	
Fluid sequestration	>6 liters	
Partial pressure of arterial oxygen∫	<60 mm Hg	
CT Severity index¶		Indicated by a total score of >6 (CT grade plus necrosis score)
CT grade		
Normal pancreas (grade A)	0 points	
Focal or diffuse enlargement (grade B)	1 point	
Intrinsic change; fat stranding (grade C)	2 points	
Single, ill-defined collection of fluid (grade D)	3 points	
Multiple collections of fluid or gas in or adjacent to pancreas (grade E)	4 points	
Necrosis score		
No pancreatic necrosis	0 points	
Necrosis of one third of pancreas	2 points	
Necrosis of one half of pancreas	4 points	
Necrosis of >one half of pancreas	6 points	
APACHE II score‡		Indicated by a score of ≥8
Initial values of 12 routine physiological measurements, age, and previous health status		

* The Atlanta criteria were adopted in 1992 by the International Symposium on Acute Pancreatitis. The presence of any condition in the five main categories indicates severe acute pancreatitis.
† The original Ranson's score is based on 11 clinical signs (5 measured on admission and 6 in the 48 hours after admission), with a higher score indicating greater correlation with the incidence of systemic complications and the presence of pancreatic necrosis.
‡ The Acute Physiology and Chronic Health Evaluation (APACHE II) score is based on initial values of 12 routine physiological measurements, age, and previous health status, with a score of 8 or more commonly used as the threshold for classification as severe pancreatitis.
∫ The test was performed without the use of supplemental oxygen.
¶ The CT severity index is a combination of the sum of the necrosis score and points assigned to five grades of findings on CT. The index ranges from 0 to 10, with higher scores indicating a greater severity of illness.

Figure 3.1 Scoring Methods for Acute Pancreatitis

Reproduced with permission from Whitcomb DC. Acute pancreatitis. *NEJM.* 2006;354:2142. Copyright © 2006, Massachusetts Medical Society. All rights reserved.

first 48 hr of presentation (Surg Gyn Ob 1974;139:69); score of 3 or higher suggests severe disease, with PPV 95% and NPV 86% in original study, but that study had high overall mortality; subsequent analysis has shown reduced PPV (~50%) for severe disease (GE 2007;132:2022).

APACHE-II scoring may also be helpful; multiple online calculators are available.

The CT severity index bases decisions on CT findings and the degree of pancreatic necrosis.

The Atlanta criteria (Arch Surg 1993;128:586) combine many of the foregoing; Atlanta classification defines severe cases as any one of the following:

- Organ failure: shock (SBP less than 90 mmHg), resp failure (PaO_2 less than 60 mmHg), renal failure (Cr more than 2 mg/dL), or GI bleeding (more than 500 cc in 24 hr)
- Pancreatic complications of necrosis, pseudo-cyst, or abscess
- Ranson score 3 or more
- APACHE-II score 8 or more

Obesity (BMI more than 30) is a risk factor for severe disease (OR 2.6) and complications, both pancreatic (OR 4.3) and systemic (OR 2.0) (Pancreatology 2004;4:42).

Cmplc: Respiratory: Pleural effusion, ARDS (in up to 20% of severe cases).

Metabolic: Severe hyperglycemia (and hypoglycemia associated with insulin therapy); hypocalcemia.

GI: Pancreatic necrosis (and associated infection), pseudocyst formation (thin-walled, fluid-filled cyst), abscess; development of chronic pancreatitis.

Possibly increased risk of pancreatic cancer with chronic pancreatitis (NEJM 1993;328:1433).

Lab: See discussion of abdominal pain in Section 3.1 for initial lab w/u; add fasting triglycerides to r/o hypertriglyceridemia (mild elevations less than 1000 mg/dL may be seen with alcoholic pancreatitis); LDH and ABG also needed for assessment of Ranson's criteria (but unnecessary in milder cases).

Amylase and lipase are the primary tests, usually 3 times normal or more in acute pancreatitis; lipase has higher sens (90%) and specif; consider salivary gland inflammation or tumors with false positive amylase; both are renally secreted and may be falsely high with CKD, but usually not to the levels seen in acute pancreatitis (J Clin Gastroenterol 2002;34:459).

Leukocytosis and hyperglycemia are common; hypocalcemia, especially in severe cases, but no evidence to show that replacement has any benefit (Section 2.4 in Chapter 2) elevated hematocrit (greater than 47%) suggests dehydration and hemoconcentration (and is associated with worse prognosis) (Am J Gastroenterol 1998;93:2130).

Elevated liver enzymes typically suggest alcoholic or biliary cause; if AST is higher, alcohol more likely; if ALT is higher, biliary more likely; PPV of ALT more than 150 IU/L for gallstone pancreatitis is 95% (Am J Gastroenterol 1994;89:1863).

Noninv: Abdominal Xrays usually done to r/o ileus, obstruction, perforated viscous, but limited help in diagnosing pancreatitis; consider CXR if resp sx, to r/o concomitant pleural effusion, ARDS.

US is performed initially on many pts to evaluate for gallstones, although limited sens to r/o CBD obstruction and pancreatic inflammation (see "Biliary Tract Disease" earlier in Section 3.3).

Contrast CT of the abdomen is the primary imaging test, but not necessary initially in most cases. Consider CT in the following cases:

- Concern for other diagnoses
- Chronic pts to r/o new complication (abscess, pseudocyst)

- Severe cases to evaluate degree of necrosis and cmplc
  - However, in severe cases, may still need to rescan 2 to 4 days later because initial test may underestimate severity.
  - Look for gland enlargement, fluid accumulation, "streaking of the fat" to suggest inflammatory changes, frank necrosis.
- Negative CT does not r/o pancreatitis; 10–15% of mild cases may have no CT findings (Radiol 2002;223:603).

MRI does not provide much more info in acute setting, but may have further value in classifying masses in severe acute or chronic pancreatitis (pseudo-cyst vs abscess vs phlegmon); MRCP can be used to noninvasively evaluate for CBD obstruction from gallstone, tumor, or strictures; endoscopic US and ERCP can also be used similarly.

Rx: Treatment approach differs for acute and chronic pancreatitis.

General therapy for acute pancreatitis

- All pts w/ acute pancreatitis require admission for further evaluation and monitoring for worsening disease (whereas some mild cases of chronic pancreatitis may be managed as outpatients).
- Aggressive IV rehydration is required for most pts; 250–500 mL/hr of crystalloids (0.9% NS or LR) to start, until showing signs of improvement with decreased tachycardia, improved BP, resumption of adequate urine output (more than 0.5 mL/kg/hr); in severe cases or with concomitant heart failure, may need PA cath to help direct fluid therapy; in younger pts without heart disease, central line with CVP monitoring should be adequate.
  - Consider albumin only if concomitant severe hypoalbuminemia (less than 2 gm/dL).
  - Provide transfusion w/ PRBCs if Hct is less than 25%, associated bleeding.

- NPO with bowel rest initially in all except the most mild cases.
  - Advance diet slowly once pt showing clinical improvement (pain and nausea resolving, enzymes returning to normal).
- Oxygen supplementation; severe cases may require intubation and mechanical ventilation.
- Pain control, usually with opiates:
  - Traditional teaching has been to avoid morphine, because of animal models and small human studies (Gut 1988;29:1402) showing sphincter of Oddi contraction, which may worsen course; subsequent reviews have argued against this (Am J Gastroenterol 2001;96:1266); previous expert opinion has suggested meperidine (Demerol) use, but now that opiate is largely avoided because of active metabolites causing undesired effects (delirium, seizures); if preference is to avoid morphine, use hydromorphone or fentanyl.
  - Can also use IV ketorolac (Toradol) but avoid prolonged use (more than 48 hr) and in severe cases, due to concern for renal dysfunction and bleeding risks.
- Nasogastric tube aspiration, if associated ileus, persistent N/V; routine NG suction not helpful (e.g., one surgical study showed no improvement in duration of pain or opiate use, with prolonged time to oral intake and LOS) (Surg 1986;100:500).
- Nutritional support, usually for severe cases, requiring pts to be NPO more than 5 to 7 days:
  - Most do not require any additional supplementation in the first few days, even in severe cases.
  - Studies have shown total enteral nutrition (TEN), especially provided by jejunal feeding tube, to be superior to TPN.
    - Small RCT of 30 pts with acute pancreatitis; randomized to TEN or TPN within 48 hr; no difference in

mortality, but TEN associated with less severity based on delayed Ranson's criteria, less risk of severe hyperglycemia, and less cost (JPEN 1997;21:14).

- Meta-analysis of six studies showed reduced infections, surgery, and LOS with enteral feeds, but no difference in mortality (BMJ 2004;328:1407).
- Meta-analysis of 27 trials showed enteral nutrition associated with reduced infections and LOS/costs, but no difference in mortality vs TPN (JPEN 2006;30:143).
- In most severe cases, where pt not likely to resume nutrition within 3 to 5 days, consider addition of enteral feeding, usually done through small bore jejunal tube (Dobhoff tube); use TPN in cases where pt unable to tolerate enteral tube or evidence of ileus/obstruction.

- Routine use of antibiotics for acute pancreatitis is a controversial subject:
  - In most pts with mild disease (80% of acute pancreatitis pts), no antibiotics are warranted.
  - In severe cases, consider therapy based on mixed data (two double-blind RCTs, multiple meta-analyses of smaller trials).
    - RCT of 74 pts with acute necrotizing pancreatitis within 72 hr of admission; randomized to imipenem 500 mg IV q 8 hr for 14 days vs placebo; abx therapy was associated with a decreased risk of sepsis/SIRS (12% vs 30%, NNT 6) (Surg Gyn Ob 1993;176:480).
    - RCT of 114 pts with acute necrotizing pancreatitis (and CRP more than 150 mg/L); randomized to ciprofloxacin 400 mg IV q 12 hr and metronidazole 500 mg IV q 12 hr vs placebo (all pts were switched to abx if documented infection, sepsis, SIRS); no difference in mortality or development of pancreatic infection (GE 2004;126:997).

- Cochrane review of five studies (~300 pts) showed reduced mortality (6% vs 15%, NNT 11), mostly driven by studies of beta-lactam therapy (Cochrane 2006;CD002941).
- Meta-analysis of eight studies (~500 pts) showed no benefit to abx for mortality, pancreatic infection, or need for surgery, but reduced rates of nonpancreatic infections (22% vs 35%, NNT 7) (Am J Surg 2009;197:806).
- Bottom line is that evidence is mixed; in cases of severe pancreatitis, and especially associated with evidence of sepsis/SIRS, consider the use of broad-spectrum abx therapy (based on current evidence, probably carbapenems, piperacillin-tazobactam, and cefepime are best) for a limited time period (usually 14 days); directed therapy if able to get diagnostic cultures from pancreatic tissue or nonpancreatic infections.
- Surgical intervention (Pancreatology 2002;2:565) involves these considerations:
  - Mainly consists of debridement of necrotic tissue.
  - Individual pt and local practice will likely dictate need and timing of surgery, but early surgical intervention is not recommended (mortality up to 65%) and if possible delay up to 2 wk with supportive care only to allow for clearer delineation of necrotic vs viable tissue.

  Some specific therapy is based on cause, as follows:
- For gallstone pancreatitis, ERCP:
  - Early ERCP is suggested for known gallstones to allow for diagnosis and therapy (sphincterotomy and stone removal).
  - Cochrane review of three trials (more than 500 pts) showed reduction in cmplc associated w/ early ERCP in severe cases of pancreatitis; no mortality differences, no improvement in mild cases (Cochrane 2004;CD003630).

- Consider cholecystectomy; early in mild cases, delayed in severe cases.
- Specifically in alcohol-induced (but also consider in "idiopathic" cases), suggest abstinence from alcohol.
- For hypertriglyceridemia: Acute plasmapharesis in severe cases (Dig Dis Sci 2006;51:2287); low-fat diet; medical therapy with fibrates, niacin, possibly statins, fish oil (consider close f/u evaluation of liver enzymes because of concerns for hepatitis); consider family screenings.
- If consider med-related, discontinuation of offending agents.

Treatment of chronic pancreatitis

(GE 2007;132:1557)

- Alcohol and tobacco abstinence is crucial.
- Pain control: Often requires long-term therapy, starting with acetaminophen and NSAIDs (although both have significant risks, especially in long-term alcohol abusers); many require intermittent or daily dosing of opiates, with a high concurrence of opiate abuse; may be some role for nonopiate pain modulators (including gabapentin, carbamazepine, SSRIs).
- Address replacement of digestive enzymes.
  - Usually required in pts with evidence of exocrine insufficiency (weight loss, diarrhea).
  - Evidence does not support significant improvement in chronic pain (Am J Gastroenterol 1997;92:2032).
  - Dosing depends on form used, usually pancreatin or pancrelipase 1–3 tabs/capsules with each meal.
  - Will also need to put on H2B or PPI to prevent gastric breakdown of enzymes.
- Diabetes: In advanced disease, many pts have islet cell endocrine insufficiency causing Type 1 DM; usually requires insulin therapy (insulin secretion stimulators and sensitizers have no role), which is often difficult to dose because of frequent hypoglycemia (especially if ongoing alcohol abuse).

- Rx of cmplc takes the following approaches:
  - Serious exacerbations often require repeat imaging to r/o new pancreatic cmplc.
  - Pseudo-cysts (Dig Dis Sci 1989;34:343): Asx can often be observed; if sx, consider endoscopic or percutaneous drainage.
  - Many pts eventually require endoscopic or surgical intervention, but long-term outcomes are usually poor.

3.4 Infectious Diseases of the Gut

Diverticulitis

(NEJM 2007;357:2057; Lancet 2004;363:631)

Cause: Inflammation (and sometimes perforation) of colonic diverticulum.

Bacterial cause is usually gut anaerobes and Gram-negative organisms.

Epidem: More than 100,000 U.S. hospitalizations per year.

Risk increases with age (as with formation of diverticula; presence of diverticulosis in pts older than 80 yr is ~70%); 80% of diverticulitis occurs in pts older than 50 yr; older pts more likely require surgery with initial bout, younger pts have higher risk of recurrence and cmplc over lifetime (Surg 1994;115:546).

Risk of diverticulosis higher in the United States, likely due to lower fiber, higher carbohydrate and fat diets (JAMA 1974;229:1068); other risk factors include sedentary lifestyle, obesity, smoking, NSAID use.

Pathophys: Diet leads to higher bulk, lower water content stools, which increases intracolonic pressure and incidence of constipation; leads to formation of colonic diverticula (85% in the sigmoid and descending colon); infection occurs, likely due to obstruction of the diverticula and subsequent edema, bacterial overgrowth.

GASTROENTEROLOGY

Sx: Lower abdominal pain, usually LLQ; may have associated fever, N/V, diarrhea, rarely hematochezia.

Elderly may present with less localized pain or no pain at all (fever, altered mental status).

Severe case may have associated sepsis/SIRS.

Si: Abdominal tenderness on exam; rebound, guarding to suggest peritoneal inflammation; may have associated mass if abscess or significant inflammation.

Crs: Hinchey's criteria used for staging; stages 1 and 2 have defined abscess (small in stage 1, large in stage 2); stage 3 has perforation; stage 4 with fecal soilage of peritoneal cavity.

Mortality low (less than 5%) for nonperforated diverticulitis, increases with need for emergent surgery and medical comorbidities.

Recurrence rates:

- Retrospective study of 3165 pts with acute diverticulitis; 20% had emergency colectomy as initial management; 7% had elective colectomy (generally younger, healthy pts who required prior abscess drainage); the remaining 74% were followed for an average of 9 yr and 13% had a recurrent episode, generally associated with younger age and more comorbid disease (Arch Surg 2005;140:576).
- Recurrent disease is not associated with an increased risk for cmplc or mortality (Ann Surg 2006;243:876).

Cmplc: Abscess formation in ~20% (Dis Colon Rectum 1992;35: 1072); bowel obstruction due to abscess/inflammatory mass; perforation with peritonitis (although many perforations do not cause abdominal spillage, 1–2% have free perforation) (NEJM 2007;357:2057).

Fistula formation: Concern for fistulae is based on sx; can image with CT or barium enema (although avoid in acute setting).

- Colovesical: Large bowel to bladder; presents with pneumaturia, recurrent UTI.

- Colovaginal: Large bowel to vagina; presents with passage of stool or flatus from vagina, frequent vaginitis.
- Coloenteric: Large bowel to small bowel; may cause obstruction, but most asx.
- Colocutaneous: Large bowel through skin; usually associated with complicated infections after surgical intervention.

Lab: See abdominal pain discussion in Section 3.1 for initial lab w/u; leukocytosis is most common finding.

Noninv: Abdominal Xrays usually done to r/o cmplc (perforation, obstruction), but not diagnostic.

Contrast CT is the best imaging test: Commonly shows thickened colonic wall, "graying of the fat" from pericolonic adipose tissue inflammation; 97% sens, 100% specif (Br J Surg 1997;84:532); CT not required in mild cases (usually treated as outpatient), but most hospitalized pts should have CT to establish diagnosis and r/o cmplc; consider repeat imaging for abscess if no clinical improvement in 3 to 4 days with adequate therapy.

US can be used if CT not available or contraindicated (due to renal failure), but less sens and specif.

Direct inspection with sigmoidoscopy/colonoscopy:

- Usually avoided due to discomfort and risk of perforation.
- Consider in atypical cases, not responding to therapy, to r/o other causes (inflammatory bowel disease, ischemic colitis, C. *diff* colitis).
- Consider f/u outpatient colonoscopy for colon cancer screening (in small study, early colonoscopy had no increased complications vs 6-wk delay) (Endoscopy 2007;39:521).

Rx: Treatment for acute diverticulitis:

- Hospitalization should be based on ability to take oral meds and fluids, pain control, compliance and f/u, presence of cmplc or exacerbation of other comorbid diseases.
- Usually NPO or clear liquids only to start; advance diet w/ clinical improvement.

GASTROENTEROLOGY

- NG tube decompression is not required, unless concomitant ileus/obstruction.
- Rx may require IV rehydration and maintenance.
- Pain control usually requires opiate therapy.
- Antibiotic therapy is directed at gut microbes; usually empiric therapy unless Cx obtained from surgical or percutaneous abscess drainage.
  - Common IV regimens include fluoroquinolone and metronidazole; 3rd generation cephalosporin and metronidazole; ampicillin-sulbactam.
  - Usual duration of treatment is 10 to 14 days, although shorter courses could be used in pts w/ rapid clinical improvement.
- Most small abscesses (less than 4 cm) do not require any invasive therapy; for larger abscesses, consider percutaneous CT-guided aspiration or surgery (Dis Colon Rectum 1992;35:1072).

  Surgical intervention for diverticulitis:

- Emergent surgery for acute disease is warranted if severe sepsis unresponsive to standard therapies, peritonitis and uncontained perforation, abscess not able to be percutaneously drained.
- 3-stage procedure (removal of inflamed colon with proximal diverting ostomy, reanastomosis of bowel, colostomy takedown) is no longer performed, except in severe cases, due to higher morbidity and mortality (Br J Surg 1997;84:380); single-stage (removal of bowel segment and primary anastomosis) or 2-stage procedure (removal of bowel with end colostomy, ostomy takedown and reanastomosis) preferred (Dis Colon Rectum 2006;49:966).
- Laparascopic surgery now used in many centers, especially for stage 1 and 2 disease.
- For recurrent disease, decision for elective partial colectomy is based on pt's age, comorbid diseases, and pt wishes.

Dietary recommendations after diverticulitis (J Fam Pract 2009;58:381):

- Traditional teaching has been to counsel pts on high-fiber diet w/ decreased intake of seeds, nuts, etc., which may lead to diverticular obstruction.
  - Only one small study (18 pts) has evaluated high-fiber diet in pts with symptomatic diverticulosis, but did show positive effect (Lancet 1977;1:664).
  - Large cohort study of male health professionals revealed intake of nuts, corn, and popcorn actually associated with reduced risk (OR 0.7–0.8) for diverticulitis (JAMA 2008;300:907); counseling pts to avoid these foods may actually lead to reduced intake of high-fiber foods and be harmful.
- Agents to treat constipation may also be effective (e.g., lactulose) (Br J Clin Pract 1990;44:314).

Appendicitis

(NEJM 2003;348:236; BMJ 2006;333:530)

Cause: Inflammation (and sometimes perforation) of the cecal appendix.

Epidem: 250,000 appendectomies per yr in the United States; most common in young pts (younger than 25 yr), but also a separate incidence spike in the elderly.

Pathophys: Obstruction of the appendiceal lumen (usually from lymphoid hyperplasia, but can also be fecal material, tumor, inflammation from Crohn's disease, *Ascaris*) leads to local edema and bacterial overgrowth, subsequently causing inflammation and infection.

Sx: Typically pain begins in the epigastrium, migrates to RLQ over time (classically, McBurney's point two-thirds of the way from the umbilicus to the anterior superior iliac spine); associated anorexia, N/V (typically after pain begins); fever and sepsis/SIRS are seen in some cases (JAMA 1996;276:1589).

In elderly pts, pain may be more diffuse, less localized, or may present without significant pain (fever, altered mental status).

Si: Abdominal exam for rebound tenderness, guarding; rectal exam may also show tenderness.

Classic signs of appendicitis include the following (none are specific or sensitive enough to diagnose appendicitis alone) (Am Fam Phys 1999;60:2027):

- Psoas sign: pain in the RLQ with extension of the right leg with pt lying in left lateral decubitus position
- Obturator sign: pain in the RLQ with internal rotation of the right leg with leg flexed at the hip and knee
- Rovsing's sign: pain in the RLQ with palpation of the LLQ
- Dunphy's sign: pain in the RLQ with coughing

Crs: Mortality rate is less than 1%; higher with delay in dx, perforation, elderly, other comorbid diseases.

Cmplc: Abscess formation, perforation (higher rates with delay in seeking care and diagnosis); post-op wound infection.

Lab: See the discussion of abdominal pain in Section 3.1 for initial lab w/u; typically have leukocytosis; make sure to get urine or serum beta-HCG in women of child-bearing age to r/o ectopic pregnancy; U/A often performed but usually to r/o other causes of pain (nephrolithiasis, UTI).

Noninv: Routine imaging has become more common in w/u of suspected appendicitis; for some time, considered a clinical dx based on history, exam, and, if needed, observation; now, CT (with oral and IV contrast) and/or US more frequently performed as part of initial w/u.

- Study of 100 pts with suspected appendicitis, with planned admission for appendectomy or observation; all pts received CT scan prior to admission; 53% of pts had final dx of appendicitis; CT had 98% sens, specif, PPV, NPV for dx of appendicitis;

59% of pts had a change in mgt due to CT results, including alternative dx by CT (11%), taken directly for appendectomy rather than delay with observation (21%), prevented appendectomy (13%), and prevented admission (18%); overall, there was a cost savings of about $500 per case associated with routine use of CT (NEJM 1998;338:141).

- Another review of CT in 650 pts with suspected appendicitis showed high specif (98%), sens (97%), and accuracy (98%), and a high rate of alternative dx seen on CT (66%) (Am J Roentgenol 2002;178:1319).

US is an alternative to CT, with accuracy of 90–94% and PPV of 89–93% (NEJM 2003;348:236), but main limitation is ability to actually visualize the appendix; used in some settings because of availability in ER; also suggested to reduce radiation risks, evaluate RLQ pain in children and women who may be pregnant.

Head-to-head studies of CT vs US have shown CT to be superior in evaluation of appendicitis (Radiol 1994;190:31; Eur J Surg 2000;166:315) and in review of 26 studies (Ann IM 2004;141:537).

Despite widespread use, one study suggested that routine imaging did not affect rates of "negative appendectomy," possibly due to false positive imaging in clinical practice, with rates as high as 20% for pts with CT or US (similar to prior population studies of 20% negative appendectomy rates based on clinical diagnosis alone) (J Am Coll Surg 2005;201:933).

Rx: Rx of pts with suspected appendicitis follows these guidelines:

- Provide supportive care; NPO for surgery; IVF for rehydration and maintenance; pain control.
- Consider perioperative broad-spectrum abx in all pts; Cochrane review of 45 studies involving more than 9,000 pts showed reduced rates of abscess formation and wound infection (Cochrane 2005;CD001439).

- Surgical appendectomy is the mainstay of rx and should be done asap once dx is made; depending on local practice, laparoscopic and mini-laparotomy approaches may be used; Cochrane review of 54 studies showed reduced LOS and time away from work associated with laparoscopy, also reduced wound infections but increased risk of abscess formation (Cochrane 2004;CD001546).

3.5 Intestinal Obstruction and Pseudo-Obstruction

(Med Clin N Am 2008;92:649; Med Clin N Am 2008;92:575)

Cause: Definitions:
- Ileus (aka paralytic ileus): Functional slowing of the GI tract due to impaired peristalsis.
- Colonic pseudo-obstruction (aka Ogilvie's syndrome): Ileus and massive dilation of the colon.
- Obstruction: Blockage of the large bowel (LBO) or small bowel (SBO), because of internal narrowing or obstruction or external compression; may be noted as partial (pt still has passage of bowel contents through the obstruction) or complete.

See **Table 3.1** for an overview of the common causes of intestinal obstruction.

Epidem: 75% of SBO is from post-op adhesions (complicates ~5% of abdominal surgeries).

Colonic pseudo-obstruction more frequent in males, elderly, and obese pts.

Pathophys: Ileus: Direct effects of trauma (surgery), illness, metabolic disturbance, or drugs; leads to inflammatory response in the gut, inhibiting bowel peristalsis; stress-related release of corticotropin-releasing factor (CRF) may also play a role (J Clin Invest 2007; 117:33).

Table 3.1   Common Causes of Ileus and Obstruction

	Upper GI Tract	Small Bowel	Large Bowel
Ileus	Postoperative Gastroenteritis Diabetic gastroparesis	Postoperative (usually bowel surgery) Meds: opiates, CCBs, anticholinergics (inc. antihistamines, TCAs) Electrolyte abnormalities: hypoMg, hyperK, hypoK, hypoNa, hypoCa, hyperCa Renal failure Other severe illnesses: infections, sepsis, DKA Gastroenteritis	Postoperative (usually bowel surgery) Meds: opiates, CCBs, anticholinergics (inc. antihistamines, TCAs) Electrolyte abnormalities: hypoMg, hyperMg, hypoK, hypoNa, hypoCa, hyperCa Renal failure Myxedema Other severe illnesses: infections, sepsis, DKA
Obstruction	Esophageal: • Foreign body (food) • Cancer • Inflammation (from esophagitis) • Hiatal hernia Gastric: • Pyloric stenosis • Foreign body (food) • Cancer • Inflammation (from gastritis or large ulcer) • Gastric volvulus	Adhesions, usually postoperative Hernias Cancer (primary small bowel rare; usually extrinsic compression from extensive intra-abdominal tumor) Inflammation (from Crohn's) Gallstone "ileus" Foreign body Intussusception Parasites (*Ascaris*)	Cancer Sigmoid/colonic volvulus Adhesions, usually postoperative Severe constipation, impaction Abscess (usually with diverticulitis)

GASTROENTEROLOGY

Obstruction: Fluid accumulates in the bowel lumen, upstream from obstruction, leading to bacterial overgrowth and gas production; 3rd spacing of fluid causes dehydration; decreased intestinal motility due to muscle fatigue; eventually leads to venous congestion and reduced arterial flow causing bowel ischemia and necrosis.

Sx: All usually present with N/V, abdominal distention; pain, if present, is usually diffuse, and more common with obstruction than ileus (if pain persists with NG suction and decompression, need to consider intestinal ischemia and compromise).

Passage of stool and flatus is important to determine complete or partial SBO vs ileus (although may have some continued loose watery stools from intestinal fluid leakage downstream from complete obstruction).

Feculent vomiting suggests large bowel obstruction.

Si: Bowel sounds may be helpful to distinguish ileus from obstruction: ileus typically has lack of (or decreased) bowel sounds; obstruction usually has hyperactive (rushing, tinkling) sounds.

Depending on severity and concomitant illness, may show signs of dehydration, sepsis/SIRS.

Crs: Postoperative ileus usually resolves quickest in upper GI and small bowel surgery; small bowel peristalsis recovers first, then gastric, then colonic (usually 2 to 3 days post-op) (Am J Physiol 1995;269:G408).

Mortality rates depend on underlying illness; post-op ileus and adhesive SBO have very low mortality (less than 1%), but mortality increases with complications (especially intestinal necrosis) or underlying cancer and other diseases.

Cmplc: Internal strangulation and bowel necrosis (aka "closed loop obstruction") can occur; also intestinal perforation and peritonitis.

SBO from adhesions has a 15% risk of recurrence within 5 yr after initial surgery (lysis of adhesions), but can occur up to 30 yr later (Med Clin N Am 2008;92:575).

Lab: See discussion of abdominal pain in Section 3.1 for initial lab w/u; check for electrolyte disturbances with calcium, magnesium, phosphorus levels; leukocytosis may suggest infection, but may also be leukemoid reaction from stress (if marked leukocytosis, more than 20K, consider C. *diff* colitis with toxic megacolon).

In ill-appearing pts, consider ABG and lactate levels to assess for metabolic acidosis from intestinal ischemia.

Noninv: (Radiol Clin N Am 2003;41:263)

AXR is the first step in imaging:

- Assess for dilated loops of bowel, air-fluid levels; r/o intestinal perforation (with free air under diaphragm).
- May be the primary diagnostic study in 50–60% of pts (South Med J 1976;69:733; Am J Roentgenol 1996;167:1451), but overall sens for SBO is limited (66%) (Am J Gastroenterol 1991;86:175).
- Definite SBO has dilated loops of small bowel with air-fluid levels and no evidence of colonic gas (suggesting decompressed bowel postobstruction); probable SBO has similar findings, but some evidence of colonic gas.
- In LBO and pseudo-obstruction, will have massive colonic distension (bowel lumen 8–12 cm in diameter) with air-fluid levels.
- In some cases, a diagnosis of complete SBO or LBO may be made with hx, physical, and AXR alone, requiring surgical intervention without need for further imaging studies.

Additional imaging may be necessary to make or confirm dx, localize obstruction, or look for underlying disease processes (cancer, IBD).

- CT scan:
  - CT is now the most utilized test in possible SBO/LBO; oral and IV contrast preferred, but can be helpful even if oral contrast cannot be given; can be done quickly and easily in all centers.

- Has high specif (93%) and sens (92%) for complete obstruction (J Gastrointest Surg 2005;9:690) and is best test to evaluate for possible strangulation and intestinal necrosis.
- Also has benefit of detecting underlying disease (e.g., cancer or IBD) or alternative diagnoses.
- Upper GI study with small bowel follow-through (SBFT):
  - Performed with barium or gastrograffin (while barium provides better imaging results, concern for barium chemical peritonitis if pt requires bowel surgery; gastrograffin is water soluble, can cause aspiration pneumonitis so usually give via NGT); pt given contrast orally or by NGT and then followed with serial radiography to assess intestinal transit time and look for evidence and level of blockage.
  - Often used in evaluation of pts with ileus or partial SBO; not appropriate for critically ill pts or if high likelihood of complete obstruction; study often takes 1 to 2 days due to slowed peristalsis.
  - Meta-analysis of six studies of gastrograffin SBFT in presumed adhesive SBO pts showed that passage of contrast to the large bowel had high specif (96%) and sens (97%) for resolution of obstruction; use of test did not decrease the need for eventual surgery (i.e., not therapeutic, as believed by some), but did reduce hospital LOS by 1.8 days (Br J Surg 2007;94:404).
- Contrast barium enema: Appropriate in pts with possible LBO to evaluate for colonic obstruction, but carries a small risk (1%) of perforation (Dis Colon Rectum 1986;29:203).
  - Gastrograffin preferred to barium in this setting because of risk of chemical peritonitis and barium-induced obstruction and obstipation.
- Other possible studies:
  - Abdominal US rarely used, probably better than plain films, but not as good as other studies; reserve for bedside eval or in pts unable to have contrast studies.

- Enteroclysis: Direct injection of contrast into small bowel from longer nasoenteral tube; requires skilled interventional radiologist.
- MRI also may be helpful, but not available for rapid assessment in many centers.

Rx: Treating intestinal obstruction can follow general procedures, as well as specific rx in some cases.

General measures for rx of intestinal ileus and obstruction

- Proper dx based on risk factors, hx, examination, and clinical imaging is key to decisions of management.
- Consider early consultation with radiology, surgery, and gastroenterology.
- Conservative therapy generally warranted for ileus (and initially for uncomplicated partial SBO).
  - NPO with bowel rest; IVF for rehydration and maintenance (many pts are volume depleted due to poor oral intake, GI fluid losses, and 3rd spacing of fluid in the bowel).
  - Consider GI stress ulcer prophylaxis depending on suspected length of NPO status and severity of illness.
  - Pain and nausea control, but consider avoiding high doses of opiates, which may worsen ileus; consider NSAIDs or APAP as appropriate; epidural analgesia may also help (Cochrane 4:CD001893).
  - Discontinue offending drugs and fix metabolic disturbances, if able.
  - NG tube suction in pts with intractable vomiting and/or severe bowel distention.
- In pts with complete obstruction, associated peritonitis and perforation, or failure to respond to conservative therapy in known partial obstruction (~10–15%), surgical evaluation and laparotomy are necessary; delaying surgery in these pts leads to increased mortality (Ann Surg 2000;231:529).

- In pts with cancer-associated obstruction, steroids may help reduce sx, but no effect on mortality (Cochrane 2:CD001219).

Specific therapies for postoperative ileus

- Motility agents are often used, but clinical evidence of benefit is lacking.
  - Metoclopramide (Reglan) has been evaluated in multiple studies, with no evidence of quicker resolution of ileus (although may help post-op N/V) (Dis Colon Rectum 1991;34:437; Ann Surg 1979;190:27; Br J Surg 1986;73:290).
  - Cisapride was shown effective when given IV, but removed from the U.S. market due to cardiotoxic effects.
  - Erythromycin also stimulates gut motility, but no evidence of clinical benefit post-op (Am J Gastroenterol 1993;88:208; Urol 2007;69:611; Dis Colon Rectum 2000;43:333).
  - Addition of oral or rectal bowel stimulants (e.g., Milk of Magnesia, Fleet's Phospho-soda, bisacodyl supp) (Gynecol Oncol 1999;73:412) may reduce ileus in posthysterectomy pts (Am J Ob Gyn 2000;182:996; Am J Ob Gyn 2007;196:311 e1), but not tested or used following bowel surgery.
  - Methylnaltrexone (mu-receptor antagonist) has been proven effective in opiate-induced constipation (NEJM 2008;358:2332), but no evidence yet for opiate-related ileus (Lancet 2009;373:1198).
- Nutrition options include the following:
  - In pts unable to resume oral intake within 3 to 5 days, consider nutritional supplementation.
  - Enteral feedings may be appropriate, if tolerated; small study (30 pts) of immediate post-op introduction of enteral feeding showed improved metabolic results and fewer

post-op complications (BMJ 1996;312:869), but no larger studies to confirm.

- TPN and PPN can also be considered.
- Gum-chewing may promote intestinal motility.
  - Meta-analysis of nine trials (437 pts) in elective post-op bowel surgery; pts showed reduced time to flatus (14 hr), first bowel movement (23 hr), and hospital LOS (1 d) (Int J Surg 2009;7:100).

Therapy for colonic pseudo-obstruction (Ogilvie's syndrome)

- Supportive rx as for SBO; most cases resolve spontaneously within 3 to 4 days with conservative mgt only.
- Consider rectal tube; however, limited efficacy and pt discomfort.
- "Log-rolling" pt (change in position by 90°) on set time intervals may be helpful.
- Rectal stimulants (bisacodyl supps) often used but no clinical evidence to support efficacy; avoid oral laxatives due to impaired peristalsis; avoid large volume enemas due to risk of perforation.
- Neostigmine rx is the preferred option in pts not responsive to conservative rx.
  - RCT of 21 pts with Ogilvie's; randomized to neostigmine 2 mg IV vs placebo; rx led to prompt colonic decompression (91% vs 0%, NNT 1) within a median time to resolution of 4 min (NEJM 1999;341:137).
  - RCT of 30 critically ill, ventilated pts with Ogilvie's; randomized to neostigmine infusion (0.4–0.8 mg/hr) over 24 hr vs placebo; rx led to colonic decompression (84% vs 0%, NNT 1) (Intensive Care Med 2001;27:822).
  - Bradycardia and bronchospasm are most concerning side effects; avoid if pt already has bradycardia or active reactive airway disorder (RAD), pregnancy, renal failure; pt should have telemetry monitoring for therapy; if significant bradycardia, rx with atropine.

- Colonoscopic decompression is warranted for pts unresponsive or not able to tolerate neostigmine rx; may require multiple colonoscopies.
- After successful decompression (by conservative, medical, or colonoscopic rx), consider daily polyethylene glycol (PEG) to reduce relapse.
  - RCT of 30 pts s/p colonic decompression of Ogilvie's (83% following neostigmine, 26% postcolonoscopy); randomized to PEG 30gm PO qd vs placebo; rx reduced rate of relapse at 7 days (0% vs 33%, NNT 3) (Gut 2006;55:638).

3.6 Intestinal Ischemia

(Arch IM 2004;164:1054; Surg Clin N Am 2007;87:1115)

Cause: Reduced blood flow to gut tissue, leading to ischemia, inflammation, and necrosis.

Categories of disease include the following:

- Acute mesenteric ischemia due to intravascular causes.
  - Arterial embolism (40–50% of acute cases): Blockage of arterial supply from upstream embolism, usually cardiac (related to AF, valvular disease, cardiomyopathy); many pts have prior hx of other vascular embolic events; small bowel most likely affected due to oblique angle of SMA off the descending aorta, leading to easier flow of emboli to mid-gut arterial supply.
  - Arterial thrombosis (25–30%): Due to rupture of chronic atherosclerotic arterial plaques in the vessel wall; most commonly seen in the proximal SMA; usually seen in pts with other vascular disease (prior MI, stroke, PVD) and may have sx consistent with chronic mesenteric ischemia.
  - Nonocclusive mesenteric ischemia (NOMI) (20%): Also called "shock bowel," usually seen in critical illness with hypotension and low-flow states leading to bowel ischemia

in the absence of underlying atherosclerotic disease; has also been noted with use of cocaine, digoxin, beta-blockers, and alpha-agonist vasopressors; may be the most difficult to recognize and diagnose because of comorbid diseases; consider in critically ill pt with abdominal distension, persistent metabolic acidosis, peritoneal signs.

- Mesenteric venous thrombosis (10%): Segmental venous thrombosis of the gut blood supply; usually related to underlying hypercoagulability (described with Factor V Leiden deficiency, protein C and S deficiency, antithrombin III deficiency, and polycythemia vera) (Med Clin N Am 2008;92:627).

- Acute mesenteric ischemia due to extravascular causes: "Closed-loop" obstructions due to incarcerated hernia, adhesions, volvulus (see Section 3.5).

- Chronic mesenteric ischemia: Progressive atherosclerosis of gut arterial supply leading to chronic sx (see below); usually presents and eval in the outpatient setting, unless admitted for chronic abd pain eval.

Epidem: Rare, only about 1 in every 1000 hospital admissions (Surg Clin N Am 2007;87:1115).

Higher incidence in women; median age 70 yr; usually concomitant cardiovascular disease.

Pathophys: Blood flow to the middle and lower GI tract:

- Superior mesenteric artery (SMA) provides gut blood flow to the small bowel (via jejunal, ileal, ileocolic arteries) and proximal large bowel (via right and middle colic arteries).

- Inferior mesenteric artery (IMA) provides flow to the distal large bowel and sigmoid (via the left colic, marginal, and sigmoid arteries).

- Internal iliac artery provides flow to the rectum.

- Splenic flexure of the colon and distal sigmoid are at high risk for injury with NOMI because they are watershed areas at the periphery of both sources of blood flow and most prone to reduced flow with hypotensive states.

Disruption or reduction in blood flow causes ischemia, initially in the mucosal layers, then subsequent edema, activation of inflammatory cascade, and subsequent tissue necrosis; severe cases eventually lead to sepsis/SIRS, multiorgan system failure.

Reperfusion injury associated with oxygen free radicals may also play a role (Crit Care Med 1993;21:1376).

Sx/Si: Most common sx of acute and chronic disease is abdominal pain, which is usually diffuse, crampy, postprandial; classic sign is pain out of proportion to exam findings; may lead to food avoidance (sitophobia), anorexia, and weight loss in chronic ischemia.

Possible associated N/V, diarrhea; may have occult GI bleeding or frank hematochezia and melena in acute cases; acute delirium often seen in elderly.

Auscultate abdomen for epigastric bruit, may be present in about 50% of cases (Surg Clin N Am 2007;87:1115).

Acute ischemia, especially embolic and thrombotic forms, usually presents with abrupt, severe sx; may have associated sepsis/SIRS; dehydration (from poor PO intake and 3rd spacing of fluids in the gut) is also seen frequently.

Crs: Acute ischemic events carry a very high mortality (up to 80%) related to multiple factors: age and comorbid disease of pts, severity of illness, difficulty with and delay to dx, limited rx options for severe disease.

Survival best when dx made within 24 hr of arrival (~50%), but drops to 20–30% with any further delay in dx.

Cmplc: Ileus/obstruction, perforation with peritonitis, GI bleeding

Lab: See abdominal pain discussion in Section 3.1 for initial lab w/u; in pts at risk for ischemic disease (elderly, h/o other vascular disease, classic sx), consider lactate and ABG (to look for anion gap metabolic acidosis) to evaluate for possible tissue necrosis/infarct; other labs are likely nonspecific (and may falsely lead to alternative dx), including elevated liver enzymes (AST/ALT), amylase, LDH, CPK; renal failure and associated hyperkalemia and hyperphosphatemia often seen.

Noninv: (Radiol Clin N Am 2007;45:593)

AXR usually done to look for evidence of cmplc (perforation, ileus), but may be normal in up to 33% of pts with acute disease (Am J Roentgenol 1990;154:99); look for thickened bowel wall ("thumbprinting"), air in the bowel wall (pneumatosis), air in the portal system (pneumobilia).

CT of the abdomen is the best and most utilized study in the acute setting; positive findings (including arterial or venous thrombosis, pneumatosis, pneumobilia, liver/splenic infarcts, lack of bowel wall enhancement) are very specific (92%), although not very sensitive (64%), so a negative CT in the setting of high clinical suspicion does not rule out disease (Radiol 1996;199:632); CT angiogram with contrast may provide best eval, but may not be available in acute setting or contraindicated due to concomitant renal failure.

Doppler US is utilized in eval of chronic ischemia, with accuracy of 96% for detection of SMA stenosis greater than 70% (J Vasc Surg 1993;17:79); however, has little to no value in acute cases, because difficult to get a good study in pt with acute pain and likely bowel inflammation, gas, ileus, etc.; also requires trained technician, as procedure is technically difficult to perform.

MRI (with angiography) may have some role in difficult cases, especially with chronic sx, but limited use in acute setting due to availability and timing.

Mesenteric angiography is the gold standard but not widely available in all centers.

Colonoscopy is often performed in subacute cases, as pts present with pain, diarrhea, hematochezia; may show inflammatory colitis consistent w/ ischemic changes, but does not allow for any visualization of the small bowel, which is more frequently affected.

GASTROENTEROLOGY

Rx: Key to effective rx is high suspicion for the dx in the proper population and facilitated w/u for dx; significant delays in dx and rx are associated with poor outcomes; only one-third of pts with mesenteric ischemia had correct dx prior to exploratory surgery or death (Eur J Surg 1999;165:203).

Overall, rx of disease is very institution-specific; given the overall rarity of disease and high mortality, there is a distinct lack of clinical trials to provide information re management; most recommendations are based on expert opinion only (Circ 2006;113:e463).

General measures for rx of intestinal ischemia are as follow:

- Treatment of acute ischemia usually requires ICU-level care.
- NPO; bowel rest; pain and nausea control.
- Aggressive IVF for rehydration and maintenance; due to significant fluid losses, critical illness, and frequency of comorbid heart disease, many require invasive monitoring with PA catheter for fluid mgt; crystalloids usually preferred, consider transfusions as necessary (and given acute ischemia, many target a goal Hgb more than 9–10 mg/dL).
- In pts with persistent hypotension despite IVF, vasopressors may be needed; dopamine preferred over norepinephrine and phenylephrine (due to vasospastic effect of alpha-agonist, which may potentiate ischemic disease); vasopressin has been suggested in anecdotal case of pt with NOMI (Anaesthesist 2006;55:283), but concern for vasospasm in arterial and thrombotic causes.
- Broad-spectrum abx targeted at gut microbes (e.g., carbapenems, cefepime, piperacillin-tazobactam) are often used in pts with evidence of sepsis/SIRS, as there is high rate of gut translocation of microbes in the setting of ischemia and necrosis.
- Unless plans for emergent surgery, consider IV unfractionated heparin to stabilize and prevent propagation of arterial (in embolic and thrombotic cases) or venous clot; contraindicated

if associated active GI bleeding or other significant coagulopathy; specifically in cases of mesenteric venous thrombosis,
heparin and long-term anticoagulation w/ warfarin is the
primary therapy (J Vasc Surg 1994;20:688).

- Glucagon (J Vasc Surg 1995;21:900) and papaverine infusions
(especially in NOMI) have shown promise in nonhuman
studies, but no human clinical evidence to support widespread
use.

Specific therapies include the following:

- Urgent surgical eval is warranted in all acute cases; if any
evidence of infarcted bowel, emergency laparotomy is usually
undertaken for bowel resection (and may require multiple
surgeries).
- Depending on the cause of ischemia, concurrent illness, and
local expertise, other available treatments can include direct
intra-arterial thrombolytics, surgical embolectomy, emergent
surgical revascularization.
- Rx of NOMI usually related to control of underlying critical
illness, volume control and pressors to alleviate hypotension
and low perfusion, surgical intervention if evidence of bowel
infarct.
- Given the severity of illness and lack of proven specific therapies, many pts receive comfort care only (with pain and sx
control), especially elderly pts with multiple comorbidities.

3.7   Liver Disease and Complications

Alcoholic Liver Disease (Including Hepatitis and Cirrhosis)

(NEJM 2004;350:1646; Med Clin N Am 2009;93:787)

Cause: Alcohol is the cause of most acute and chronic liver disease
in the United States, including acute alcoholic hepatitis and
alcoholic cirrhosis.

Alcohol accounts for about 80% of U.S. cases of cirrhosis; other causes of cirrhosis include the following:

- Chronic viral hepatitis: Mainly hepatitis B and C; A and E are self-limited acute diseases; D is only seen as co-infection with B.
- Nonalcoholic fatty liver disease (NAFLD), aka nonalcoholic steatohepatitis (NASH): An emerging cause of cirrhosis in the United States with obesity epidemic.
- Autoimmune hepatitis: Affects pts of any age; dx based on presence of auto-antibodies and ruling out other causes (NEJM 2006;354:54).
- Primary biliary cirrhosis (PBC): Occurs mostly in young women; associated with pruritus and arthritis, elevated serum alk phos (NEJM 2005;353:1261).
- Primary sclerosing cholangitis (PSC): More common in young men; similar to PBC with fatigue, pruritus, elevated alk phos (NEJM 1995;332:924).
- Alpha-1 antitrypsin deficiency: Rare genetic disorder with early-onset liver disease and COPD (Lancet 2005;365:2225).
- Wilson's disease: Rare genetic disorder that leads to copper overload, with progressive liver failure and neurologic sequelae (Hepatol 2008;47:2089).
- Hereditary hemochromatosis (HH): Genetic disorder that leads to iron overload, with liver failure, diabetes, arthritis, cardiomyopathy (Hepatol 2001;33:1321, NEJM 1993;328:1616).
- Others: Vitamin A intoxication (GE 1991;100:1701), drugs and poisons (methotrexate, amiodarone, carbon tetrachloride), infections (intestinal schistosomiasis, syphilis).

Epidem: Cirrhosis accounts for 25,000 deaths and more than 300,000 hospitalizations per year in the United States; more common in males.

Pathophys: Inflammation and subsequent fibrosis of liver tissue, causing increased venous pressures (portal hypertension); leads to collateralization of blood flow to the systemic circulation; subsequent drop in arterial flow leads to activation of RAA system, with arterial vasoconstriction, fluid and sodium retention; this further exacerbates fluid balance; increased venous pressures (varices, ascites) and loss of arterial pressures (hypotension, renal failure) cause many of the cmplc.

Good review of pathophys of alcoholic hepatitis is in NEJM 2009;360:2758.

Sx: Early stages usually asx; may be recognized based on routine labs for liver function.

Initial sx may be constitutional: weight loss, weakness, anorexia, fatigue; most sx develop with decompensation and cmplc.

Si: Liver may be enlarged (hepatomegaly) or small, depending on stage of disease.

Signs based on presumed cause include:

- Elevated bilirubin: jaundice and scleral icterus
- Portal hypertension: splenomegaly, ascites, "caput medusa" (prominent subcutaneous abdominal veins), Cruveilhier-Baumgarten syndrome (venous hum on abdominal auscultation due to portal vein to umbilical vein collateral flow) (JAMA 1982;248:831)
- Elevated estrogen levels: spider angiomas and telangiectasias, palmar erythema, gynecomastia, testicular atrophy
- Diminished clotting factors: bruising/ecchymoses, GI bleeding
- Portosystemic shunting: asterixis (see "Hepatic Encephalopathy" later in Section 3.7), fetor hepaticus (pungent breath) (Lancet 1994;343:483)

Crs: Six-month mortality of acute alcoholic hepatitis is about 40% (NEJM 2009;360:2758).

Mortality in cirrhosis low in early stage (median survival from time of dx is 10–12 yr) (Hepatol 1987;7:122), but high when associated with cmplc (annual risk of progression to decompensated disease is 5–7%) (J Hepatol 2006;44:217); presence of ascites has 6-yr mortality of about 50% in compensated pts and about 80% in pts w/ cmplc (unless pt undergoes liver transplant) (Dig Dis Sci 1986;31:468).

Course of sx important in determination of dx; cirrhosis generally has indolent, slowly developing sx over long period of time; acute sx of jaundice, ascites suggest acute alcoholic hepatitis and/ or acute fulminant hepatitis from variety of causes.

Estimating severity of disease involves the following factors:

- Presence of hyponatremia: a predictor of poor prognosis (NEJM 2008;359:1018)
- Child-Pugh-Turcotte (CPT) classification (see **Table 3.2**):
  - Used to predict life expectancy (Hepatol 1987;7:660) and perioperative mortality for significant abdominal procedures (Br J Surg 1973;60:646)
- MELD score (Model for End-Stage Liver Disease) (Hepatol 2001;33:464):
  - Primary determinant for liver transplant; based on severity of liver and renal disease
  - $(11.2 \times \ln[\text{INR}]) + (9.57 \times \ln[\text{Cr}]) + (3.78 \times \ln[\text{Bilirubin}]) + 6.43$
  - Multiple online calculators available (www.unos.org/resources/MeldPeldCalculator.asp)
  - Range of scores: 6–40, w/ higher scores indicating increased severity of illness
- Maddrey's discriminant function:
  - Determinant of severity for acute alcoholic hepatitis, to determine need for steroids
  - $(4.6 \times [\text{PT}_{\text{patient}} - \text{PT}_{\text{control}}] + \text{Bilirubin})$
  - Consider steroids for severe hepatitis with score greater than 32 (GE 1978;75:193)

Cmplc: Evidence of severe acute liver disease or decompensated cirrhosis, as indicated by the following:

- Ascites (see "Ascites and Spontaneous Bacterial Peritonitis" later in Section 3.7 for details)

Table 3.2 Child-Pugh-Turcotte Classification for Cirrhosis

	Assign points based on clinical criteria		
	1	2	3
Encephalopathy	None	Controlled with meds	Poor control
Ascites	None	Controlled with meds	Poor control/resistant
Total bilirubin (mg/dL)	<2.0	2.0–3.0	>3.0
Serum albumin (gm/dL)	≥3.5	2.8–3.5	<2.8
INR	<1.7	1.7–2.2	>2.2

	Assign class (and prognosis) based on points		
	A (Mild)	B (Moderate)	C (Advanced)
Points	5–6	7–9	10–15
1-yr survival rates	100%	80%	45%
Perioperative mortality	10%	30%	80%

GASTROENTEROLOGY

- Spontaneous bacterial peritonitis (SBP) (see "Ascites and Spontaneous Bacterial Peritonitis" later in Section 3.7 for details)
- Esophageal and gastric varices with GI bleeding (see Section 3.2 for details)
- Hepatorenal syndrome (HRS) (see "Hepatorenal Syndrome" later in Section 3.7 for details)
- Hepatic encephalopathy (see "Hepatic Encephalopathy" later in Section 3.7 for details)

Lab: Initial labs usually include CBC with plt, metabolic panel, renal and liver function tests, PT/PTT.

Common lab findings include the following:

- Abnormal liver enzymes:
  - Especially AST/ALT with acute alcoholic hepatitis; adequate for screening, but no role in determining severity of disease; AST/ALT ratio of more than 2:1 suggests alcoholic liver disease (Dig Dis Sci 1979;24:835).
  - In cirrhotic pts, elevated bilirubin may be the most common finding.
- Thrombocytopenia (J Hepatol 2008;48:1000): Likely from multiple causes including splenic sequestration, peripheral destruction, and marrow suppression; plt less than 160K has a sens of 80% and specif of 58% for chronic liver disease; plt more than 260K has NPV of 91% (J Hepatol 1999;31:867).
- Associated renal failure can be from multiple causes (see "Hepatorenal Syndrome" later in Section 3.7).
- Low albumin and elevated PT are cardinal signs of reduced hepatic synthetic activity.

Once liver abnormalities are confirmed, consider eval of other hepatic comorbid diseases (Am Fam Phys 2006;74:756), as follows:

- Acetaminophen levels, if acute liver failure (but may be normal by the time liver failure develops)

- Screening for hepatitis B and C
- ANA, anti-smooth muscle ab, and immunoglobulin levels for autoimmune disease
- Alk phos and antimitochondrial ab for primary biliary cirrhosis
- Alk phos and antineutrophil cytoplasmic antibody (ANCA) for primary sclerosing cholangitis
- Fasting iron studies (iron/TIBC/ferritin), genetic testing for hemochromatosis
- Ceruloplasmin and copper levels for Wilson's disease
- Alpha-1-antitrypsin levels for deficiency

Noninv: Abdominal US is often the first test to eval for ascites (physical exam can be limited, especially in obese pts), liver appearance, portal and hepatic blood flow; high sens (91%) and specif (94%) for cirrhosis (Br J Radiol 1999;72:29).

CT imaging is not necessary, but can show liver nodularity, varices, ascites.

MRI most helpful in evaluating liver masses to r/o hepatocellular carcinoma and portal vein thrombosis (using MRA).

Liver biopsy is the gold standard confirmatory test for cirrhosis; decision for need based on certainty of dx from clinical situation and other testing, as well as likelihood of changing mgt (probably most helpful in settings of viral hepatitis).

Rx: Most management issues pertain to specific cmplc of cirrhosis, as covered later in Section 3.7 and in Section 3.2.

General treatment issues for cirrhosis include:

- Avoidance of alcohol immediately on dx and lifelong (GE 1981;80:1405); may require counseling and multiple interventions; no definitive medical therapies available.
- Interferon and antiviral therapy for active hepatitis B and C, if present.
- Consider vaccination for hepatitis A and B if no prior infection; acute disease carries more risk if underlying cirrhosis.

- Evaluation for transplant based on MELD scoring and complications.

  Treatment of acute alcoholic hepatitis requires the following additional steps:

- Supportive care: IV rehydration (avoid saline solutions and overhydration once initial deficits repleted)
- Nutritional support: thiamine, folate, MVI; may require enteral or parenteral feedings in severe cases
- Rx of alcohol withdrawal syndromes: usually within 48 to 72 hr of last ETOH ingestion; potential for tachycardia, hypertension, tremors, delirium, agitation; quantify sx w/ CIWA scoring
  - Benzodiazepines, usually lorazepam or diazepam, acutely
  - Beta-blockers and clonidine for tachycardia and hypertension
  - In severe cases, intubation and mechanical ventilation with IV lorazepam drip (or propofol)
- Corticosteroids:
  - Meta-analysis of 11 trials showed 33% reduction in mortality of alcoholic hepatitis associated with steroid rx, but effect limited to pts with hepatic encephalopathy (Ann IM 1990;113:299).
  - Meta-analysis of 15 trials (more than 500 pts) showed no mortality benefit, except for pts with hepatic encephalopathy or severe hepatitis (defined as Maddrey's score higher than 32) (Aliment Pharmacol Ther 2008;27:1167).
  - If used for pts w/ severe disease, common dosing is prednisolone 40 mg qd for up to 4 wk, but can discontinue after 7 d if not showing improvement (associated with poor prognosis); 40% of pts are unresponsive to steroids (NEJM 2009;360:2758).
- Pentoxifylline:
  - A phosphodiesterase inhibitor, is often used in pts w/ peripheral vascular disease.

- RCT of 101 pts with severe alcoholic hepatitis (Maddrey's score 32 or higher); randomized to pentoxifylline 400 mg tid vs placebo for 4 wk; rx reduced incidence of hepatorenal syndrome (50% vs 92%, NNT 2) and mortality (25% vs 46%, NNT 5) (GE 2000;119:1637).
- Cochrane review of five trials did not support the use of pentoxifylline based on lack of mortality benefit and possible adverse effects (Cochrane 2009;CD007339).
- No head-to-head studies of pentoxifylline vs steroids to determine best 1st-line therapy; most would use steroids based on preponderance of evidence; one study showed no benefit to switching to pentoxifylline in steroid nonresponders (J Hepatol 2008;48:465).
- Treatment of hepatitis-related complications as described in separate sections
- Liver transplantation: usually not an option in this population because of recent alcohol use, risk for relapse, and course of disease

Acute Liver Failure (Including Acetaminophen Overdose)

(Med Clin N Am 2008;92:761)

Cause: As determined by Acute Liver Failure Study Group (ALFSG), causes in 1033 consecutive pts with ALF across 23 sites (Ann IM 2002;137:947; Med Clin N Am 2008;92:761):

- Acetaminophen (APAP) overdose (46%):
  - Consider with any ingestion of more than 4 gm in 24 hr.
- Drug reaction (12%):
  - Many drugs have been implicated, including isoniazid, sulfa drugs, propylthiouracil, phenytoin, valproate (Liver Transpl 2004;10:1018); herbal medications, especially difficult with multiple herbal formulations and lack of FDA control over preparations; mushrooms (*Aminita phalloides*)
  - For a good review of drug-related liver disease, see NEJM 2006;354:731.

- Hepatitis A and B (10%)
- Autoimmune (5%)
- Ischemic (4%)
- Other causes (8%), including Wilson's disease, pregnancy-related, Budd-Chiari syndrome
- Idiopathic (15%)

Epidem: Fewer than 3,000 cases per year in the United States; much less common reason for hospitalization than cmplc of cirrhosis and acute hepatitis; about 60,000 cases of APAP overdose every year (Pharmacoepidemiol Drug Saf 2006;15:398).

Pathophys: APAP toxicity (NEJM 2008;359:285): With normal dosing, more than 90% of APAP is metabolized to glucuronide and sulfate forms; cytochrome P-450 enzymes convert some to N-acetyl-p-benzoquinone imine (NAPQI), which is toxic to the liver, but in normal circumstances is converted to nontoxic form with glutathione as a cofactor; with toxic doses, there is more NAPQI formed and liver quickly depletes its stores of glutathione, leading to hepatic cellular necrosis; treatment with acetylcysteine increases glutathione stores and reduces buildup of toxic NAPQI.

Sx: May be asx in early phase; then N/V, abd pain

Si: Jaundice

Crs: ALF has 33% 3-week mortality, 46% with spontaneous recovery and 25% with liver transplant (Ann IM 2002;137:947).

Cmplc: Complications are similar to chronic liver failure: ascites, encephalopathy, hepatorenal syndrome; high rates of concomitant bacterial and fungal infections.

Lab: Initial lab w/u usually include CBC with diff, metabolic panel, renal and liver function tests, PT/PTT; APAP, alcohol, and salicylate levels; urine or serum toxicology screen.

Hepatitis profile for acute infection: acute hep B infection diagnosed with positive hep B surface antigen (HBsAg) and anti-hep B core antibody (anti-HBcAb); acute hep A infection by anti-HAV antibody.

APAP levels may be low immediately after initial ingestion or if delayed presentation; typically check every 4–6 hr for 12–24 hr to best assess for treatment; use the Rumack-Matthew nomogram (**Figure 3.2**) to assess need for NAC treatment.

AST, ALT may be very elevated (10–400 times normal); more than 1000 IU/L typically suggests APAP overdose or ischemic cause of hepatitis.

Rx: Treatment of acute liver failure (and APAP overdose) includes the following:

- Initial therapy is supportive care; see discussion of cirrhosis earlier in Section 3.7 for details.
- Recognize and treat cmplc as detailed elsewhere in this chapter.
- Hypotension is common in ALF, requiring vasopressor therapy.
- Comorbid infections are common; low threshold for broad-spectrum abx.
- Coagulopathy is common; vit K and FFP often used (24% of cirrhotic pts discharged with vit K in one European study) (Eur J Clin Pharmacol 2002;58:435), but no data to support efficacy (Cochrane 2008;CD004792).
- Activated charcoal, gastric lavage, ipecac may all be considered for acute APAP overdose.
- NAC for APAP overdose (NEJM 2008;359:285):
  - Evidence for use:
    - Report (not RCT, compared to historical data) of more than 2,500 pts treated w/ oral NAC showed 6% risk of hepatotoxicity when given within 10 hr of ingestion, 26% when given within 10–24 hr; overall mortality was 0.4% (82% when liver enzymes up prior to NAC therapy, no deaths if NAC given within 16 hr of ingestion) (NEJM 1988;319:1557).

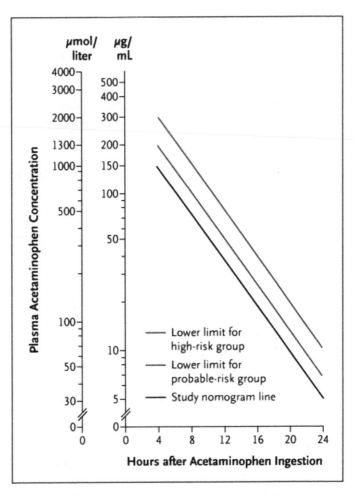

Figure 3.2 Rumack-Matthew Nomogram for Acetaminophen Ingestion
Reproduced with permission from Heard KJ. Acetylcysteine for
acetaminophen poisoning. *NEJM*. 2008;359:285. Copyright © 2008,
Massachusetts Medical Society. All rights reserved.

- For pts w/ presence of ALF on arrival: RCT of 50 pts w/ ALF from APAP overdose; randomized to IV NAC rx vs IV dextrose (placebo); NAC rx reduced mortality (52% vs 80%, NNT 4), as well as cerebral edema and pressor-requiring hypotension (BMJ 1991;303:1026).
- Cochrane review of evidence showed limited clinical data for NAC use, but based on available evidence, NAC is the best therapy to reduce mortality in APAP overdose (Cochrane 2006;CD003328).
- Who should receive NAC therapy?
  - Known acute APAP overdose of more than 4 gm, despite initial APAP levels, pending repeat APAP levels to allow risk stratification per nomogram
  - Elevated ALT with h/o APAP ingestion, despite timing of ingestion
  - Possibly effective for non-APAP-related acute liver failure?
    - RCT of 173 pts w/ non-APAP-related ALF; rx w/ IV NAC showed improved transplant-free survival in pts with grade I–II encephalopathy (no effect in III–IV) (52% vs 30%, NNT 5) (GE 2009;137:856).
- Oral regimen:
  - 140 mg/kg loading dose, then 70 mg/kg q 4 hr for 17 doses.
  - Adverse effects include N/V; may require NGT administration for persistent vomiting or uncooperative pt.
- IV regimen:
  - 150 mg/kg loading dose over 15–60 min, then 12.5 mg/kg/hr for 4 hr, then 6.25 mg/kg/hr for 16 hr.
  - May not be long enough in some pts; if persistently elevated ALT or measurable APAP levels after 20 hr of rx, consider continuing IV infusion.

GASTROENTEROLOGY

- Not FDA approved for use in the United States, but still used in most centers, especially in pts w/ evidence of liver disease.
- No head-to-head studies of efficacy of IV vs PO regimens.
- Adverse effects include N/V, flushing, angioedema, bronchospasm; if occurs, can hold infusion for 1 hr and rx with IV diphenhydramine, methylprednisolone, and/ or bronchodilators as needed; consider switch to PO if appropriate.

Ascites and Spontaneous Bacterial Peritonitis (SBP)

(NEJM 2004;350:1646; Clin Liver Dis 2001;5:833)

Cause: 75% of ascites due to cirrhosis; other causes include the following (BMJ 2001;322:416):

- Cardiac: CHF, constrictive pericarditis
- Vascular: IVC obstruction; Budd-Chiari syndrome (hepatic vein obstruction)
- Cancer: peritoneal carcinomatosis, ovarian, colorectal, lymphoma, other metastatic disease
- Hypoalbuminemia: critical illness, nephrotic syndrome; protein-losing enteropathies
- Other: pancreatitis, myxedema, Meigs syndrome (ovarian fibroma with ascites and pleural effusion), systemic lupus erythematosus (SLE)
- Pseudo-ascites from obesity, bowel ileus/obstruction, solid tumors, pregnancy, bladder distension (especially elderly men with BPH)

SBP is ascitic fluid infection without another obvious source of intra-abdominal infection or perforation; common organisms include *E. coli, Streptococcus sp.*

Epidem: SBP occurs in 10–30% of pts with ascites (J Hepatol 2000;32:142).

Pathophys: Ascites is result of fluid loss from one of the following:

1. Intestinal loss by splanchnic vasodilation (from portal HTN)
2. Hepatic loss from increased sinusoidal pressures

SBP is due to translocation of gut microbes through edematous bowel from portal hypertension.

Sx: Ascites: Predominant sx is increasing abdominal girth (may have associated pain, dyspnea).

SBP may be asx in many cases; fever, abdominal pain, sepsis/SIRS may be present, but consider in all cases of new or worsening ascites, encephalopathy, renal failure, or GI bleeding associated with cirrhosis.

Si: Flank and shifting dullness on abdominal exam; not very specific, but absence of flank dullness is 90% accurate to r/o ascites (JAMA 1982;247:1164).

Crs: In-hospital mortality associated with SBP is as high as 30%.

Cmplc: Ascites: Hepatic hydrothorax (recurrent pleural effusions); hyponatremia is common.

SBP is commonly complicated by hepatorenal syndrome in about 33% of cases (Hepatol 1994;20:1495).

Lab: All pts with new-onset, or abruptly worsening, ascites (especially if signs of sepsis, encephalopathy, or GI bleeding) should undergo paracentesis:

- Diagnostic:
  - Evaluate cause of ascites if not apparent.
    - Send fluid for cell count and diff, total protein and albumin, culture (Gram stain has low yield) (GE 1988;95:1351).
    - In specific cases, can also send for cytology (low yield, unless high concern for neoplasm) (Hepatol 1988;8:1104), AFB stain and culture (tuberculosis), amylase (pancreatitis); if bloody ascites, consider trauma or hepatocellular carcinoma.

- Serum-ascites albumin gradient (SAAG) helpful to determine cause.
  - (Serum albumin – Ascites albumin); if more than 1.1 gm/dL, most likely cause is portal hypertension (97% accuracy) (Ann IM 1992;117:215).
- Rule out spontaneous bacterial peritonitis (SBP).
  - There is concern for SBP with fluid WBC more than 250 cells/mm^3.
  - Start empiric abx while waiting for confirmatory Cx.
- Therapeutic: See discussion of large-volume paracentesis (LVP) under Rx below.
- Main risks of procedure are bleeding (although usually does not require vit K or FFP prior to procedure), infection, and perforation (reduced by use of US guidance) (Arch IM 1986;146:2259).

Noninv: US to eval for amount of ascites and assist with paracentesis.

If concern for acute peritonitis, may require AXR (looking for pneumoperitoneum) or CT.

Rx: Treatment of ascites:

- Reduce sodium intake: 1500–2000 mg Na qd.
- Fluid restriction: 1000 mL qd, in pts w/ dilutional hyponatremia (less than 130 mEq/L), unless concomitant hypovolemia and hypotension (aggressive initial fluid resuscitation for sepsis/shock states); if maintenance IVF required, avoid isotonic solutions (0.9% NS, LR) as high sodium concentrations will exacerbate fluid overload.
- Diuretic therapy:
  - Spironolactone is most effective; start at 100 mg qd (or 50 mg bid) and titrate up to 400 mg qd max; main side effect is hyperkalemia, which can be reduced by addition of furosemide.
  - Furosemide is also effective, but avoid as monotherapy because of risk of precipitating renal failure and hypokalemia

(J Clin Gastroenterol 1981;3 Suppl 1:73); start at 20–40 mg qd and titrate up based on response, trying to keep ratio of 100 mg spironolactone to 40 mg furosemide, to balance potassium response.

- Goal weight loss initially is 1 kg qd; in hospitalized pts, PO diuretics still preferred, but can use IV if needed.
- If initial response not adequate, measure urine sodium; if remains low, increase diuretics or consider paracentesis.
- Main side effects of diuretic therapy are renal failure (avoid with Cr more than 2.0 mg/dL, usually resolves with discontinuation and IV fluids), hyponatremia, and potassium abnormalities.
- Avoid NSAID use because attenuates natriuretic effect and increases risk for renal failure.

- Large-volume paracentesis (LVP):
  - A therapeutic procedure to remove large volumes of ascitic fluid, sometimes up to 10 L.
  - LVP is associated with better outcomes than diuresis in tense ascites.
    - RCT of 117 pts with cirrhosis and tense ascites; randomized to dual diuretic therapy vs daily LVP and albumin infusion; LVP/albumin was associated with more resolution of ascites (73% vs 97%, NNT 4) and fewer complications including encephalopathy, renal failure, and electrolyte disturbances (61% vs 17%, NNT 2) and reduced hospital LOS (GE 1987;93:234).
  - With LVP of more than 5 L, IV albumin should be given to reduce circulatory dysfunction and renal failure.
    - Give IV albumin 6–8 gm per L of fluid removed.
    - RCT of 105 pts with cirrhosis and ascites; randomized to LVP (4–6 L qd) with and without albumin (40 gm IV after the procedure); albumin infusion was associated with less renal dysfunction or hyponatremia (21% vs 2%, NNT 5) (GE 1988;94:1493).

- Albumin is preferred over crystalloid solutions or other plasma expanders (dextran, polygeline) (GE 1996;111:1002).
- Start diuretics once LVP has achieved resolution of ascites, as long as renal failure is not present.
- Rx for refractory ascites (ascites unresolved with chronic high-dose diuretics or associated with side effects of therapy, including renal failure, encephalopathy, hyperkalemia, hyponatremia):
  - LVP with albumin infusion is the preferred therapy.
  - Placement of a percutaneous or peritoneovenous shunt can be considered, but is associated with cmplc, including blockage (NEJM 1991;325:829); usually reserved for palliative care circumstances.
  - Transjugular intrahepatic portosystemic shunt (TIPS) procedure:
    - Consists of intravascular placement of a metal shunt from hepatic vein to the portal vein through the liver tissue to reduce portal hypertension.
    - Although multiple studies have shown reduced ascites, data about survival benefit are mixed; one study showed improved survival with TIPS vs repeat LVP for refractory ascites (NEJM 2000;342:1701), but two subsequent studies did not corroborate that finding (GE 2002;123:1839; GE 2003;124:634).

  Treatment of SBP:

- Most important first step is high degree of suspicion for SBP in cirrhotic pts w/ new-onset or worsening ascites, encephalopathy, renal failure, or acute variceal bleeding; administering early paracentesis and empiric abx is key to survival.
- Antibiotics:
  - Cefotaxime 2 gm IV q 12 hr or ceftriaxone 1 gm IV q 24 hr are the most common choices.

- Other broad-spectrum agents (carbapenems, piperacillin-tazobactam, ampicillin-sulbactam) are also acceptable; avoid aminoglycosides due to nephrotoxicity (GE 1998;114:612).
- If pt stabilizes, can switch to preventive doses of oral norfloxacin (400 mg PO qd) in 3 to 5 days.
- Due to high rate of recurrence, antibiotic prophylaxis for SBP is warranted in the following pts:
  - Prior episode of SBP (long-term)
    - 40–70% risk of recurrence (Hepatol 1988;8:27).
    - RCT of norfloxacin prophylaxis vs placebo in 80 cirrhotic pts w/ prior SBP reduced 1-yr recurrence of SBP (20% vs 68%, NNT 2); recurrent SBP in pts on abx less likely to be typical gut Gram-negative rods (Hepatol 1990;12:716).
  - Cirrhotic pts w/ prior variceal bleeding (regardless of presence of ascites)
    - Administer norfloxacin 400 mg PO (or NGT) bid for at least 7 days.
    - 1999 meta-analysis of five trials (534 pts) w/ GI bleeding and cirrhosis given prophylaxis for SBP showed reduced rates of infection, SBP, and improved survival (Hepatol 1999;29:1655).
  - Consider in pts w/ low-protein ascites (less than 1 gm/dL), high bilirubin (more than 2.5 mg/dL) and low platelets (less than 98K), as they have high risk for SBP (55% at 1 yr) (GE 1999;117:414), but no RCTs to show benefit of prophylaxis yet.
- Albumin infusion:
  - Administer IV albumin 1.5 mg/kg on admission or at time of paracentesis, then 1 mg/kg 48 hr later.
  - RCT of 126 pts with ascites and SBP; randomized to abx plus IV albumin vs abx alone; addition of albumin associated w/ reduced renal failure (10% vs 33%, NNT 4)

and reduced in-hospital (10% vs 29%, NNT 5) and 3-mo
mortality (22% vs 41%, NNT 5) (NEJM 1999;341:403).

- Avoid aggressive treatment of ascites (repeated LVP, high-dose diuretics) in initial phase to avoid hepatorenal syndrome.

Hepatic Encephalopathy

(NEJM 1997;337:473)

Cause: Related to acute or chronic liver failure.

Common precipitants of HE include the following:

- Meds/dietary: benzodiazepines, barbiturates, other CNS depressants; high-protein diet
- Metabolic: acute renal failure, hypokalemia, hyponatremia, metabolic or respiratory alkalosis
- Concomitant illnesses: dehydration, constipation, GI bleeding, anemia, infection, hypoxemia
- Iatrogenic: TIPS or surgical portosystemic shunting

Epidem: Encephalopathy, to some degree, may be present in up to 70% of cirrhotics, but many may be asx except on psychometric testing (J Hepatol 1986;3:75)

HE accounts for 30–50% of cirrhosis-related admissions (Med Clin N Am 2008;92:795).

Pathophys: Reduced liver function and portosystemic shunting leads to higher serum concentrations of ammonia (and possibly other substances).

Sx: Symptoms range from subtle personality trait changes to frank delirium and coma.

Si: Asterixis: tremor or flapping of the wrist when dorsiflexed; not necessarily specific for hepatic encephalopathy; hyper-reflexia also seen.

Focal neuro signs: A prospective study of 34 cirrhotic pts with HE showed 17% with focal neuro sx on presentation (most were hemiplegia or hemiparesis), increased risk in females, sx were reversible w/ acute therapy, and no evidence of worse prognosis with focal deficits (Am J Gastroenterol 2001;96:515).

Crs: Onset may be insidious in cirrhosis; more often seen acutely due to acute liver failure, hepatitis, or decompensated chronic cirrhosis; see **Figure 3.3.**

Cmplc: Acute cases may have cerebral edema; look for other cmplc of liver disease (ascites, SBP, variceal bleeding, hepatorenal syndrome); ventilatory failure, which may require intubation for airway control and mechanical ventilation; hypoglycemia is often present and may require rx.

Lab: Serum ammonia level used as initial screening; older studies suggested poor correlation between ammonia levels and severity of disease, but more recent studies suggest good correlation (Am J Med 2003;114:188); normal ammonia in the setting of severe encephalopathy suggests another cause, but pts w/ cirrhosis may have elevated ammonia without symptomatic encephalopathy.

Noninv: Consider intracranial imaging (CT, MRI) if concern for other comorbidities (CVA, intracranial mass), especially if focal neuro sx or low ammonia levels.

EEG also employed for staging or to r/o underlying seizure disorder (seizures uncommon in HE).

Rx: Treatment of HE follows these guidelines:

- Treat or remove precipitating causes.
- Restrict dietary protein, up to 1–1.5 gm/kg of daily protein.
- Administer lactulose therapy in most pts (NEJM 1969;281:408).
  - Cathartic action leads to rapid removal of protein and ammonia from GI tract.
  - Lactitol is an alternative, but not available in the United States.
  - Usually start at 30 mL PO tid–qid, titrate to lowest dose that produces 2–4 loose stools qd and controls HE sx.
  - In obtunded pts, may be given by NGT or enema form.

GASTROENTEROLOGY

GRADE	LEVEL OF CONSCIOUSNESS	PERSONALITY AND INTELLECT	NEUROLOGIC SIGNS	ELECTROENCEPHALOGRAPHIC ABNORMALITIES
0	Normal	Normal	None	None
Subclinical	Normal	Normal	Abnormalities only on psycho-metric analysis	None
1	Inverted sleep pattern, rest-lessness	Forgetfulness, mild confusion, agitation, irritability	Tremor, apraxia, incoordination, impaired handwriting	Triphasic waves (5 cycles/sec)
2	Lethargy, slow responses	Disorientation as regards time, amnesia, decreased inhi-bitions, inappropriate behavior	Asterixis, dysarthria, ataxia, hypo-active reflexes	Triphasic waves (5 cycles/sec)
3	Somnolence but rousability, confusion	Disorientation as regards place, aggressive behavior	Asterixis, hyperactive reflexes, Babinski signs, muscle rigidity	Triphasic waves (5 cycles/sec)
4	Coma	None	Decerebration	Delta activity

Figure 3.3 A Grading System for Hepatic Encephalopathy

Reproduced with permission from Riordan SM, Williams R. Treatment of hepatic encephalopathy. *NEJM.* 1997;337:473. Copyright © 1997, Massachusetts Medical Society. All rights reserved.

- In some pts, consider abx therapy as detailed:
  - Reduce urease-producing gut bacteria to inhibit production of intestinal ammonia.
  - Neomycin 6 gm PO qd is as effective as lactulose (GE 1977;72:573; Am J Dig Dis 1978;23:398); rifaximin and metronidazole are alternatives.
  - RCT of 299 pts with HE; randomized to rifaximin 550 mg BID vs. placebo (~90% of pts in both arms on lactulose rx); rx reduced the risk of a breakthrough episode of HE (22% vs 46%, NNT 4) and reduced risk of hospitalization for HE (OR 0.50) (NEJM 2009;362:1071)
  - Usually a 2nd-line agent to lactulose rx because of side effects and antimicrobial resistance.
- Acutely, most pts require only the addition of lactulose and close monitoring w/ supportive care; in ALF or severe disease, there may be concern for increased ICP with cerebral edema (which requires ICU monitoring and consideration of mannitol therapy).

Hepatorenal Syndrome

(NEJM 2009;361:1279; Med Clin N Am 2008;92:813)

Cause: Common causes of renal failure in pts with cirrhosis are:

- Prerenal:
  - Hypoperfusion associated with hypovolemia from GI bleeding, 3rd spacing of fluids, diuretics.
- Intrinsic:
  - Hepatorenal syndrome (HRS)
  - Sepsis, particularly with SBP
  - Medication-induced, particularly NSAIDs and aminoglycosides
  - Glomerulonephritis from hep B, hep C, alcoholic cirrhosis
- Postrenal:
  - Obstruction of ureters, bladder outlet

Diagnosis of HRS requires:

- Presence of acute or chronic liver disease w/ portal hypertension
- Serum Cr greater than 1.5 mg/dL (lower threshold due to normally low Cr in malnourished pts w/ decreased muscle mass)
- Must be off diuretics for at least 2 days and must have received fluid challenge with IV albumin (1 mg/kg) to r/o prerenal cause
- No recent use of nephrotoxic drugs
- No evidence of shock
- No evidence of intrinsic or obstructive renal disease (normal kidneys on imaging, no hematuria or proteinuria on urinalysis)

Epidem: HRS develops in 40% of pts with cirrhosis and ascites within 5 yr (GE 1993;105:229).

Occurs in 15–20% after LVP unless albumin given as well; occurs in 10% of cirrhotics with GI bleed (Lancet 2003;362:1819).

Pathophys: Systemic vasodilators released by the splanchnic vasculature in response to portal hypertension; causes reduced systemic vascular resistance and renal blood flow; there may be some component of inflammation related to gut bacterial translocation.

The kidney does not show irreversible cellular damage; kidney function returns to normal with liver transplant; kidneys from pts with HRS have been successfully transplanted in others.

Sx/Si: Usually asx until severe renal failure w/ complications.

Crs: Four types of HRS (based on cause and course) are:

- Type 1: Rapidly progressive, serum Cr rises to more than 2.5 mg/dL within 2 wk; high mortality.
- Type 2: Less progressive, slow rise in Cr; usually associated with refractory ascites.
- Type 3: HRS in setting of prior chronic kidney disease.
- Type 4: HRS associated with acute fulminant liver failure.

Very high mortality: 50% 1-mo and 80% 6-mo mortality, unless liver transplant performed; type 1 HRS in-hospital mortality may be as high as 90% (GE 1993;105:229).

Lab: Serum creatinine is the best test; renal failure in cirrhosis is defined as Cr more than 1.5 mg/dL; generally have FE_{Na} less than 1.0%.

Urinalysis for protein, blood to suggest intrinsic renal disease; check for pyuria, bacteruria to r/o infection.

Hyponatremia is present in almost all cases; if not present, consider other causes.

Given high rate of HRS with SBP and other infections, should always have paracentesis with ascitic culture; blood and urine cultures if no evidence of SBP to r/o other infections.

Noninv: Renal US to r/o obstruction with hydronephrosis.

Rx: General treatment measures for HRS:

- R/o other causes, as previously outlined.
- Avoid aggressive fluid resuscitation after initial challenge with albumin (described earlier in Section 3.7), due to concern for sodium overload and worsening ascites.
- Avoid nephrotoxic drugs (NSAIDs, aminoglycosides, ACEIs, ARBs); CT contrast dye can be used if absolutely necessary in cirrhotics, but consider pretreatment with IVF, sodium bicarbonate, or N-acetylcysteine (Hepatol 2004;40:646); see Section 8.4 in Chapter 8 for details.
- Hold diuretic rx; if ascites requires rx, use LVP with albumin as described in the discussion of ascites earlier in Section 3.7.
- Consider vasopressors:
  - The most evidence for benefit is with terlipressin (vasopressin analog).
    - Meta-analysis of 10 trials of vasopressors in HRS showed terlipressin associated with improved 15-d mortality (but no longer-term benefit) (Hepatol 51:576); similar results in Cochrane Reviews, but limited data

Table 3.3 Hepatic and Nonhepatic Causes of Abnormal Liver Function Tests

Test	Common Hepatic Causes	Common Nonhepatic Causes	Considerations
Aminotransferases (ALT/AST)	Alcohol use and abuse Cirrhosis and alcoholic hepatitis Nonalcoholic fatty liver disease (NAFLD) Drug toxicity (APAP overdose, other drugs) Acute and chronic viral hepatitis (A, B, C) Liver congestion from CHF Primary or metastatic liver cancer Hemochromatosis Autoimmune hepatitis Wilson's disease Alpha-1-antitrypsin deficiency	AST can be elevated from muscle disorders: • Myocardial infarction • Rhabdomyolysis • Myositis/myopathy Both can be elevated in celiac sprue (*Hepatol.* 1999;29:654)	Check CPK to r/o muscle causes if elevated AST Screen for alcohol use Review meds Lab testing as detailed in cirrhosis discussion under "Alcoholic Liver Disease (Including Hepatitis and Cirrhosis)" Consider imaging for NAFLD or other liver disease
Alkaline phosphatase	Cirrhosis and alcoholic hepatitis CBD obstruction (see "Biliary Tract Disease") Primary or metastatic liver cancer Primary biliary cirrhosis Primary sclerosing cholangitis Drug toxicity	Bone disorders: • Metastatic or primary bone cancers • Paget's disease • Normal growth in adolescents Intestinal disorders: • Inflammatory bowel disease Placental source during pregnancy	Check GGTP; if elevated, suggests hepatic cause Fractionated alk phos to determine liver, bone, intestinal fractions Imaging of liver and CBD if liver cause of elevated alk phos

Bilirubin	Indirect/unconjugated: • Gilbert's syndrome Direct/conjugated: • Cirrhosis and alcoholic hepatitis • CBD obstruction (see "Biliary Tract Disease") • Primary or metastatic liver cancer • Primary biliary cirrhosis • Primary sclerosing cholangitis • Drug toxicity	Indirect/unconjugated: • Hemolysis of RBCs • Transfusion-related Direct/conjugated: • Sepsis • TPN	Get direct and indirect bilirubin If concern for hemolysis, check LDH, haptoglobin, direct and indirect Coomb's (see Section 4.1 "Anemia"), peripheral smear Imaging of liver and CBD in direct hyperbilirubinemia of uncertain etiology
Albumin (reduced levels)	Reduced liver synthetic function due to cirrhosis	Malnutrition (dietary, malabsorption, critical illness) Nephrotic syndrome Pregnancy	• PT/INR to evaluate for liver synthetic function • U/A for proteinuria • Nutritional analysis

did not allow for definite recommendation for use (Co-chrane 2006;CD005162).
- Not yet available in the United States.
- Norepinephrine and midodrine/octreotide have also been studied, but limited data.
  - Norepinephrine (Levophed) 0.5–3 mg/hr infusion, goal to increase MAP by 10 mmHg.
  - Two small pilot studies (40 and 22 pts) have shown equivalent outcomes with norepinephrine vs terlipressin for type 1 HRS pts (J Hepatol 2007;47:499; Am J Gastroenterol 2008;103:1689).
- Albumin: Little evidence for improved outcomes when used alone in HRS (usually the control arm in vasopressor studies), but most pts receive albumin because of concomitant SBP or need for LVP; typically dosed 1–1.5 gm/kg initially, then 20–40 gm/day.
- Consider TIPS, but definitive evidence of survival benefit is lacking.
- Hemodialysis is not definitive therapy, and has a high rate of complications (bleeding, infection, hypotension); can be used as a bridge to liver transplant; usually reserved for pts w/ pulmonary edema, severe metabolic acidosis, or resistant hyperkalemia.
- Evaluation for liver transplantation is based on MELD score.

Evaluation of Abnormal LFTs

Cause: See **Table 3.3** (NEJM 2000;342:1266; GE 2002;123:1367).

Pathophys: Gilbert's syndrome is a genetic disorder in which defects of uridine diphosphate-glucuronyl transferase lead to isolated elevated levels of unconjugated bilirubin in setting of fasting, illness; usually does not exceed indirect bilirubin of 2–3 mg/dL (NEJM 1995;333:1171).

Lab: Refer again to **Table 3.3.**

Noninv: Initial imaging usually with US or CT; study of inpatients with elevated LFTs showed higher yield with CT as initial test (57% significant findings vs 25% on US); most common findings were CBD obstruction, cholecystitis, liver masses (Arch IM 2001;161:583).

Rx: Rx based on underlying cause; in asx pts with abnormal liver enzymes unexplained by illness causing hospitalization, consider deferring to outpatient setting after repeat testing.

Chapter 4

Hematology

4.1 Anemia (Including Transfusion Practices)

(Mayo Clin Proc 2003;78:1274)

Cause: Major causes of hospital-identified anemia in adults, classified by mean corpuscular volume (MCV), are as follows:

- Microcytic (MCV less than 80 fL) anemia includes the following types:
  - Iron deficiency anemia (IDA) (Am Fam Phys 2007;75: 671): Related to nutritional deficiency (rare in the United States); also caused by chronic blood loss (particularly GI loss from cancer, menorrhagia, and other sources)
  - Anemia of chronic disease (ACD): Associated with microcytosis in about 30% of cases (see the discussion of anemia of chronic disease under "Normocytic" below)
  - Thalassemia: Genetic hemoglobinopathy; usually a known condition in inpatients, but may be unrecognized in younger, asx pts
  - Lead poisoning
- Normocytic (MCV 80–100 fL) anemia has several causes including the following (Am Fam Phys 2000;62:2255):
  - Dilutional effect from hydration: Consider in hospitalized pts, especially in first few days of admission; clues include acute proportional drop in all cell lines with hydration but no evidence of acute blood loss or other factors.
  - Iatrogenic anemia: Due to phlebotomy, especially in critically ill; ICU pts generally have 40–65 mL of blood

removed daily from arterial and venous blood draws (JAMA 1973;223:73; JAMA 2002;288:1499), especially when blood removed from central venous lines.

- Acute blood loss anemia from a variety of sources is commonly seen in hospitalized pts, with an obvious or obscure source.
- Anemia of chronic disease (NEJM 2005;352:1011): 70% of ACD is normocytic; related to a variety of underlying illnesses, including connective tissue diseases, cancer, diabetes.
    - Anemia of critical illness: Similar to ACD, but develops acutely with severe illness; probably a combination of peripheral RBC destruction, acute blood loss, and inflammation-related marrow suppression
    - Anemia of chronic kidney disease (CKD)
- Hemolytic anemia can be caused by any of the following (Am Fam Phys 2004;69:2599):
    - Autoimmune: Cold- or warm-induced; drug-induced (penicillins and other abx, quinine, hydrochlorothiazide, methyldopa, NSAIDs)
    - Microangiopathies: TTP, DIC, HELLP syndrome
    - Transfusion reaction (Blood Rev 2001;15:69): Very rare with proper pretransfusion testing and policies to prevent misadministration; acute reaction with fever, shock, ARDS based on ABO-incompatibility; delayed reactions milder and suggest antibodies to minor RBC antigens
    - Infections: *Mycoplasma, Bartonella,* babesiosis, malaria
    - Others: G6PD deficiency, hereditary spherocytosis, sickle cell disease
- Bone marrow disorders that cause normocytic anemia include aplastic anemia, myelodysplasia, myelophthistic disorders (infiltration of bone marrow from cancer, other diseases), viral or drug-induced myelosuppression.

- Splenic sequestration with hypersplenism is rare cause of normocytic anemia.
- Macrocytic (MCV more than 100 fL) anemia includes these causes (Am Fam Phys 2009;79:203):
  - Alcohol use and abuse
  - Vitamin B12 deficiency: Due to poor nutrition (including alcoholism, vegan diet) or atrophic gastritis (autoimmune, H. pylori infection, Zollinger-Ellison syndrome)
  - Folate deficiency: Due to poor nutrition (especially in alcohol abuse), drug effect (methotrexate, hydroxyurea, AZT, trimethoprim, phenytoin)
  - Reticulocytosis: Due to larger reticulocytes, leading to elevated MCV level; can confirm with high random distribution of width (RDW) and reticulocyte count
  - Myelodysplasia or other primary bone marrow disorder
  - Chronic liver disease
  - Hypothyroidism

Epidem: Normal Hgb varies with age, sex, and ethnicity; typically normal Hgb in white males is 12.7–17.0 gm/dL; in females is 11.6–15.6 gm/dL; African ancestry is about 1gm/dL lower than normal levels (Mayo Clin Proc 2005;80:923).

Anemia present in about 10% of all people older than 65, 20–40% in pts older than 85 (most are mild, 2% with Hgb less than 10 gm/dL) (Blood 2004;104:2263; Mayo Clin Proc 1994;69:730).

Higher rates in hospitalized elderly pts (up to 40%) (CMAJ 1996;155:691); almost universally present in critically ill (95%) (Crit Care Med 2003;31:S668).

Pathophys: Variable, based on underlying cause, but all related to decreased bone marrow production of RBC precursors or peripheral loss/destruction of mature RBCs.

Sx: Usually asx in mild to moderate cases; as severity worsens, may have fatigue (very nonspecific; anemia as cause of fatigue in fewer

HEMATOLOGY

than 5% of outpatient evaluations) (Am J Med 1992;93:303), exertional dyspnea; chest pressure if associated coronary ischemia.

If associated bone marrow disorder, may have weight loss, night sweats.

Si: Tachycardia, pallor (good PPV, but low NPV even in severe anemia) (J Gen Intern Med 1997;12:102); look for lymphadenopathy, splenomegaly to suggest underlying cancer or bone marrow disorder.

B12 deficiency associated with peripheral neuropathy, ataxia, loss of proprioception and vibratory sense.

Crs: If dx of IDA made in adults, must consider GI eval to r/o occult GI bleeding from cancer (especially because dietary iron deficiency is rare in the United States); in one series of 100 pts older than 60 yr with IDA, 62% had bleeding source found on endoscopy (37% upper, 26% lower) and 11% had colon cancer (NEJM 1993;329:1691); see Section 3.2 in Chapter 3 for details on w/u of occult and obscure GI bleeding.

Cmplc: Severe anemia may contribute to acute coronary ischemia, especially in pts with underlying CAD.

Lab: Initial dx based on CBC with diff; abnormalities in other cell lines may suggest cause (neutropenia and thrombocytopenia associated with underlying bone marrow disorder, thrombocytosis associated with iron deficiency).

Consider eval of peripheral blood smear in all cases of anemia, when cause is not readily apparent by history (NEJM 2005;353:498); **Table 4.1** summarizes peripheral blood smear findings.

F/u eval of anemia in hospitalized pts without evident cause includes serum ferritin, B12, folate, reticulocyte levels.

Further eval for specific causes includes testing for the following:

- Microcytic anemia

Table 4.1   Peripheral Blood Smear Findings

Abnormal RBC Findings on Peripheral Smear	Diagnostic Considerations
Reticulocytes	Rapid RBC turnover due to acute blood loss, hemolysis, recovery stage of nutritional deficiency
Microcytes	(See causes of microcytic anemia at beginning of chapter)
Nucleated RBCs	Immature RBC precursors; seen in rapid blood loss (from acute bleeding, hemolysis) or with marrow disorders
Basophilic stippling	Hemolysis; thalassemias; alcohol abuse
Target cells	Liver disease; thalassemias
Spiculated (Burr) cells	Chronic kidney disease (CKD); liver disease
Spherocytes	Hereditary spherocytosis; G6PD deficiency; autoimmune hemolysis
Schistocytes	Microangiopathic hemolysis (DIC, TTP)
Bite cells	G6PD deficiency
Sickle cells	Sickle cell anemia
Tear drop cells	Thalassemias; bone marrow disorders
Howell-Jolly bodies	Remnant of cell nucleus; seen in post-splenectomy and functional asplenic pts
Heinz bodies	G6PD deficiency

- Initial screen is serum ferritin for iron deficiency.
  - In elderly population with IDA causing about 20% of anemia, a ferritin level of less than 18 mcg/L had a PPV of 95% for IDA; levels 18–45 mcg/L still strongly suggestive of IDA; levels greater than 100 mcg/dL found in IDA in fewer than 10% of cases (Am J Med 1990;88:205).
  - Although ferritin is an acute phase reactant (high levels with acute or chronic inflammation), pts with IDA still should not be able to mount significant ferritin response even in acute illness.

- Additional iron studies (serum iron, total iron-binding capacity [TIBC], transferrin) are often performed.
  - IDA has low serum iron, high TIBC (with low % of transferrin saturation).
  - ACD has low serum iron, normal to low TIBC (with variable % of transferrin saturation).
  - Overall, serum iron and TIBC add little to dx of IDA over serum ferritin level, although may help in confirmation of ACD.
- If w/u for IDA is negative, most likely cause in hospitalized setting is ACD; in appropriate pts, consider hemoglobin electrophoresis for thalassemia and lead level.
- Normocytic anemia
  - Because of possibility of mixed disorders (especially if concern for nutritional deficiency), consider serum ferritin, B12, folate levels.
  - Serum BUN/Cr for CKD; should be elevated in anemia of CKD, but does not correlate well with severity of anemia.
  - Consider serum erythropoietin (EPO) levels, which should be inappropriately normal in setting of anemia, but may only be low if Hgb is less than 10 gm/dL (NEJM 1990;322:1689).
  - Could consider CRP/ESR for underlying inflammatory disorder in ACD, but is usually evident based on pt hx and clinical sx.
  - Look for si/sx of acute or chronic bleeding; usually prompts stool testing for occult blood, but high rates of false positives and negatives in hospitalized pts.
  - Concern for acute hemolysis; look for the following lab abnormalities:
    - Marked reticulocytosis: Usually 4–6%; sign of significant cell turnover due to rapid destruction from hemolysis; may be lower if associated nutritional deficiency or bone marrow disorder that blunts marrow response
    - Elevated serum LDH: Sign of cell destruction

- Low haptoglobin: Serum binder of free hemoglobin; low levels indicate increased free hemoglobin from hemolysis
- Increased indirect bilirubin
- Coomb's test
  - Direct Coomb's tests pt's RBCs for adherent anti-RBC antibodies; positive in hemolytic anemia, except for microangiopathies (TTP, DIC).
  - Indirect Coomb's tests pt's serum for circulating antibodies against RBC antigens; evaluation prior to RBC transfusion to determine blood compatibility.
- Urinary hemosiderin to distinguish intravascular hemolysis
- Macrocytic anemia
  - Reticulocyte count to r/o reticulocytosis
  - Screen for B12 and folate deficiency:
    - Initial test is serum B12 and folate levels.
    - Serum folate variable based on recent diet; deficient pts may falsely elevate serum levels in the hospital with one folate-rich meal; screen to confirm folate deficiency if normal serum levels, but high clinical suspicion:
      - Can perform RBC folate level: Folate bound to RBC, so provides folate level at the time of RBC production (within the last 3 mo).
      - Increased homocysteine level: Lack of folate inhibits homocysteine to methionine conversion, raising serum levels (also seen in B12 deficiency and hereditary hyperhomocysteinemia).
      - Therapeutic trial of folate replacement: Some argue that routine folate replacement is cheaper and easier than lab eval when concern for folate deficiency (Am J Med 2001;110:88), but still need to r/o B12 deficiency (as neuro sx will not improve with folate replacement).

- Serum B12 level is fairly good indicator of deficiency, but may have low to normal levels in some elderly pts with deficiency; consider deficiency if less than 400 pg/mL.
    - Confirm with serum methylmalonic acid (MMA) level: B12 is cofactor in conversion of MMA to succinyl coenzyme A, so deficiency will lead to elevated MMA levels.

Noninv: Bone marrow bx is a consideration, but usually reserved when high likelihood of primary bone marrow disorder; can be considered in severe IDA (showing depleted marrow iron stores), but most recommend serum testing only, and then a therapeutic trial of iron.

Rx: Treatment of anemia is based on cause.
- Acute blood loss anemia: See Section 3.2 in Chapter 3 for details.
- Iron deficiency anemia (Am Fam Phys 2007;75:671):
    - Typically replace iron via oral route; ferrous sulfate 325 mg qd to tid.
    - May require addition of stool softeners, laxatives because of constipation effects.
    - Vitamin C co-therapy may enhance intestinal absorption, but is not necessary in all cases.
    - IV iron rx reserved for pts w/ severe IDA or no response to oral rx (due to malabsorption, inability to take or tolerate PO iron); also often used in chronic dialysis pts; available types include iron dextran (Dexferrum), ferrous gluconate, iron sucrose (Venofer); IV dosing based on weight and pre-rx hemoglobin; use initial test dose and watch for serious drug reaction; 5% of pts had drug reaction in one study (0.7% were deemed serious; most were itching, dyspnea, chest pain, nausea), higher risk if other prior drug allergies (Am J Kidney Dis 1996;28:529).
    - Can monitor response to rx with reticulocyte count, which should increase within 1 wk of effective therapy.

- Duration of rx depends on cause and risk factors; if related to chronic blood loss that is stopped, can discontinue rx once anemia is resolved and ferritin repleted.
- B12 deficiency anemia:
  - Traditionally, B12 1 mg im qd for 1 wk, then 1 mg weekly for 1 mo, then 1 mg monthly long-term.
  - PO dosing of B12 at 1–2 mg qd may be as effective (Blood 1998;92:1191; Clin Ther 2003;25:3124).
  - Duration of rx usually lifelong, unless clearly related to nutritional deficiency with reversible risk factors.
- Folate deficiency:
  - Folate 1 mg PO qd, although can use higher doses if concerns for malabsorption.
  - Duration of rx depends on cause and risk factors for ongoing deficiency.
- Anemia of chronic disease and critical illness:
  - Main rx is supportive and directed at underlying cause.
  - In chronic disease and cancer pts, can consider erythropoiesis stimulators (epoetin, darbepoetin).
    - Has not been rigorously studied for this indication; available data in pts with rheumatoid arthritis (RA) (Am J Med 1990;89:161), hematologic cancers (J Clin Oncol 2002;20:2486), CHF (Eur Heart J 2007;28:2208) show improved Hgb and QOL scores with rx.
    - Manufacturers suggest treatment only up to Hgb of 12 gm/dL because of concerns for increased morbidity/mortality with higher Hgb goals.
    - If used, consider co-rx with iron (J Clin Oncol 2004;22:1301).
  - In critically ill, use of erythropoiesis stimulators is unproven.
    - Use of erythropoietin (300 units/kg qd from ICU day 3 through day 7, or 40,000 units weekly) may reduce need for transfusion (Crit Care Med 1999;27:2346;

JAMA 2002;288:2827), but no effect on mortality in medical pts (possibly mortality effect in posttrauma pts) with an increased risk of thrombotic events (NEJM 2007;357:965).

- RBC transfusion may be appropriate in severe cases (see RBC transfusion practices below).
- Anemia of chronic kidney disease: Mainly outpatient therapies; national guidelines suggest addition of erythropoiesis stimulators to goal Hgb 11–12 gm/dL (Am J Kidney Dis 2006;47:S16).
- Hemolytic anemia (Semin Hematol 2005;42:131):
  - Hematology consultation is appropriate, to suggest proper rx based on cause.
  - If underlying precipitant (drug, transfusion, etc.), remove offending agent if possible or treat infection.
  - Steroid therapy, usually with oral prednisone, is the 1st-line agent for most autoimmune causes; in severe or resistant cases, may require splenectomy, IV immunoglobulin, plasmapheresis.
  - Transfusion therapy may be problematic due to difficulty finding compatible blood.

RBC transfusion practices (Crit Care Med 2003;31:S668; Crit Care Med 2009;37:3124) require consideration of the following issues:

- Evolving field of study; traditional practice of "transfusion triggers" (typically Hgb of 9–10 gm/dL) is no longer considered appropriate rx based on risks and benefits.
- Risks of blood transfusion therapy include the following:
  - Do blood transfusions increase mortality?
    - SOAP study: Multicenter European trial of more than 3,000 ICU pts; 33% received blood transfusion; transfused pts had higher initial APACHE scores, and were older pts with higher rates of sepsis and surgery;

transfused pts had higher ICU mortality (23% vs 16%) and ICU LOS (6 vs 2.5 d), but no difference when controlled for age, severity of illness, and other factors (Anesthesiology 2008;108:31).

- Seems improbable that transfusions cause significant mortality, but more likely that they are a marker of severe illness.
- Transfusion-related acute lung injury (TRALI) (Crit Care Med 2006;34:S114; Crit Care Med 2005;33:721): ARDS that occurs during or within 6 hr after blood transfusion.
- Transfusion-related infectious diseases, including HIV, hepatitis B and C, syphilis, West Nile: Risks now extremely low (ranging from 1 in 250,000 to 1 in 2 million, depending on agent) due to universal blood product screening.

- Aggressive transfusion has not shown improvement in outcomes and may be related to increased mortality; TRICC study showed "restrictive" transfusion policy (only for Hgb less than 7 gm/dL) vs "liberal" (Hgb less than 9 gm/dL) in critically ill pts was associated with reduced in-hospital mortality (22% vs 28%, NNT 16), especially in pts younger than 55 yr and with APACHE-II scores of 20 or less (NEJM 1999;340:409).
- Consider RBC transfusion in the following settings (also see **Figure 4.1**):
  - Patients with true hemorrhagic shock (based on hemodynamics, not just acute blood loss)
  - All critically ill pts with Hgb less than 7 gm/dL (some may tolerate lower Hgb levels, but unable to determine)
  - Patients with acute coronary syndromes (unstable angina, acute MI) and Hgb less than 8–9 mg/dL
    - Most data based on retrospective reviews; no large RCTs to guide decision-making.
    - Retrospective study of 79,000 Medicare pts w/ acute MI; 4.2% had initial Hct less than 30%, 4.7% had

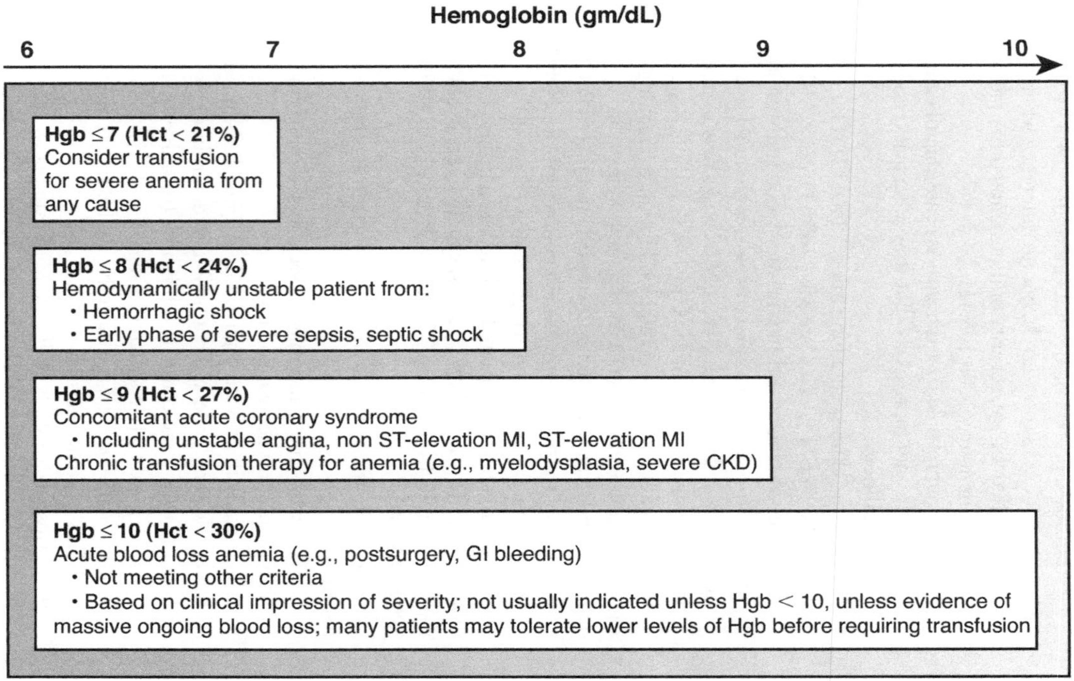

Hemoglobin (gm/dL)

Hgb ≤7 (Hct < 21%)
Consider transfusion for severe anemia from any cause

Hgb ≤8 (Hct < 24%)
Hemodynamically unstable patient from:
- Hemorrhagic shock
- Early phase of severe sepsis, septic shock

Hgb ≤9 (Hct < 27%)
Concomitant acute coronary syndrome
- Including unstable angina, non ST-elevation MI, ST-elevation MI
Chronic transfusion therapy for anemia (e.g., myelodysplasia, severe CKD)

Hgb ≤10 (Hct < 30%)
Acute blood loss anemia (e.g., postsurgery, GI bleeding)
- Not meeting other criteria
- Based on clinical impression of severity; not usually indicated unless Hgb < 10, unless evidence of massive ongoing blood loss; many patients may tolerate lower levels of Hgb before requiring transfusion

Figure 4.1 Indications for RBC Transfusion

blood transfusion during hospital stay; blood transfusion was associated with reduced adjusted mortality in pt cohorts with Hct 5–24% (OR 0.22), 24–27% (OR 0.48), 27–30% (OR 0.60), and 30–33% (0.69); for pts w/ Hct more than 36%, transfusion was associated with worse mortality (NEJM 2001;345:1230); these results seem to lend credence to the "transfusion trigger" of Hgb/Hct 10/30 for pts with acute coronary syndromes.

- Sub-analysis of TRICC data showed no difference between liberal and conservative transfusion strategies in pts w/ primary or secondary dx of cardiac disease (~20% of pts) (NEJM 1999;340:409).

- Given the lack of definitive data in this population, the critical care guidelines suggest that pts w/ ACS and Hgb 8 gm/dL or less may benefit from transfusion (although many still employ the trigger of 10 gm/dL).

- Patients with severe sepsis and septic shock, with evidence of reduced mixed central venous oxygen saturation ($ScvO_2$ less than 70%), after treatment with appropriate fluid resuscitation and pressors during early goal-directed rx (see "Sepsis and Septic Shock" in Section 5.3 for details)

- Post-op pts w/ Hgb 7 gm/dL or less (JAMA 1988;260:2700)
  - Similar to medical pts, no controlled RCTs are available in routine perioperative pts to guide transfusion policies.
  - Study of post-op pts who refused transfusion showed no increase in mortality rates until Hgb was less than 7 gm/dL, with mortality increasing by about 2.5 times with every subsequent 1 gm/dL decrease in Hgb below 7 (pts with Hgb 4–5 gm/dL had mortality rate of 34%) (Transfusion 2002;42:812).
  - Ongoing FOCUS trial may help; enrolling hip fracture pts older than 50 yr with h/o CAD or multiple risk factors; randomized to transfusion for Hgb 10 gm/dL or less

HEMATOLOGY

vs transfusion for symptomatic anemia or Hgb 8 gm/dL or less (Transfusion 2006;46:2192).

- For pts requiring chronic transfusion rx (for myelodysplasia, leukemias, etc.), consider transfusions if Hgb is less than 9 gm/dL.
- Transfusion for significant acute blood loss (from surgery or other bleeding source) may be difficult to assess; should certainly transfuse for Hgb less than 7 gm/dL, but may use higher level if massive ongoing bleeding.
- When choosing to transfuse, better to use 1 unit PRBC at a time and assess response than to routinely transfuse 2 units, unless severely anemic or ongoing blood loss.

4.2 Thrombocytopenia

(South Med J 2006;99:491; Am J Respir Crit Care Med 2000;162:347)

Cause: Defined as platelet count less than 150,000/mcL, but 2–3% of population will have "normal" platelet count outside that range; mild 100–150K, moderate 50–100K, severe less than 50K.

Causes of thrombocytopenia in hospitalized pts include:

- "Pseudo-thrombocytopenia": Commonly seen clumping of platelets due to EDTA anticoagulant added to phlebotomy tube; accounts for 15% of ICU episodes of thrombocytopenia (South Med J 2006;99:491); large clumped plt will not be adequately read by automated CBC machines; confirm with peripheral smear verifying clumping or repeat plt count with blood collected in non-EDTA tube.
- Due to peripheral destruction, sequestration, or dilution:
  - Sepsis-induced: Most common form of thrombocytopenia seen in ICU setting; probably multifactorial with plt destruction, marrow suppression, splenic sequestration.

- Disseminated intravascular coagulation (DIC) (NEJM 1999;341:586): Excessive production of thrombin due to underlying critical illness, causing consumption of plt and paradoxical bleeding and thrombosis; seen w/ many critical illnesses including sepsis, severe trauma and burns, obstetrical emergencies, cancers.
- Drug-induced (NEJM 2007;357:580): Multiple mechanisms, but usually due to cross-reactivity of antigens leading to antiplatelet antibodies, similar to idiopathic thrombocytopenic purpura (ITP); consider in new-onset isolated, severe thrombocytopenia (commonly less than 20K) within 1–2 wk of new drug administration; many drugs have been implicated, as follows:
  - Heparin-induced thrombocytopenia (HIT): Consider in pts on any unfractionated or low-molecular-weight heparin with new drop in plt counts within 5 to 14 d (or sooner if prior use); see "Heparin-Induced Thrombocytopenia" later in Section 4.2 for details.
  - Glycoprotein IIb/IIIa inhibitors (Chest 2005;127:53S): Consider if new thrombocytopenia in pts on these agents for ACS and PCI, about 2% of pts; usually mild, self-limited with removal of agent.
  - Other commonly used drugs: Potential causes of thrombocytopenia include quinine (now off the U.S. market but still found in tonic water), linezolid (especially with long-term use) (Clin Infect Dis 2002;34:695), sulfa drugs, vancomycin, NSAIDs, APAP, thiazide diuretics, anticonvulsants (for full list of implicated meds, see Ann IM 2005;142:474).
- Idiopathic thrombocytopenic purpura (ITP) (NEJM 2002;346:995): Autoimmune disease due to antiplatelet antibodies; seen more commonly in children (usually postviral illness), but also in adults (~50 cases per 1 million

HEMATOLOGY

people in the United States) (Blood 1999;94:909); more common in women; usually isolated (although occasionally associated w/ connective tissue diseases); sometimes severe (fewer than 20K) thrombocytopenia, but often asx and found on CBC done for other reasons.

- Thrombotic thrombocytopenic purpura (TTP) (also termed TTP-HUS, as hemolytic uremic syndrome previously thought to be separate entity is now considered the same) (NEJM 2006;354:1927): Often confused for ITP w/ similar name, but TTP is a very rare (~10 cases per 1 million people in the United States) (J Thromb Haemost 2005;3:1432) and more severe microangiopathy; cause is enzyme deficiency of ADAMTS-13 (von Willebrand factor-cleaving protease) (NEJM 1998;339:1578), idiopathic, or due to meds (clopidogrel, ticlopidine, quinine, chemotherapeutics), infections (*E. coli* O157:H7, HIV), or cancer; classic pentad (but only first two seen commonly or required for dx):
  - Hemolytic anemia: See description and w/u in Section 4.1.
  - Thrombocytopenia: Median plt about 20K.
  - Acute renal failure: Usually only mild and transient in most cases.
  - Fever: Usually low-grade; if higher than 102°F, consider infection.
  - Acute neurologic sx: In about 50% of cases, includes delirium, seizures, focal stroke-like neuro deficits.
- HELLP syndrome (Ob Gyn 2004;103:981): Microangiopathy of pregnancy w/ hemolysis, elevated liver enzymes, low plt; in spectrum of disease w/ severe preeclampsia.
- Mechanical destruction: Can result from prosthetic cardiac valves, CABG surgery.
- Posttransfusion purpura (Am J Med 1985;78:361): Rare cmplc of RBC transfusion w/ autoimmune reaction to P1[A1] platelet antigens.

- Gestational thrombocytopenia (J Am Board Fam Pract 2002;15:290): Possibly autoimmune, peripheral destruction, and dilutional drop in plt seen in fewer than 5% of pregnancies; typically, asx and moderate (plt 70–100K), returns to normal postpartum; no rx is necessary other than monitoring.
- Hypersplenia w/ sequestration: Usually seen in cirrhosis w/ portal hypertension, lymphoma; associated w/ mild to moderate thrombocytopenia.
- Massive blood loss w/ high-volume transfusions (Am J Clin Path 1991;96:770): Replacement of large volume RBCs alone will lead to dilutional thrombocytopenia due to lack of replaced platelets; rx w/ platelet transfusion as needed.
- Due to impaired production (i.e., bone marrow suppression):
  - Chronic alcohol abuse: Common cause of mild to moderate thrombocytopenia in hospitalized pts
  - Aplastic anemia, myelodysplasia, myelophthistic disorders
  - Leukemia, lymphoma, metastatic cancer
  - Chemotherapy-induced: Commonly seen with many chemo or immunosuppressive agents; usually associated with concomitant anemia and neutropenia; typically have nadir of myelosuppression within 5–10 d and recovery within 2–3 wk
  - Radiation induced
  - Infections: HIV, CMV, EBV, malaria, ehrlichiosis
  - Vitamin B12, folate, iron deficiency (although latter usually associated with thrombocytosis)

Select pts may have plt dysfunction without actual thrombocytopenia (Chest 2009;136:1622).

- Usually present with abnormal bleeding, ecchymoses.
- Drug-induced: Commonly occurs with ASA, clopidogrel, ticlopidine.
- Chronic kidney disease: Usually occurs in pts with uremia and stage V CKD; renal consultation suggested in acute bleeding;

HEMATOLOGY

consider rx with dialysis, IV desmopressin, IV estrogens, cryo-precipitate transfusion.

- Von Willebrand disease: Common genetic disorder (~1% of population) (Blood 1987;69:454) with lack or decreased function of von Willebrand factor, which binds to and prevents rapid breakdown of Factor VIII.

Epidem: Thrombocytopenia present in fewer than 1% of all hospitalized pts (South Med J 2006;99:491), but much higher rates in critically ill (20–40%) (Ann Pharmacother 1997;31:285); moderate to severe plt count (less than 50K) in 10–20% (Chest 1999;115:1363); of inpatients, half will present with thrombocytopenia, half will develop while hospitalized (Crit Care Med 2002;30:753).

Pathophys: Platelets are formed by fragmentation of megakaryocytes in the bone marrow; one-third of all plt are usually sequestered in the spleen (higher in pathologic splenomegaly); typical plt circulate for 7–10 d in the absence of bleeding/disease.

Platelets play major role in hemostasis, as both physical part of clot formation and release of vasoactive substances to assist in clotting.

Sx: Most cases are asx (especially if plt are more than 100K); diagnosed incidentally on lab eval for other reasons.

Chronic thrombocytopenia may be associated with easy bruising; excessive bleeding with trauma, surgery, or menses.

If associated neurologic sx, consider TTP.

If fever, chills, N/V, consider sepsis, TTP, drug-induced.

Si: Lymphadenopathy, splenomegaly depending on underlying cause.

Crs: Thrombocytopenia correlates with longer ICU and hospital LOS, increased mortality (Chest 2009;136:1622).

Mortality rate typically related to underlying cause.

- Sepsis-induced thrombocytopenia is based on severity of disease (see "Sepsis and Septic Shock" in Section 5.3 for details).
- Drug-induced usually has low mortality if recognized early.

- ITP is usually chronic disease (except in children) with low mortality, unless severe thrombocytopenia; 5-yr mortality is 2.2% in those younger than 40 yr, up to 50% in those older than 60 (Arch IM 2000;160:1630).
- DIC is usually a predictor of poor outcomes, high mortality due to underlying critical illness.
- TTP has high mortality rate without therapy (~90%) (Blood 2000;96:1223), but improved rate (~20%) with appropriate early rx.

Cmplc: Spontaneous bleeding usually only with plt less than 10–20K, including epistaxis, mucocutaneous bleeding, non- or mildly traumatic ecchymoses; lethal GI bleeding and intracranial hemorrhage in severe cases.

Lab: Once true thrombocytopenia is diagnosed (i.e., r/o pseudothrombocytopenia), further lab eval includes the following:

- Peripheral blood smear to look for evidence of other underlying disease; schistocytes to suggest TTP, DIC; reticulocytes to suggest TTP (due to hemolytic anemia)
- Renal function to look for ARF with TTP, sepsis
- Liver function to look for underlying cirrhosis, alcohol abuse
- Concomitant anemia
    - If microcytic anemia, check serum ferritin for iron deficiency.
    - If normocytic anemic, get reticulocyte count, LDH, bilirubin, haptoglobin for hemolytic anemia (with TTP); if neutropenic as well, consider marrow biopsy.
    - If macrocytic anemia, check B12 and folate levels.
- Direct Coomb's test
    - Tests pt's RBCs for adherent anti-RBC antibodies.
    - Will be neg in TTP, DIC.
    - Will be pos in rare ITP-associated hemolytic anemia (aka Evans syndrome); use Coomb's test to differentiate from TTP (South Med J 2006;99:491).

- DIC profile, including PT, PTT, D-dimer, fibrinogen, fibrin split products (FSP); especially to distinguish from sepsis-induced and TTP; DIC will show:
  - Increased D-dimer due to either fibrinolysis from activation of clotting cascade or underlying inflammation; nonspecific as also elevated in many other critical illnesses, thrombosis, infection
  - Increased PT/PTT (also consider recent use of anticoagulants)
  - Decreased fibrinogen levels (less than 100 mg/dL) and increased FSP due to fibrinolysis
  - DIC score developed by International Society of Thrombosis and Haemostasis (ISTH) suggests presence of DIC (Crit Care Med 2004;32:2416) using the following system:
    - 0 points for plt more than 100K, 1 point for plt 50–100K, 2 points for plt less than 50K
    - 0 points for normal FSP, 1 point for moderate FSP elevation, 2 points for strong FSP elevation
    - 0 points for prolonged PT 0–3 sec, 1 point for prolonged PT 3–6 sec, 2 points for prolonged PT more than 6 sec
    - 0 points for fibrinogen more than 100 mg/dL, 1 point for fibrinogen less than 100 mg/dL
    - Score of 5 or more suggests DIC; if less than 5, consider other dx or follow daily score for progression
- If concern for TTP, can directly measure ADAMTS-13 enzyme activity (reduced in TTP), but may not add further to clinical dx, and certainly should not delay appropriate therapy awaiting testing.
- If concern for ITP, can directly measure antiplatelet antibodies, but has limited PPV (80%) (Blood 1996;88:194) and poor NPV to r/o disease.

Noninv: Bone marrow bx not necessary in most cases, unless concern for infiltrative bone marrow disease (based on concomitant anemia, neutropenia).

Rx: General approach to treatment of thrombocytopenia is as follows:

- Determination of underlying cause is crucial, especially with severe disease; need to r/o HIT and TTP in particular, given high rates of morbidity and mortality.
- Mild thrombocytopenia (100–150K) in hospitalized mostly due to sepsis, other critical illness, alcohol use, meds; does not usually require further therapy other than regular monitoring.
- In pts with plt less than 50K, avoid unnecessary invasive procedures (additional CVC access, arterial lines) unless plan to transfuse platelets first.
- Platelet transfusion therapy involves these issues:
  - Random donor plt are standard; single donor reduces risks of infection from pooled random donors; HLA-matched plt from single donors in pts with anti-HLA antibodies.
  - Typically dosed 1 U per 12 kg of body weight; in average-size adult, 6 U is standard dose ("6-pack of platelets"); 6 U will typically increase serum plt count by about 30K, enough to provide adequate hemostasis in most situations; if plt do not rise to that degree, need to consider "platelet resistance" due to autoimmune disease (can consider pre-treatment with IVIG to reduce plt loss in some cases).
  - Suggestions for consideration of platelet transfusion:
    - Plt more than 50K: Usually unnecessary unless high-risk surgery (eye, neuro) or significant bleeding
    - Plt less than 50K: Consider if active bleeding or if plan for surgery
    - Plt less than 15–20K: Consider if known coagulopathy, high bleeding risk, infection, critical illness
    - Plt less than 10–15K: Prophylactic transfusion due to high risk of spontaneous bleeding
  - Platelet transfusions are relatively contraindicated in HIT and TTP, as may worsen thrombosis (and usually unnecessary due to lack of severe thrombocytopenia).

Treatment of specific causes of thrombocytopenia

- Sepsis-induced: Appropriate rx of sepsis; see "Sepsis and Septic Shock" in Section 5.3 for details.
- DIC (NEJM 1999;341:586):
  - Mainly requires supportive therapy, with rx of underlying illness.
  - If serious bleeding, will require transfusions of FFP and plt.
  - If associated thrombosis, consider IV unfractionated heparin therapy, but use is usually limited by concomitant bleeding.
- Drug-induced (NEJM 2007;357:580):
  - HIT: See "Heparin-Induced Thrombocytopenia" later in this section.
  - Chemotherapy-induced: Requires supportive care only; plt transfusions as needed.
  - Proper recognition and prompt removal of drug: This is most difficult aspect, especially in critically ill, as there may be multiple potential offending agents.
  - Platelet transfusions: Administer as indicated, based on guidelines listed previously.
  - Steroid therapy (oral or IV): Often used, but no evidence to support efficacy; in severe cases without improvement after drug removal (and consideration of other causes), can consider IVIG or plasma exchange.
  - Usually resolves with drug removal within 1–2 wk.
  - If concern for multiple drugs, can attempt low-dose testing of single agents for recurrent thrombocytopenia, but should be reserved for special circumstances with hematology consultation.
- ITP (NEJM 2002;346:995):
  - If asx and mild to moderate thrombocytopenia (plt more than 50K), may follow without therapy; otherwise, rx warranted; counsel re bleeding risks if plt are less than 50K, especially if physical labor or contact sports.

- Prednisone 1–1.5 mg/kg PO qd; response in up to 67%, usually within 2–3 wk (Blood 1996;88:3; Am J Med 1980;69:430); can usually slowly taper off once plt count returns to normal.
- In severe cases with acute bleeding or need for emergent surgery, use IV methylprednisolone 1 gm/d for 2–3 d, IVIG 1 gm/kg/d for 2–3 d, and plt transfusions given after IVIG (Ann IM 1997;126:307).
- In chronic or recurrent cases, primary rx is splenectomy (for a good review of other investigational therapies and options, see Mayo Clin Proc 2004;79:504).
- TTP (NEJM 2006;354:1927):
  - Early dx is essential to effective rx and reduced mortality.
  - Plasmapheresis (aka plasma exchange therapy) (NEJM 1991;325:393) of 1 to 1.5 times predicted plasma volume of the pt; reduced 6-mon mortality as compared to FFP therapy (22% vs 37%, NNT 7); half of pts treated with plasma exchange had normal plt count and no new neuro sx within 1 wk; continue qd rx until 2 d after plt count returns to normal.
  - If delay to plasmapheresis, consider FFP infusions as initial rx.
  - Look for possible causes (drugs, infections) and treat as appropriate.
  - Consider IV or PO steroids in idiopathic or resistant cases.
- B12, folate, iron deficiency: See the discussion of anemia in Section 4.1 for details.

Heparin-Induced Thrombocytopenia (HIT)

(NEJM 2006;355:809; Chest 2009;135:1651)

Cause: HIT is a clinical spectrum of disease characterized by thrombocytopenia, and in many cases thrombosis, following administration of heparin products; some use the term HITTS (HIT thrombotic syndrome) to distinguish simple thrombocytopenic response (aka "isolated" HIT) vs HIT with thrombotic cmplc; in confirmed HIT, thrombosis occurs in 50–75% of cases (Crit Care Med 2007;35:1165).

HIT is defined as having the following characteristics:

- Drop in plt count to less than 150,000/mcL, *or* decrease in plt count by 50% from baseline (even if plt still more than 150K).
- Median nadir of plt count in HIT is 50–70K (Semin Hematol 1998;35:9), and 20% have plt that remain greater than 100K (Crit Care Med 2006;34:2898); if very severe thrombocytopenia (less than 20K), consider other causes as more likely.
- Typically develops within 5 to 14 d after heparin dosing (~70% of cases), unless pt has had prior sensitization with heparin in the past 100 d (and then may have immediate drop in plt); as a rule, if thrombocytopenia develops while on heparin for fewer than 5 d without confirmed prior use, look for another cause (see the general thrombocytopenia discussion earlier in Section 4.2 for differential diagnosis).
- Occurs with any form of heparin (UFH or LMWH), in therapeutic or prophylactic doses; however, risk is about 10 times higher with UFH (Blood 2005;106:2710), prolonged therapeutic dosing, and postsurgical pts (Br J Haematol 2002;118:1137).

Presentation of HIT in hospitalized pts is as follows:

- Most commonly, drop in plt count in pts on heparin rx, usually asx at the time of identification.
- New thrombosis in hospitalized pt with recent exposure to heparin products (consider in pts who develop VTE despite appropriate prophylaxis).
- Rarely, acute syndrome similar to anaphylaxis with fever, delirium, shock in pts given IV heparin bolus with circulating HIT antibodies from recent prior exposure.

- Delayed-onset HIT: Develops after discontinuation of heparin, usually 3–4 wk after initial exposure (consider in post-op pts who return with new-onset VTE and thrombocytopenia despite appropriate prophylaxis); characterized by very high titers of anti-PF4 antibody, which bind plt even without heparin (Ann IM 2001;135:502).

Epidem: Develops in 1–3% of medical pts on UFH, 0.1–1% on LMWH.

HIT results in increased LOS of about 14 days and additional cost of about $14,000 for the hospitalization (Chest 2008;134:568).

Pathophys: Development of antibodies against platelet-factor 4 (PF4), released by platelets and that naturally binds heparin and cell surfaces; antibodies lead to an immune response against PF4-heparin complex, leading to platelet activation, causing thrombocytopenia and thrombosis (Crit Care Med 2006;34:2898); typically, the PF4 antibody remains circulating for only up to 3 mo, and in most pts will not cause immediate repeat clinical response to heparin after 100 days postexposure (NEJM 2001;344:1286).

Sx/Si: Usually asx, until development of cmplc; usually lack typical sx of thrombocytopenia, as rarely severe drop in plt.

Crs: Mortality up to 20%; severity of thrombocytopenic response is strong predictor of thrombosis and mortality (Blood Coagul Fibrinolysis 2008;19:471).

Can use HIT scoring system to determine pretest probability and r/o low-risk pts (Curr Hematol Rep 2003;2:148):

- Also called the "4 T's": **T**hrombocytopenia, **T**iming, **T**hrombosis, and o**T**her causes.
- Thrombocytopenia:
  - 0 points for plt nadir less than 10K (remember, severe plt drop rare in HIT) or plt drop less than 30%
  - 1 point for plt nadir 10–19K or drop 30–50%
  - 2 points for plt nadir more than 20K or drop more than 50%

- Timing:
  - 0 points for plt drop within 4 d of first heparin dose
  - 1 point for plt drop more than 10 d after first heparin dose or less than 1 d with remote prior heparin exposure
  - 2 points for "classic" timing of 5–10 d after first dose or less than 1 d if recent (less than 30 d) prior exposure
- Thrombosis:
  - 0 points for no evidence of new thrombosis
  - 1 point for erythematous skin lesions, new thrombosis in pt with prior hx of VTE
  - 2 points for confirmed new thrombosis or necrotic skin lesions
- Other causes:
  - 0 points for definite alternative cause of thrombocytopenia
  - 1 point for possible other cause
  - 2 points for no other obvious cause
- 6–8 points means HIT is likely dx; 4–5 pts intermediate risk; 3 pts or less means HIT unlikely (fewer than 1% of pts had pos HIT ab with score of 3 or less) (J Thromb Haemost 2006;4:759).

Cmplc: Thrombotic and other cmplc of HIT (30 times increased risk) (Chest 2005;127:1857), including these:

- Venous thromboembolism: DVT and PE; most commonly lower extremity DVT, but can occur anywhere, especially at sites of trauma, venous access (Blood 2003;101:3049)
- Arterial thrombosis: Especially in pts with vascular and cardiac surgery
- Thrombotic and embolic CVA, cerebral venous thrombosis
- Acute MI
- Skin erythema and necrosis at the sites of heparin injection
- Limb gangrene (especially with concomitant warfarin therapy)
- Adrenal insufficiency from adrenal vein thrombosis and hemorrhage (similar to Waterhouse-Friderichsen syndrome)

Lab: Concern for HIT based on absolute or relative drop in plt count (as described above); because usually asx, plt monitoring recommended before initiation (baseline) and at least qod in pts on UFH or LMWH (Chest 2004;126:311S).

Definitive diagnosis of HIT requires the following:

- Anti-PF4 antibodies (aka "HIT antibody"): ELISA recommended as initial test; high sens (up to 97%) and NPV (95%), but poor PPV, as some postoperative pts can have ab in 15–50% despite no evidence of thrombocytopenia or thrombosis; most commonly seen in orthopedic and CABG surgery (Blood 2000;96:1703), may be pos in 20% of pts on UFH and 8% of pts on LMWH (Am J Hematol 1996;52:90); given the high false positive rate, guidelines recommend against screening pts for HIT without thrombocytopenia, thrombosis, or other suggestive sx (Chest 2004;126:311S).
- Functional HIT assay, (aka serotonin release assay, or heparin-induced platelet activation assay): Mix pt serum with donor plt and heparin to look for ab binding and receptor activation, causing serotonin release from the plt; high PPV (89–100%) to rule in disease, but limited NPV (81%) (Am J Clin Path 1999;111:700).
- General approach to confirming HIT (NEJM 2006;355:809):
  - Neg HIT ab has high enough NPV to r/o disease in almost all pts (unless very high pretest probability based on clinical scenario; then recommend repeat testing in a few days or consider functional assay).
  - In pts with high pretest probability of HIT (using clinical scoring), a pos HIT antibody will confirm disease.
  - In pts with intermediate to low pretest probability, a pos HIT ab may be a false positive (especially in postsurgical pts); perform functional assay and if positive, HIT is present; if neg, consider other possibilities.

- In many centers, testing results are delayed; unless HIT felt to be very unlikely, discontinue heparin and treat for HIT until results available.

Noninv: No imaging tests assist in dx of HIT, but once definitively diagnosed should get lower extremity venous dopplers to r/o DVT (even in the absence of sx) because of the high rate of thrombosis (Chest 2004;126:311S); other imaging tests for thrombotic cmplc based on sx.

Rx: (Crit Care Med 2007;35:1165; Chest 2004;126:311S)

General approach to treatment of presumed HIT is as follows:

- Initially should have high index of suspicion for new drop in plt count in any pts on heparin therapy.
- Must immediately stop all sources of heparin (UFH or LMWH, therapeutic or prophylactic, and any line flushes or locks with heparin); however, cessation of heparin rx alone is not adequate therapy for HIT because of high risk of thrombosis.
    - In one study, up to 50% of pts with HIT who did not receive proper non-heparin anticoagulation after dx developed thrombosis within 1 mo (Blood 2004;104:3072).
    - 6% of untreated pts in another study developed thrombotic cmplc while awaiting results of confirmatory HIT testing (compared with 0.6% treated with alternative anticoagulants) (Blood 2000;96:846).
- Add heparin to pt's allergy list to avoid further exposure.
- Except in lowest risk pts based on HIT scoring, start alternative non-heparin anticoagulant rx until test results available (see "Non-heparin anticoagulants for the treatment of HIT" below for alternatives); switch to LMWH is not appropriate, as risk for HIT remains (even if lower than UFH).

- If HIT testing is neg, can resume heparin as appropriate and search for other causes of thrombocytopenia.
- If HIT testing is pos, continue anticoagulation and screen for lower extremity DVT; monitor closely for other si/sx of thrombosis; IV rx should be continued until plt count returns to normal (usually 5–7 d).
- Follow these guidelines for long-term anticoagulation with warfarin rx:
  - Should be considered for up to 4 wk in all pts with confirmed HIT; longer duration of rx in pts with documented thrombosis, based on type and risk factors; may require lifelong rx in some cases.
  - Unlike rx of non-HIT-related VTE, do not start warfarin rx at the time of dx; initial procoagulant effect of warfarin (by reducing proteins C and S levels) may cause in situ thrombosis and limb gangrene (Ann IM 1997;127:804); if pt already recently started on warfarin rx, consider administering vit K to reduce risk of gangrene.
  - Start warfarin at 5 mg qd once plt count normalized (greater than 150K).
  - Should have therapeutic overlap of warfarin and non-heparin IV anticoagulation for at least 5 d and at least 48 hr of therapeutic INR before discontinuation of IV rx
  - Monitoring of INR can be difficult because of PT prolongation from IV anticoagulants (unlike with heparins, which do not affect PT); see "Non-heparin anticoagulants for the treatment of HIT" below for details.
- Avoid plt transfusions; in most cases, unnecessary as plt count is usually more than 50K and bleeding cmplc rare (as thrombosis predominates); addition of extra plt may worsen thrombotic episodes; consider only in cases of severe thrombocytopenia associated with active bleeding.

Non-heparin anticoagulants for the treatment of HIT

- Argatroban
  - Probably the most commonly used agent in the United States for rx of HIT.
  - Direct thrombin inhibitor with rapid onset and short half-life (45 min); cleared by the liver.
  - Dose: Start IV infusion at 2 mcg/kg/min (no bolus required), except in pts with impaired hepatic function (0.5 mcg/kg/min), as determined by Child-Pugh score greater than 6 (see discussion of cirrhosis in Section 3.7 for details).
  - Monitor PTT; requires adjustment of dosing to maintain PTT 1.5 to 3 times normal.
  - Bleeding is major adverse effect; no direct inhibitor or reversal agent; if bleeding occurs, stop infusion and transfuse RBCs as appropriate.
  - Causes prolongation of PT, and therefore makes initiation of warfarin more difficult.
    - Obtain baseline PT/INR on argatroban prior to starting warfarin.
    - Start warfarin rx once plt count is normalized and pt taking adequate PO.
    - Target INR is (2 + baseline INR on argatroban); e.g., if baseline INR on argatroban is 2.3, target INR with addition of warfarin is 4.3.
    - Once target INR is reached, stop argatroban infusion for 2 hr and recheck INR (will now reflect only warfarin effect); if INR is greater than 2, can discontinue argatroban and continue warfarin monotherapy; if INR is less than 2, restart argatroban and continue overlapping therapy for another day.
    - Target long-term INR goal is 2–3.

- Lepirudin
  - Direct thrombin inhibitor with rapid onset and short half-life (60 min); is cleared by kidneys.
  - Dose: Start IV infusion at 0.1 mg/kg/hr; can give IV bolus of 0.2–0.4 mg/kg but reserve for limb- or life-threatening thrombosis; in pts with acute or chronic renal failure, start infusion at 0.01 mg/kg/hr (Crit Care Med 2007;35:1165).
  - Monitor PTT; requires adjustment of dosing to maintain PTT 1.5 to 2 times normal.
  - Bleeding is major adverse effect; no direct inhibitor or reversal agent; if bleeding occurs, stop infusion and transfuse RBCs as appropriate.
  - Can cause mild prolongation of PT, but not to degree of argatroban; check baseline INR prior to starting warfarin rx and manage as described for argatroban above.
  - Can lead to immune reaction with anti-lepirudin antibodies in up to 30% with first exposure (and 70% with second exposure) (Blood 2000;96:2373; J Thromb Haemost 2005;3:2428), especially with bolus and higher dosing; if antibodies develop, repeat dosing can cause life-threatening anaphylaxis (many advocate for single lifetime use only, which limits its widespread use as primary agent for HIT) (Circ 2003;108:2062).
- Bivalirudin
  - Direct thrombin inhibitor with rapid onset and short half-life (25 min).
  - Current evidence and FDA approval only for peri-PCI therapy in pts with active or prior HIT.
- Danaparoid
  - Inhibits Factor Xa.
  - Has been widely tested and used in Europe for HIT but was removed from U.S. market by manufacturer in 2002 (because of drug shortage).

- Fondaparinux
  - Inhibits Factor Xa.
  - Administered SQ at doses of 5–10 mg qd for VTE rx and 2.5 mg qd for VTE prophylaxis.
  - Has not been tested or approved for use in HIT rx, but mentioned here because drug can be safely used for VTE prophylaxis in pts with prior hx of HIT or as alternative anticoagulant in low-risk pts (by HIT scoring) until HIT can be safely ruled out by lab testing (Thromb Haemost 2008;99:208).

Future anticoagulation in patients with prior episode of HIT

- With hx of HIT, pts will likely have increased risk for VTE with subsequent hospitalizations, surgery, etc.
- If already anticoagulated on warfarin, continue therapy unless bleeding risk or surgical procedures prohibit.
- Fondaparinux should be 1st-line agent for VTE prophylaxis; low-dose SQ lepirudin (15 mg bid) can also be considered, but concerns for repeat use as described above.
- If IV therapy required, consider use of argatroban or other alternative non-heparin agent.
- If any heparin therapy considered (UFH or LMWH), follow these guidelines:
  - Absolutely avoid within 3 mo of acute HIT (because of risk of anaphylactic shock-like episode).
  - Consider pretesting for HIT ab (and possibly HIT functional assay); if neg, can consider closely monitored, short-term heparin use.

4.3 Neutropenia

(Cancer 2005;103:1103)

Cause: Defined as low absolute neutrophil count (ANC), either from bone marrow suppression or peripheral destruction of cells;

leukopenia denotes low total WBC, lymphopenia means reduced lymphocyte count; norms based on age and race; typically not clinically significant unless ANC is less than 1000/mcL, and criterion for febrile neutropenia guidelines is less than 500/mcL.

ANC calculation: (% of Neutrophils + % of Bands) × Total WBC

Causes of leukopenia include the following:

- Neutropenia
  - Chemotherapy (Cancer 2004;100:228): Most common cause in hospitalized pts due to direct bone marrow suppression; typically, WBC nadir from chemo is within 5–10 d of rx and lasts 2–3 wk; usually associated with concomitant anemia and thrombocytopenia.
  - Infection: Sepsis, many viral diseases (including EBV, VZV, CMV); usually mild to moderate neutropenia and does not clinically affect immunity or require specific rx, other than monitoring.
  - Drug-related (non-chemotherapy) (Ann IM 2007;146:657): Many drugs have been implicated; common drugs/classes include clozapine (antipsychotic, requires regular CBC monitoring due to risk of neutropenia), ticlopidine (use largely replaced by clopidogrel due to neutropenic risk), many abx, anticonvulsants (phenytoin, carbamazepine, valproate), antithyroid drugs, cimetidine, pain meds including APAP, salicyclates, NSAIDs.
  - Cancer-related: Acute leukemia, myelodysplasia.
  - Congenital causes: Very rare as new presentation in adults, unlike in children (J Clin Pathol 2001;54:7).
- Lymphopenia (Mayo Clin Proc 2005;80:923)
  - Infections: HIV/AIDS, tuberculosis, other viral infections, sepsis (mild, similar to neutropenia)
  - Drugs: Corticosteroids and other immunosuppressant drugs; alcohol

- Chronic disease: Autoimmune disorders, including SLE, RA; sarcoidosis
- Idiopathic, especially in pts older than 80 yr; possibly related to nutritional deficiency (Lancet 1996;347:328).

Microbial causes of febrile neutropenia include the following:

- Most cases presumed to be bacterial or fungal; although microbe isolated in only about 30–40% of cases.
- Traditionally, concern has been for Gram-negative organisms, specifically *Pseudomonas*, but recent studies have shown that most cases related to Gram-positives (~75% of isolates), with predominant organisms including MRSA and coagulase-negative staphylococci (CNS) (Clin Infect Dis 2003;36:1103).
- Common Gram-positives: *S. aureus* (including MRSA), CNS, *Enterococcus* (including VRE), *Streptococcus* spp.
- Common Gram negatives: *P. aeruginosa*, *E. coli*, *Klebsiella*, *Enterobacter*, *Acinetobacter*, *Citrobacter*, *Stenotrophomonas maltophilia* (Clin Infect Dis 1992;15:824).
- Fungal: *Candida*, *Aspergillus*.

Epidem: Febrile neutropenia admission associated with mortality rate of about 10% per episode, average LOS of 11 days, total costs of $20,000 (Cancer 2006;106:2258); infection is the cause of death in about 50% of pts with solid and blood-related tumors (Am Fam Phys 2006;74:1873).

Pathophys: Neutrophils are derived in the bone marrow from pluripotent stem cells; colony-stimulating factors direct the progression from myeloblast to promyelocyte to myelocyte, which then mature to metamyelocyte and then to band neutrophil and to polymorphonuclear neutrophil (PMN, mature cell); typically, PMNs predominate in peripheral circulation, but leukamoid reaction due to stress, critical illness, or steroids may lead to marrow release of immature forms (metamyelocytes and bands);

presence of other progenitor cells in circulation suggests leukemia or bone marrow infiltration, usually from cancer (J Clin Pathol 2001;54:7).

Sx/Si: Fever (temp higher than 101°F, 38°C) may be the only si present in many pts with febrile neutropenia; look for sx/si of focal infection (respiratory, GI, GU, oral ulcers, sinus disease); consider line infection if central venous catheter (CVC) in place (see "Central Venous Catheters and Associated Infections" in Section 5.3 of Chapter 5 for details).

Crs: Risk assessment models have been developed to determine low-risk pts with febrile neutropenia who may tolerate home rx with oral abx (Talcott, J Clin Oncol 1992;10:316; MASCC, J Clin Oncol 2000;18:3038); generally, pts at low risk for mortality and cmplc are young (younger than 60 yr), have minimal or no sx (other than fever) and unremarkable initial w/u, lack other comorbid diseases or prior episodes of fungal infection, and have no associated hypotension, dehydration, or respiratory distress.

Cmplc: Infections due to blunted immune response can occur with severe neutropenia.

Lab: W/u of febrile neutropenia includes CBC with diff, metabolic panel, liver and renal function tests; blood cultures (preferably two or more sets; if CVC present, may draw one set from line; at least 20% will have bacteremia) (Am J Med 1986;80:13); urinalysis and urine Cx (due to neutropenia, only ~10% of UTI pts will have pyuria) (Arch IM 1975;135:715); sputum culture (Gram stain usually neg for PMNs as well) (Med 1977; 56:241).

Stool studies and lumbar puncture in specific cases if suggested by hx, sx.

Avoid invasive procedures, unnecessary needle sticks or LP, digital rectal exams, which may increase risk of bacteremia.

Noninv: W/u of febrile neutropenia should include CXR in all cases, but normal CXR does not r/o pneumonia (up to 33% of neutropenic pts with pneumonia had normal initial CXR in one study, likely due to blunted immune response from neutropenia) (Med 1977;56:241); consider CT for further eval in pts with sx suggestive of pneumonia and normal CXR (NPV of ~90% if no findings of pneumonia on high-res CT) (J Clin Oncol 1999;17:796).

Rx: Mild to moderate isolated neutropenia generally requires no specific therapy except for rx of underlying infection, removal (if possible) of offending agents, and monitoring for progression to severe disease; no role for prophylactic abx or colony-stimulators in this group of pts.

For pts with lymphopenia, consider prophylaxis for *Pneumocystis* infection; see "*Pneumocystis* Pneumonia" in Section 5.6 for details.

Treatment of febrile neutropenia (Clin Infect Dis 2002;34:730) includes the following:

- If source is clear, please refer to specific sections in Chapter 5 for details (pneumonia, UTI, meningitis, etc.).
- Prior recommendations were for empitic rx with two-drug abx regimens, because of the primary concern for drug-resistant *Pseudomonas*; however, the presence of single agents with broad-spectrum coverage (including *Pseudomonas*) has now led to recommendation for single-drug therapy in most pts.
- Initial IV therapy:
  - Start with extended-spectrum penicillin (cefepime, ceftazidime), carbapenem (imipenem-cilastatin, meropenem, doripenem), or piperacillin-tazobactam.
  - If additional concern for drug-resistant Gram-negatives, based on pt hx or local resistance patterns, add aminoglycoside to above.
  - Addition of vancomycin (Clin Infect Dis 1999;29:503):

- Specifically for coverage of MRSA or resistant pneumococcus.
- Consider in the following pts: Known MRSA or resistant pneumococcus, frequently hospitalized pt with high rates of MRSA in facility, suspected CVC infection, critically ill/septic shock, Gram-positive organisms on initial blood Cx results (MMWR Recomm Rep 1995;44:1).
- Assess renal function for initial and subsequent dosing; consider pharmacy consult.
- Vancomycin not indicated for empiric therapy in all cases of febrile neutropenia (J Infect Dis 1991;163:951).
  - RCT of 428 stem cell transplant pts with febrile neutropenia; randomized to imipenem alone vs imipenem and vancomycin as initial rx; addition of vancomycin led to higher rate of resolution of fever without adjustment to initial rx (69% vs 55%, NNT 7), but no difference in overall time to fever resolution or mortality (Biol Blood Marrow Transplant 2009;15:512).
  - RCT of 747 pts with febrile neutropenia; randomized to ceftazidime/amikacin/vancomycin vs ceftazidime/amikacin only; addition of vancomycin showed no difference in fever duration or mortality, but vancomycin addition was associated with increased risk of renal failure (6% vs 2%, NNH 25) (J Infect Dis 1991;163:951).
  - Widespread use in this population would certainly contribute to increase in VRE rates.
- Linezolid has similar indications and efficacy for MRSA (Clin Infect Dis 2006;42:597).
- Initial antifungal rx recommended only in pts with prior hx or current si/sx suggestive of invasive fungal disease.

HEMATOLOGY

- Initial oral therapy:
  - Consider only for low-risk pts based on risk assessment described above; commonly used in outpatients, but can be considered for low-risk inpatients admitted for observation, or other conditions.
  - Common regimen is fluoroquinolone (ciprofloxacin, moxifloxacin, levofloxacin) plus amoxicillin-clavulanate (Augmentin) (NEJM 1999;341:305; NEJM 1999;341:312).
- Inadequate response to initial therapy:
  - Typical course is little improvement in fevers or neutropenia for about 3–5 d after initiating appropriate empiric therapy (J Clin Oncol 2000;18:3699).
  - Await results of Cx to identify microbe, if possible, and adjust abx therapy based on sensitivities.
  - If no response in 3–5 d, consider the following:
    - Continue close monitoring for sx to suggest source of infection or other causes of fever.
    - Addition of vancomycin, for reasons stated above, but no direct evidence to suggest this improves outcome unless MRSA or resistant pneumococcus detected.
    - Addition of antifungal agent, usually directed at *Candida* or *Aspergillus*; amphotericin B most commonly used and most evidence for benefit (Am J Med 1989;86:668); fluconazole (Am J Med 2000;108:282) and itraconazole (Ann IM 2001;135:412) are options (with safer side effect profile), but avoid if high institutional rates of resistant *Candida* or if suspected *Aspergillus* with respiratory or sinus disease (does not cover, use voriconazole).
  - If CVC in place, can consider removal, but not necessary in all cases; see "Central Venous Catheters and Associated Infections" in Section 5.3 for details.
- Duration of antibiotic therapy:
  - If confirmed source, treat based on guidelines for specific disease.

- Otherwise, continue empiric or directed rx until clinical response (afebrile for 48 hr) and resolution of neutropenia (ANC more than 500).
- If clinically improved, but neutropenia persists, can consider transition to oral regimen as above.
- Colony-stimulating factors (CSFs) include granulocyte colony-stimulating factor (G-CSF, filgrastim) and granulocyte-macrophage colony-stimulating factor (GM-CSF, sargramostim).
  - IDSA (Clin Infect Dis 2002;34:730) and American Society of Clinical Oncology (J Clin Oncol 2000;18:3558) recommend against routine use of CSFs in febrile neutropenia.
  - Multiple studies have shown improvement in neutropenia, but no significant effects on other clinical outcomes, including fever duration, mortality, or cost of care (Clin Infect Dis 2002;34:730).
  - Consider in cases of critical illness with febrile neutropenia (sepsis, shock, overwhelming pneumonia), especially if not expecting rapid improvement in neutropenia (as expected s/p chemotherapy).
  - Dose: Filgrastim 5 mcg/kg SQ qd until ANC normalized.

4.4 Multiple Myeloma

(Mayo Clin Proc 2005;80:1371, Am Fam Phys 2008;78:853)

Cause: Bone marrow cancer affecting plasma cells, with elevated serum levels of monoclonal protein (immunoglobulin chains). Definitions and diff dx:

- Multiple myeloma (MM): Presence of typical sx, confirmed with laboratory evidence of myeloma (monoclonal protein spike of more than 3 gm/dL, more than 10% plasma cells on marrow aspirate).
- Monoclonal gammopathy of undetermined significance (MGUS) (NEJM 2006;355:2765): Presence of monoclonal

protein spike (less than 3 gm/dL) with no clinical si/sx of MM; progresses to MM in about 1–2% of cases per yr (NEJM 2002;346:564), but most cases of MM do not have prior documented MGUS.

- "Smoldering" (asx) MM (NEJM 2007;356:2582): Laboratory evidence of myeloma, but lack of end-organ damage (see CRAB in Cmplc below); progresses to sx at rate of about 10% per yr.
- Nonsecretory MM: Due to abnormal light chain disease only; may present with classic sx and cmplc, but neg SPEP/UPEP and diagnose by serum free light chains (FLC) assay.
- Waldenstrom's macroglobulinemia (WM) (Blood 2007;109:5096): Rare disorder of lymphoplasmacytic lymphoma associated with monoclonal gammopathy with IgM proteins; can present in similar fashion as MM, but differentiate by signs of hepatosplenomegaly, bleeding cmplc (Br J Haematol 2001;115:575), lack of bone lesions; presence of IgM spike (rare in MM).
- Amyloidosis: Particularly, amyloid light chain (AL) amyloidosis (Mayo Clin Proc 2006;81:693); rare disorder with overproduction of Ig light chains leading to tissue deposition with neuro, cardiac, renal, bone marrow cmplc; differentiate from MM by presence of light chain disease only, lack of bone disease and amyloid deposition (by Congo red staining) in affected tissues.
- Metastatic carcinoma: Can lead to similar sx as MM, including monoclonal gammopathy, but differentiate by lack of significant plasma cells on marrow aspirate.
- Other hematologic cancers include chronic lymphocytic leukemia (usually presents with massive leukocytosis), lymphoma, plasmacytoma.

Epidem: Median age at dx is 65–70 yr; fewer than 2% of cases in pts younger than 40 yr (Mayo Clin Proc 2003;78:21).

Annual U.S. incidence 15,000 to 20,000 new cases; prevalence 50,000 to 60,000 cases; more common among African Americans (2:1) in the United States (Am J Med 1998;104:439).

Pathophys: Plasma cells (form of B-lymphocytes) predominantly in bone marrow (but also in circulation and lymph nodes) produce large amounts of immunoglobulins (Ig, aka antibodies) as part of the humoral immune response; Ig can take the form of IgG (most commonly), IgM (acute ab formed in response to new antigen), IgA (found predominantly in gut and respiratory mucosa), IgE (associated with allergic response), IgD; but all composed of two heavy chains and one light chain.

In MM, overproduction of Ig leads to elevated serum protein levels, activation of cytokines to stimulate osteoclasts and suppress osteoblasts (causing lytic bone lesions), and angiogenesis factors causing new blood vessel growth; renal disease is a manifestation of cast nephropathy (intrinsic tubular damage from high protein loads).

Sx: Will be asx in early stages (MGUS, smoldering MM); found incidentally with presence of elevated serum total protein.

Constitutional sx of fatigue, weakness, night sweats, anorexia, and weight loss; lytic bone lesions can lead to diffuse or localized bone pain.

Si: If hepatosplenomegaly, mucocutaneous bleeding, consider WM.

Crs: Median survival after dx is 3 yr; 5-yr survival about 33%.

Cmplc: Main complications of MM follow the CRAB mnemonic (hyper**C**alcemia, **R**enal failure, **A**nemia, **B**one lesions); percentages listed below are based on Mayo review of ~1000 new cases of MM (Mayo Clin Proc 2003;78:21):

- Hypercalcemia (13% with serum Ca 11 mg/dL or more): See "Hypercalcemia" in Section 2.4 for more details.
- Renal failure (19% with serum Cr 2 mg/dL or more): Also called "myeloma kidney."

- Anemia (73% with Hgb less than 10 gm/dL): Typically normocytic; r/o concomitant iron, B12, folate deficiencies.
- Bone lesions (79%): Lytic lesions of the bone, can lead to bone pain and pathologic fractures in up to 33% (Mayo Clin Proc 2003;78:21); most commonly vertebral compression and femur fx.
- Other potential cmplc include the following:
  - Myeloma pts have an increased risk of infections.
  - Peripheral neuropathy (including carpal tunnel syndrome) can occur.
  - Tumor lysis syndrome (Mayo Clin Proc 2006;81:835): More commonly seen in aggressive hematological malignancies (leukemias, lymphomas) than in MM; due to release of cell contents in rapidly dividing and dying cells (especially after therapies); suggested by serum findings of increased uric acid, increased potassium, increased phosphate, decreased calcium (due to hyperphosphatemia), and elevated LDH; may lead to acute renal failure, cardiac arrhythmias (due to electrolyte disturbances), seizures, coma; see Rx below.
  - Hyperviscosity syndrome (Mayo Clin Proc 2006;81:835; J Intensive Care Med 1995;10:128): More commonly seen in WM and acute leukemias than in MM; increased serum viscosity due to protein leads to stasis/sludging, ischemia, and bleeding cmplc; sx can include spontaneous bleeding, CNS disturbances (delirium, stroke, coma), visual deficits, CHF; diagnose by clinical sx in at-risk pts and by serum viscosity of more than 4–5 cP (Am J Med 1985;79:13).

Lab: Initial w/u for possible MM should include the following:

- CBC with diff: Look for anemia; presence of neutropenia or thrombocytopenia might suggest other bone marrow disorder.
- Electrolytes: Hypercalcemia suggests MM or other disease causing bone destruction; hyperphosphatemia,

especially if renal disease, tumor lysis syndrome, or may have "pseudo" hyperphos due to binding to high levels of serum protein.

- Renal function: Elevated BUN/Cr suggest intrinsic renal disease, although concomitant dehydration not uncommon; see Section 8.3, "Acute Renal Failure," for differential dx.
- SPEP: Required to assess for monoclonal protein spike (3 gm/dL or more).
- UPEP: Will corroborate SPEP in most cases; but may be pos in some cases of MM with neg SPEP due to predominant light chain disease; can also do 24-hr urine protein assessments and check for Bence Jones protein (light chains).
- Serum FLC assay in pts with strong suspicion for MM, but neg SPEP/UPEP (nonsecretory MM).
- Uric acid: Screen for hyperuricemia after dx made and before starting rx to reduce risk of worsening ARF and tumor lysis syndrome.
- ESR: Should be more than 50 mm in almost all cases (except nonsecretory forms), but little value in overall eval.

Noninv: Skeletal survey for lytic lesions; should be pos in majority of cases of MM; if none, consider "smoldering" MM if no other cmplc present, WM, amyloid, other dx; if cmplc present and lytic lesions seen on other studies (e.g., head CT), not necessary to get skeletal survey and base further imaging on concern for pathologic fx.

Imaging with CT or MRI based on assessment of cmplc, particularly fx (MRI may help determine new vertebral compression fx amenable to therapy); avoid contrast dye due to nephrotoxicity in setting of ARF.

Consider EKG if severe electrolyte disturbances.

Bone marrow bx required for proper dx, should reveal plasma cell concentration greater than 10% (if less than 10% with clinical si/sx, consider metastatic disease from other primary cancer as cause of sx).

Rx: General approach to MM therapy (NEJM 2004;351:1860) includes these guidelines:

- Once dx suspected or confirmed, should get oncology consultation as inpatient (or accelerated outpatient) for decisions on rx.
- Almost all cases of MGUS and "smoldering" MM do not require immediate therapy, other than close monitoring; however, these cases are rarely seen as inpatients (unless hyperproteinemia found incidentally while evaluating for other disease).
- Management of cmplc:
  - Hypercalcemia: See "Hypercalcemia" in Section 2.4 for details.
  - Renal failure: Hydrate initially because newly diagnosed MM pts may have dehydration related to age, weakness, poor PO intake; avoid nephrotoxic drugs (NSAIDs, aminoglycoside, CT contrast dye); see "Acute Renal Failure," Section 8.3, for details.
  - Anemia: Most require monitoring only, unless additional nutritional deficiency; transfusions should be given in most cases only if Hgb is 7 gm/dL or less (see discussion of transfusion practices in Section 4.1); consider erythropoietin-stimulating agents; epoetin beta 150 U/kg 3 times weekly for 16 wk decreased transfusions, severe anemia, and improved QOL scores in pts with hematological malignancies (33% of pts had MM) and baseline Hgb less than 10 gm/dL with prior transfusions (J Clin Oncol 2002;20:2486); epoetin alfa also effective with same dosing (Br J Haematol 2001;113:172).
  - Bone lesions: Pain control, usually with opiates (try APAP first, avoid NSAIDs); rx of associated hypercalcemia and consider long-term bisphosphonate rx (Cochrane 2002; CD003188); if long-bone fx, manage according to orthopedic

consultation; if vertebral compression fx, consider MRI or bone scan to evaluate acute vs chronic and if acute, consider vertebroplasty (direct injection of bone cement into the collapsed vertebral body) (Am J Neuroradiol 2008;29:642) or kyphoplasty (balloon expansion of the vertebral body followed by injection of methyl methacrylate) (Eur Spine J 2009;18(suppl)1:115); bone pain without fx can be treated with focused radiotherapy (Cochrane 2004;CD004721).

- Tumor lysis syndrome (Mayo Clin Proc 2006;81:835): Main rx is prevention by checking pretreatment electrolytes and uric acid; treat hyperuricemia with allopurinol 600 mg loading dose, then 300 mg qd (reduced dosage in renal failure, low body weight; IV dosing available if unable to take PO); or in most severe cases, IV rasburicase 0.05–0.2 mg/kg qd; in acute tumor lysis syndrome, aggressive IVF with isotonic saline and rx hyperK, hyperphos, hypoCa as described in separate sections.
- Hyperviscosity syndrome (Mayo Clin Proc 2006;81:835): Avoid RBC transfusions as may worsen disease; treat underlying disease as appropriate; plasmapheresis in severe cases (Semin Thromb Hemost 2003;29:535).

- Concern for concomitant infections, even if not neutropenic; consider vaccination for influenza, pneumococcus, H. influenzae; if on long-term steroid rx, consider prophylaxis against Pneumocystis (see Section 5.6 for details).
- Primary therapy for MM: All therapies are palliative, as cure not possible, even with transplantation procedures; however, as therapies have evolved many pts may die with, not from, MM (for an excellent review and consensus guidelines, see Mayo Clin Proc 2009;84:1095).
  - Consider autologous or allogeneic stem cell transplantation (SCT) based on age, functional status, other comorbid diseases.

- Initial chemotherapy depends on whether pt is considered a candidate for SCT (NEJM 2004;351:1860).
  - Induction therapy with plan for SCT: Would base decision on local oncology expertise and pt factors; options for rx include combinations of the following:
    - Dexamethasone (Decadron): Corticosteroid; common adverse effects include weight gain, adrenal suppression, Cushing's-like syndrome, hyperglycemia, euphoria, depression, cataracts.
    - Thalidomide (Thalomid): Initially used in the 1950s as sedative and antiemetic, until withdrawn from the market for severe teratogenicity; likely antiangiogenesis effects in MM; common adverse effects include sedation, constipation, peripheral neuropathy; VTE in 1–3% with monotherapy, but about 25% in combination regimens (NEJM 2001;344:1951; Blood 2001;98:1614), so guidelines recommend LMWH or warfarin qd with combo regimens (Mayo Clin Proc 2009;84:1095); absolutely contraindicated in women of child-bearing age, although MM very unlikely in this population.
    - Lenalidomide (Revlimid): Analog of thalidomide; antiangiogenesis effects; oral therapy; common side effects include fatigue, thrombocytopenia; VTE risk and recommendations similar to thalidomide.
    - Bortezomib (Velcade): Proteasome inhibitor with antiangiogenesis effects; given as cycles of IV infusion; common adverse effects include bone marrow suppression (especially thrombocytopenia), fatigue, diarrhea, peripheral neuropathy.
    - Prior chemotherapy regimen with vincristine, doxorubicin, and dexamethasone (VAD regimen) not used as frequently due to toxicity, need for

continuous central access, and likelihood that most effect from steroids.

- Therapy in non-SCT pts: Melphalan and prednisone orally on 6-wk cycles; meta-analysis showed no difference in response rates with traditional chemotherapy regimens, with less toxicity (J Clin Oncol 1998;16:3832); recent guidelines suggest addition of thalidomide or lenalidomide (Mayo Clin Proc 2009;84:1095).

Chapter 5
Infectious Disease

5.1 Antimicrobial Medications

Following is a brief overview of widely available antimicrobial agents, mainly focusing on those available in IV form for inpatient use; please confirm antibacterial coverage with your local resistance patterns.

1st generation penicillins

- Covers streptococci and oral anaerobes
- Penicillin G 250K–400K U/kg/d IV split q 4–6 hr
- Oral meds: penicillin V

2nd generation penicillins

- Penicillinase-resistant, antistaphylococcal
- Nafcillin 1–2 gm IV q 4 hr; adverse effects: ASA-like plt impairment (NEJM 1974;291:265); dose-dependent neutropenia; hard on veins
- Oxacillin 1–2 gm IV q 4 hr; adverse effects: reversible anicteric hepatitis, occurs at greater than 1 gm qd (Ann IM 1978;89:497); hard on veins
- Oral meds: dicloxacillin

3rd generation penicillins

- Streptococci and some Gram-neg coverage
- Ampicillin 1–2 gm IV q 4–6 hr; penicillinase-sensitive
- Ampicillin-sulbactam (Unasyn) 1.5–3 gm IV q 6 hr
- Oral meds: amoxicillin, ampicillin, amoxicillin-clavulanate (Augmentin)

4th generation penicillins

- Extended spectrum, antipseudomonal
- Piperacillin 3–4 gm IV q 4 hr
- Piperacillin-tazobactam (Zosyn) 3.375–4.5 gm IV q 6 hr; good single broad-spectrum coverage agent
- Ticarcillin-clavulanate (Timentin) 3.1 gm IV q 4–6 hr; spectrum includes staph, Gram-negs, and anaerobes

1st generation cephalosporins

- Good staph/strep coverage (except MRSA, *Enterococcus*), some Gram-negs; some cross-reactivity with PCN allergy (for whole class)
- Cefazolin (Ancef) 1–1.5 gm IV q 6–8 hr
- Oral meds: cephalexin (Keflex), cefadroxil (Duricef)

2nd generation cephalosporins

- Better Gram-neg and some anaerobic coverage
- Cefoxitin (Mefoxin) 1–2 gm IV q 6–8 hr; spectrum includes anaerobes
- Cefuroxime (Zinacef) 750–1500 mg IV q 8 hr; spectrum includes H. flu and *Moraxella catarrhalis*
- Oral meds: cefaclor (Ceclor), cefprozil (Cefzil), cefuroxime (Ceftin)

3rd generation cephalosporins

- Better Gram-neg and anaerobic coverage, but not consistent antipseudomonal and not as much antistaphylococcal activity as 1st generation
- Ceftriaxone (Rocephin) 1–2 gm IV q 12–24 hr; good cerebrospinal fluid (CSF) penetration, hence best for blind rx of meningitis (NEJM 1990;322:141); can be used for penicillin-sensitive strep SBE, useful as outpatient drug (JAMA 1992; 267:264); adverse effects: pseudo-cholecystitis and true gallstones (Ann IM 1991;115:712), very rare severe acute

hemolysis (Med Lett Drugs Ther 2002;44:100); im formulation good bridge in pts with inadequate IV access
- Cefotaxime (Claforan) 1–2 gm IV q 6–8 hr
- Ceftazidime (Fortaz) 1–2 gm IV q 6–8 hr; good vs *Pseudomonas* but high MIC for staph so not reliable for it
- Ceftizoxime (Cefizox) 1–2 gm IV q 8–12 hr
- Oral meds: cefdinir (Omnicef), cefixime (Suprax), cefpodoxime (Vantin), ceftibuten (Cedax)

4th generation cephalosporins

- Broad spectrum, antipseudomonal coverage
- Cefepime (Maxipime) 1–2 gm IV q 12 hr

Aminoglycosides

- Work well vs Gram-neg bacilli; some activity against staph, penicillin-resistant diphtheroids, enterococci with a penicillin; all renal and vestibular toxic; once daily dosing reasonable and perhaps less toxic (BMJ 1996;312:338; Ann IM 1996;124:717; Ann IM 1992;117:693)
- Amikacin 15 mg/kg/d IV divided q 8–12 hr; useful for resistant Gram-negs
- Gentamicin 5–7 mg/kg IV q 24 hr (or 3–5 mg/kg/d IV divided q 8 hr); get peak level 30 min after dose (6–9 mcg/mL) and trough 30 min before dose (less than 2 mcg/mL); vestibular toxicity is worse than auditory nerve toxicity
- Tobramycin: same dosing as gentamicin, more expensive; less renal toxicity, monitor levels with goal peak level 5–10 mcg/mL; also in nebulized form for CF/bronchiectasis pts

Carbapenems

- Broad spectrum, antipseudomonal coverage; some cross-reactivity with PCN allergy
- Imipenem-cilastatin (Primaxin) 500–1000 mg IV q 6 hr; resistant to penicillinase; broader spectrum than 3rd

generation cephalosporins; good vs strep, staph, anaerobes; resistant *H. influenzae*, most Gram-negs; gets into CSF; *Pseudomonas* resistance develops; inadequate vs penicillin-resistant pneumococcus, MRSA, *Enterococcus*, *Mycoplasma*, *Chlamydia*; adverse effects: seizures

- Doripenem (Doribax) 500 mg IV q 8 hr
- Meropenem (Merrem) 500 mg IV q 8 hr; similar to imipenem/cilastatin but a little better vs Gram-negs and a little less coverage of Gram-pos organisms; ok vs *Listeria*; renal excretion
- Ertapenem (Invanz) 1 gm IV q 24 hr; can be used for CAP like ceftriaxone daily in elderly (J Am Ger Soc 2003;51:1526); similar spectrum to other carbapenems but not for *Pseudomonas* and *Acinetobacter spp.* (avoid for nosocomial infections)

2nd generation fluoroquinolones

- Staphylococcal, atypical, and Gram-neg coverage, but poor pneumococcal coverage
- Avoid all in pregnant women and children younger than 18 (due to cartilage damage) (NEJM 1991;324:384)
- Ciprofloxacin (Cipro) 400 mg IV q 12 hr; no coverage of anaerobes, *Enterococcus*, *Chlamydia*, staph (resistance develops quickly) (Ann IM 1991;114:424), or strep, but gets all else including gonorrhea and other Gram-negs including *Pseudomonas aeruginosa* in UTIs, nosocomial infections (as 2nd-line agent), bronchiectasis and CF pts; as prophylaxis in leukemias (Ann IM 1987;106:1; Ann IM 1987;106:7); adverse effects: causes increases in theophylline levels
- Oral meds: ciprofloxacin, norfloxacin (Noroxin), ofloxacin (Floxin)

3rd generation fluoroquinolones

- Covers same as 2nd generation but with better antipneumococcal coverage and same antipseudomonal coverage

- Levofloxacin (Levaquin) 500–750 mg IV qd; like others, is active isomer component of ofloxacin, better than Cipro vs Gram-pos cocci; covers atypicals, resistant pneumococcus, H. flu, and *Moraxella*, but not as good as Cipro vs Gram-negs; 750 mg dosing (for 5 d) is preferred for CAP coverage; can prolong QT interval
- Oral meds: levofloxacin

4th generation fluoroquinolones

- Covers same as 3rd generation with better antipneumococcal coverage, but without adequate antipseudomonal activity
- Gatifloxacin (Tequin) 400 mg IV qd; like levofloxacin, covers atypicals, resistant pneumococcus, H. flu, and *Moraxella*, but not as good as Cipro vs Gram-negs; may prolong QT; dysglycemias (i.e., hypoglycemia and rarer hyperglycemia) in nondiabetic pts (NEJM 2006;354:1352)
- Moxifloxacin (Avelox) 400 mg IV qd; can prolong QT interval
- Oral meds: gatifloxacin, gemifloxacin (Factive), moxifloxacin

Macrolides

- Beware cardiotoxic effects (prolonged QT) when given with terfenadine and other nonsedating antihistamines (JAMA 1996;275:1339), or alone especially in women (JAMA 1998;280:1774)
- Azithromycin (Zithromax) 500 mg IV qd (may switch to 250 mg after first dose); fewer GI sx than erythromycin; less coverage for staph and strep than erythromycin; long half-life, 5-day course may have measurable levels past 10 days (which may be a factor in developing resistance)
- Oral meds: azithromycin, erythromycin (E-mycin), clarithromycin (Biaxin)

Monobactams

- Aztreonam (Azactam) 500–2000 mg IV q 6–12 hr; used vs aerobic Gram-negs; consider for CAP coverage in pts with severe PCN allergy

Oxazolidinones

- Linezolid (Zyvox) (Ann IM 2003;138:135) 600 mg IV q 12 hr; mainly for MRSA and other vancomycin-resistant organisms; adverse effects: GI sx, MAO inhibitor so avoid with tyramine-containing foods and several antidepressants, myelosuppression with prolonged use
- Oral meds: linezolid

Sulfonamides

- Trimethoprim-sulfamethoxazole (Septra, Bactrim) 15–20 mg/kg/d IV divided q 6–8 hr; adverse effects: severe allergic reactions; renal failure and hemolysis, especially in elderly; resistance develops in GI tract organisms with prophylactic use; neutropenia with azathioprine (Imuran) due to folate metabolism interference (Ann IM 1980;93:560); hyperkalemia (Ann IM 1993;119:291; Ann IM 1993;119:296; Ann IM 1996; 124:316)
- Oral meds: trimethoprim-sulfamethoxazole

Tetracyclines

- Doxycycline (Vibramycin) 100 mg IV q 12 hr; adverse effects: photosensitivity, fatty liver in pregnancy (Ann IM 1987;106:703), GI intolerance
- Tigecycline (Tygacil) 100 mg IV loading dose, then 50 mg IV q 12 hr; broad-spectrum coverage including Gram-pos and Gram-neg organisms, anaerobes, and MRSA for abdominal and skin infections, but not *Pseudomonas* or *Proteus*
- Oral meds: doxycycline, minocycline (Minocin), tetracycline

Miscellaneous

- Chloramphenicol (Chloromycetin) 500 mg/kg/d IV divided
  q 6 hr; im as good as IV (NEJM 1985;313:410); vs anaerobes,
  E. coli, Salmonella, Rickettsia; liver excretion; adverse effects:
  aplastic anemia, dose-related or allergic; rarely used in developed world
- Clindamycin (Cleocin) 600–900 mg IV q 8 hr; vs anaerobes,
  especially with gentamicin, as well as soft tissue and bone
  infections with staph and strep; adverse effects: high rates of
  C. difficile colitis
- Metronidazole (Flagyl) 500 mg IV q 6 hr; vs *Trichomonas,
  Giardia*, amoebic abscess, most anaerobes especially *B. fragilis;*
  adverse effects: Antabuse effect (GI sx with concomitant
  alcohol use), decreased warfarin metabolism
- Quinupristin-dalfopristin (Synercid) 7.5 mg/kg IV q 8 hr; active vs MRSA and vancomycin-resistant enterococci; numerous drug interactions; very expensive
- Vancomycin 1 gm IV q 12 hr (may underdose larger pts with
  normal renal function; consider 15–20 mg/kg q 12 hr); IV
  form mainly for MRSA and *Enterococcus;* tissue penetration
  not as good as other antistaph drugs for MSSA, so use another
  drug once MRSA excluded; monitor trough levels just before
  dosing with goal level of at least 10 mg/L (15–20 mg/L for
  severe infections), especially in pts with renal failure; does not
  cross gut lumen, so IV form ineffective for *C. diff* colitis (and
  PO form is not effective for any other indication); adverse
  effects: "red man" syndrome (diffuse erythema with rapid infusion) (Med Lett Drugs Ther 2009;51:25)

5.2 Gastrointestinal Infections

Acute Diarrhea and Gastroenteritis

(Am J Med 1999;106:670; NEJM 2009;361:1560)

Cause: Defined as loose stools, more than 200 gm/d, present for less than 4 weeks.

Most cases are viral, but bacteria more prevalent in pts requiring hospitalization because of severe disease.

Infectious causes include the following:

- Viral: Includes rotavirus, norovirus (aka Norwalk-like virus), adenovirus, among others (NEJM 1991;325:252)
- Bacterial: *Shigella, Salmonella, Campylobacter, E. coli* (five different subtypes: enterotoxigenic and enteropathogenic cause watery diarrhea; enteroinvasive, enterohemorrhagic, enteroaggregative cause inflammatory diarrhea), *Clostridium difficile, Bacillus cereus, Staphylococcus aureus, Vibrio*
- Parasitic: *Giardia, Cryptosporidium* (NEJM 2002;346:1723), *Entamoeba histolytica*

The following are noninfectious causes of acute diarrhea to consider in the differential diagnosis:

- Medication (including abx) side effects
- Inflammatory bowel disease (Crohn's, ulcerative colitis)
- Radiation or ischemic colitis
- Bacterial overgrowth syndromes
- Functional bowel disorders (i.e., "irritable bowel")
- Diet-related: high-sugar diets, dumping syndrome, food intolerances
- Carcinoid syndrome: secretory tumor causing flushing, diarrhea, other sx (JAMA 1988;260:1602)

Traveler's diarrhea associated with travel to Mexico, Central and South America, southeast Asia, Middle East, usually due to bacterial cause.

Hospital-acquired diarrhea is *C. difficile* until proven otherwise; new-onset diarrhea in pt hospitalized more than 3 days is very unlikely to be any other infectious cause (aka "3-day rule" to prevent unnecessary stool cultures); consider nosocomial infections, med effects (including standing bowel regimens), tube feedings; however, pts with risk factors of age older than 65, significant comorbidities, neutropenia, or HIV infection may benefit from stool Cx, even after 3 days in hospital (JAMA 2001;285:313).

Epidem: U.S. incidence of about one episode per person per year, although rates of hospitalization are much lower.

Pathophys: Most causative organisms obtained by fecal-oral route; mechanisms to prevent infection include (1) gastric acidity, (2) gut-associated lymphoid tissue (GALT), (3) GI motility.

Sx/Si: Differentiate two main types: noninflammatory, watery diarrhea vs inflammatory diarrhea with mucous, blood.

Large volume, watery stools with associated dehydration suggest viral, cholera (*Vibrio*), parasitic infections.

Inflammatory diarrhea with fever, abdominal pain, hematochezia, mucous suggests bacterial causes including *Salmonella*, *Shigella*, *Campylobacter*, *E. coli*, *C. difficile*.

Crs: Most cases, with or without active treatment, are self-limited, less than 7 days; longer course suggests nonviral infectious or noninfectious causes.

Cmplc: Severe dehydration; anemia if significant hematochezia.

Rare cmplc of Guillain-Barre syndrome (GBS) (especially with *Campylobacter* infections; see Section 6.3), reactive arthritis, hemolytic uremic syndrome (HUS) (associated with treatment for *E. coli* O157:H7), toxic megacolon (*C. difficile*).

Lab: Usually history (travel, sick contacts, food exposure, other recent or chronic illnesses, antibiotic use, etc.) is much more important to determining etiology than routine lab testing.

Reserve dx testing for sick pts with inflammatory diarrhea, requiring hospitalization, or with persistent sx; or those at high-risk given recent travel or immune compromise.

Stool cultures for bacteria; ova and parasite examinations; direct assays for *C. diff* toxin, *Giardia*, *E. coli* O157:H7.

In cases associated with dehydration, consider electrolytes, renal function testing.

Yield of stool cultures (Ann IM 1997;126:505):

- 30,000 inpatients with stool Cx; 5.6% yielded at least one bacterium.
- *Campylobacter* 41%; *Salmonella* 32%; *Shigella* 19%; *E. coli* O157:H7 7%.
- Fever was more commonly associated with *Salmonella* and *Shigella* on Cx.
- Visible or occult blood in stools more commonly associated with *E. coli*.

Fecal leukocytes typically suggest inflammatory, bacterial cause.

Carcinoid tumor with elevated urinary 5-hydroxyindoleacetic acid (5-HIAA) levels.

Noninv: Imaging (plain films, CT, US) may not prove helpful, unless concern for cmplc like ileus/obstruction, intestinal perforation; if used routinely, may show nonspecific bowel wall thickening of uncertain significance (which may prompt further unnecessary testing).

Endoscopy should be considered if concern for *C. diff* colitis with neg toxin assays (see "*Clostridium difficile* Colitis" later in Section 5.2) or noninfectious cause such as IBD or ischemic colitis.

Rx: (Gut 2004;53:296)

For most pts, treatment is only supportive, with IV fluid hydration or oral replacement therapy; many cases, especially in children, associated with a non-anion gap metabolic acidosis, which does not require bicarbonate replacement.

Also consider antispasmodics (opiates, loperamide [Imodium]) except in severe, inflammatory diarrheas, and bismuth subsalicylate (Pepto-Bismol) to stimulate fluid resorption in gut and toxin-binding.

Empiric antibiotics for community-acquired inflammatory diarrhea:

- Swedish study of 598 pts with acute diarrhea (70% had recent travel); randomized to norfloxacin 400 mg bid for 5 days vs placebo; rx reduced diarrhea sx by 1 day (3 vs 4 d for placebo), but only in pts with pos stool Cx and severe disease (Ann IM 1992;117:202).
- RCT of 173 pts with acute diarrhea randomized to ciprofloxacin 500 mg bid for 5 d vs placebo; rx reduced sx and rates of carriage in f/u stool Cx (Clin Infect Dis 1996;22:1019).
- IDSA guidelines (Clin Infect Dis 2001;32:331) suggest abx treatment for:
  - Traveler's diarrhea, which carries a high rate of bacterial causes, particularly enterotoxigenic *E. coli*
  - Severely ill or immunocompromised pts
- Avoid abx in these settings:
  - Known cases of enterohemorrhagic *E. coli,* because of the risk of hemolytic-uremic syndrome associated with treatment
  - Non-typhoid *Salmonella,* which does not improve with therapy, and abx may actually prolong shedding (GE 2000;118:S48)
- Empiric therapy for acute inflammatory diarrhea (except C. *diff*) can be a fluoroquinolone for 3 to 5 days; macrolides can be used if concern for allergy or FQ resistance.

Targeted abx therapies in specific types of diarrhea (GE 2000;118:S48) include:

- C. *difficile* colitis: vancomycin or metronidazole (see "*Clostridium difficile* Colitis" later in Section 5.2).
- Enteric fever (*S. typhi* and *paratyphi*): depends on local resistance patterns, usually FQ, 3rd or 4th generation cephalosporins
- *Vibrio cholerae:* tetracycline 500 mg qid for 3 d, doxycycline 300 mg single dose rx

- Giardiasis: metronidazole 250 mg PO tid for 5 d
- Cryptosporidiosis in pts with HIV/AIDS: paramycin, azithromycin, nitazoxonide (NEJM 2002;346:1723)
- CMV colitis in immunocompromised pts: IV gancyclovir, foscarnet

Clostridium difficile Colitis

(NEJM 2008;359:1932; Ann IM 2006;145:758)

Cause: Due to infection and toxins produced by *C. difficile* in the colon of the host; aka antibiotic-associated diarrhea; was originally thought to be related to *S. aureus* colitis, until *C. difficile* was isolated.

Other causes of diarrhea associated with abx therapy include (NEJM 2002;346:334):

- Other bacterial pathogens (see "Acute Diarrhea and Gastroenteritis" earlier in Section 5.2)
- Direct drug effects on the intestinal mucosa
- Bacterial overgrowth syndromes
- Irritable bowel syndrome

Classically associated with clindamycin and cephalosporin rx, but recent strains also seem to be linked to excessive use of fluoroquinolones; at this point, almost all antibiotics have been linked to cases of *C. diff*.

Risk factors for disease, in addition to abx use, include elderly pts, severe comorbidities, presence of NG tube, ICU care, long hospital LOS, long duration of abx use or multiple abx (BMJ 2005;331:498).

Use of antiulcer meds is controversial; some studies have shown correlation (JAMA 2005;294:2989), but others have argued this is just a marker of severe disease (i.e., use of GI prophylaxis in critically ill pts); spores are not affected by GI tract pH.

Epidem: Incidence has greatly increased over the past 10 years: from 31/100K in 1996 to 84/100K in 2005.

Have also encountered an increase in severe infections and associated mortality in recent years associated with a new strain of bacteria (NAP-1/027 strain).

Pathophys: Antibiotic therapy in a susceptible host, exposed to C. *diff* spores, allows for bacterial growth and production of toxins A and B, which cause the sx of disease.

Some pts can have asymptomatic colonization (probably less than 5%) (J Infect Dis 1985;151:476), but may be higher in hospitalized pts (J Hosp Infect 1999;43:317).

Sx/Si: Frequent, watery diarrhea; occasional hematochezia; crampy abdominal pain.

Severe cases present with signs of hypovolemia (dizziness, thirst, oliguria, dry mucous membranes), sepsis/SIRS (fever, tachycardia, diaphoresis), delirium.

Crs: Most cases respond to initial abx therapy, but rates of recurrence after abx are quite high: 20% after first episode, 40% after second, 60% after multiple recurrences (Am J Gastroenterol 2002;97:1769); most occur within 2 weeks of stopping abx therapy.

In cases of recurrent disease, about 50% are relapses of initial infection not fully treated and about 50% are new exposure to spores; does not generally represent resistance to abx therapy.

Marked leukocytosis (WBC greater than 35K) may be a marker of severe disease (South Med J 2004;97:959).

Mortality low in younger pts (except with more recent, severe strains), but can approach 25% in elderly pts.

Cmplc: Ileus and toxic megacolon; protein-wasting enteropathy, leading to hypoalbuminemia.

Lab: Initial lab work to include CBC with diff, metabolic panel, glucose; can cause a marked leukocytosis, especially with severe cases (and in some inpatients, a rapid rise in WBC, leukemoid reaction, may be the first sign of disease, even before diarrhea).

Stool sample for C. *diff* toxins (A and B); in hospitalized pts with acute diarrhea, this may be the only necessary test (as other bacterial or parasitic causes of diarrhea are very unlikely in pts in hospital more than 3 days).

Most samples require loose stool for analysis; do not send formed stool to "screen" for C. *diff*, especially with risk for asx carriage.

Should test initially to confirm dx; if neg test, but high clinical suspicion, would still consider treating until three stool samples can be tested.

Do not need to repeat testing once the dx is established or when the treatment is complete; "testing for cure" does not have any bearing on risk of relapse/recurrence.

In critically ill pts, consider blood Cx to r/o secondary bacterial infection with sepsis.

Noninv: Imaging only if concern for ileus/megacolon or to r/o other diseases or intestinal perforation in severe cases.

Endoscopy can be done to look for "pseudo-membranes" caused by colonic wall sloughing, but not necessary in all cases; reserve for pts with resistant disease or high clinical suspicion with neg lab testing.

Rx: Basic steps to C. *diff* therapy include:

- Supportive care
- Cessation of prior abx therapy, if possible
- Directed abx therapy for C. *diff* infection
- Treatment of severe, resistant disease
- Treatment of recurrent disease

Supportive rx generally includes aggressive IV fluid therapy for hypovolemia; antispasmodics (loperamide, opiates) are generally avoided early in the course of disease to avoid cmplc of ileus/megacolon, although studies have not actually been done that show harm.

If possible, discontinue all offending abx, or switch to those not as likely to be related to disease: sulfa drugs, macrolides, tetracyclines, aminoglycosides

Toxin sequestrants can be used, but limited efficacy in trials; most common is cholestyramine 4 gm tid–qid.

Probiotics have also been suggested as a way to reintroduce normal intestinal flora, but mixed results in clinical trials; a Cochrane review of four trials concluded no benefit to probiotics as monotherapy, and insufficient evidence to use as adjunctive therapy (Cochrane 2008;CD004611); however, their safety and ubiquity still lead to significant use, especially in nonhospitalized pts.

Antimicrobial therapy for C. *diff* is as follows:

- Oral therapy is the preferred route for almost all cases.
- Metronidazole 500 mg PO tid for 10–14 d *or* vancomycin 125 mg PO qid for 10–14 d (in severe cases, can increase dose to 250 mg).
- In older studies, both therapies considered equal and metronidazole often used because of lower cost; prior to 2000, failure rates were about 3% for both drugs (NEJM 2008;359:1932).
- However, more recent studies have shown better results with vancomycin therapy, particularly in severe cases.
  - Observational study of 207 pts with C. *diff* colitis, rx with metronidazole; 22% had no improvement in sx after 10 days of rx (representing treatment failure) and 28% responded to rx but relapsed within 90 days (Clin Infect Dis 2005;40:1586).
  - Major outbreak of C. *diff* in Quebec (from new strain described above) was associated with high rates of metronidazole failure (26%) (Clin Infect Dis 2005;40:1591).
  - One RCT compared therapies directly; 172 pts with C. *diff*, randomized to metronidazole 250 mg PO qid vs vancomycin 125 mg PO qid; in pts classified with mild

disease, no difference in cure rates, both better than 90%; in pts with severe disease (defined as two or more of the following: older than 60 yr, temp higher than 38.3°C, serum albumin less than 2.5 mg/dL, WBC more than 15K; or any pts with endoscopic evidence of pseudo-membranes or ICU care), vancomycin had higher cure rates at 21 d (97% vs 76%, NNT 5) (Clin Infect Dis 2007;45:302).

- In pts initially unable to take oral abx, use a combination of IV metronidazole (500 mg IV q 6 hr) and vancomycin (either through enteral route or by enema); IV vancomycin is ineffective because does not pass into the gut lumen.
- In pts with severe sx of sepsis and C. *diff*, consider the possibility of a secondary bacterial infection from translocation of gut microbes; consider broad-spectrum abx in addition to directed C. *diff* therapy until blood Cx and clinical course can further direct therapy.

To treat severe, resistant C. *diff* disease, follow these guidelines:

- Consider additional antibiotics.
  - Rifaximin 400 mg PO bid for 2 wk; shown to be effective in one small case series (8 pts) (Clin Infect Dis 2007;44:846).
  - Rifampin has also been used as adjunctive therapy, but one small study (39 pts) revealed no improvement in outcomes with addition of rifampin to metronidazole and an unexplained increase in mortality (Clin Infect Dis 2006;43:547).
- Intravenous immunoglobulin therapy (IVIG) has been reported effective in case series only; 400 mg/kg for 1–5 doses.
- Fecal enemas from donated stool have been reported effective to restore normal gut flora, but not used regularly for obvious reasons.

- Colectomy, but associated with very high mortality rates (36%, Colorectal Dis 2006;8:149; 48%, Dis Colon Rectum 2004;47:1620); usually done only in life-threatening infections.
- Monoclonal antibodies against C. *diff* toxins shown to reduce the risk of recurrent disease in pts also treated with abx therapy (NEJM 2010;362:197).

For treatment of recurrent C. *diff* disease, follow these guidelines (GE 2009;136:1899):

- Can use the same abx as for prior events, but consider vancomycin as primary choice, given better results with severe disease as described above.
- Generally treat a first recurrence as initial infection with 10–14 days of therapy.
- Use tapered dosing for a second (or more) recurrence:
  - Vancomycin 125 mg qid for 2 wk, then bid for 2 wk, then qd for 2 wk, then qod for 1 wk, then every 3 d for 2 wk
- One study of multiple therapies for recurrent episodes showed tapered dosing (31%) and pulse dosing (14%) better than all other therapies (50% recurrence rates) (Am J Gastroenterol 2002;97:1769).
- In elderly pts with frequent, severe recurrences, can consider lifelong daily vancomycin rx or frequent pulse dosing.

For all hospitals, the most important step is prevention with pt isolation, barrier precautions for all visitors and staff, adequate hand-washing with soap and water (alcohol-based gels do not kill C. *diff* spores).

5.3   Systemic Infections

Sepsis and Septic Shock

(NEJM 2006;355:1699, Crit Care Med 2008;36:296)

Cause: Definitions:

- Sepsis: Infection with systemic inflammatory response syndrome (SIRS)
  - SIRS can be seen without underlying infectious cause (e.g., pancreatitis, post-op, trauma), but is only called sepsis when presumed or proven due to infection.
  - Si/sx of SIRS (two or more of the following):
    - Fever higher than 38.3°C (101°F) or hypothermia lower than 36°C (97°F)
    - Tachycardia: HR more than 90 bpm
    - Respiratory: tachypnea (RR more than 20/min), respiratory alkalosis with $PaCO_2$ less than 32 mmHg, or respiratory failure requiring mechanical ventilation
    - Abnormal WBC: leukocytosis (more than 12K), leukopenia (less than 4K), or more than 10% bandemia
- Severe sepsis: Sepsis plus acute organ dysfunction
  - Examples of organ dysfunction include:
    - Neurologic: delirium, altered mental status, coma
    - Circulatory: hypotension (SBP less than 90 mmHg, MAP less than 70 mmHg, or drop in SBP by more than 40 mmHg from established baseline), demand myocardial ischemia, CHF
    - Respiratory: hypoxemia, respiratory failure
    - Renal: acute renal failure by oliguria (urine output less than 0.5 mL/kg/hr) or elevated serum creatinine (more than 0.5 mg/dL over baseline)
    - Hematologic: elevated PT/INR, thrombocytopenia
    - Gastrointestinal: ileus, acute liver dysfunction by elevated liver enzymes, jaundice
- Septic shock: Persistent hypotension despite adequate fluid resuscitation, usually requiring addition of vasopressors
- Proper terminology is important for decisions on pt status, care, and billing/coding.

Sepsis can be caused by almost any type of infection (viral, bacterial, parasitic, fungal); common offenders include:

- Respiratory: pneumonia, empyema, influenza
- Urologic: pyelonephritis, complicated cystitis, urolithiasis with obstruction, perinephric abscess, pelvic inflammatory disease
- Gastrointestinal: colitis (including C. *difficile*); diverticulitis; appendicitis; biliary tract diseases including cholecystitis, ascending cholangitis; liver and other occult abscesses; peritonitis including acute due to bowel perforation, SBP with liver disease
- Cardiac: endocarditis
- Skin: cellulitis, fasciitis, wound infection; septic arthritis
- CNS: meningitis, brain abscess
- Other: systemic parasitic or viral infections; infected hardware or CVCs

Epidem: Incidence of 750K cases per year in the United States.
Mortality rates approach 30% for severe sepsis; 70% for septic shock.

Pathophys: Complex interplay of microbial factors and the host immune response including: activation of inflammatory factors (TNF-alpha, interleukins), humoral and cell-mediated immunity, and coagulopathy due to activation of procoagulants (tissue plasminogen activator, TPA) and suppression of anticoagulants (antithrombin III, proteins C and S).

Sx/Si: SIRS criteria and organ dysfunction as described above; specific sx related to cause.

Crs: Risk factors for poor prognosis include the following:

- Advancing age (Crit Care Med 2006;34:15)
- Presence of multiple comorbidities, including cancer (Chest 2006;129:1432)

- Higher severity scores, including APACHE-II scoring (Crit Care Med 1985;13:818); multiple online calculators available (e.g., www.mdcalc.com/apache-ii-score-for-icu-mortality)
- Multiple organ system failure
- Presence of coagulopathy, particularly elevated PT (Crit Care 2004;8:R82)
- Elevated plasma lactate levels (Crit Care Med 2004;32:1637)

Cmplc: Watch for complications including:

- Acute respiratory failure due to ARDS, or cardiogenic pulmonary edema from prior or sepsis-induced LV dysfunction
- Acute renal failure with oliguria, elevated serum creatinine
- "Shock" liver with extremely high AST/ALT levels
- Coagulopathies including thrombocytopenia, elevated PT/PTT
- Malnutrition; DVT/PE; gastric "stress" ulcers

Lab: Initial lab w/u often includes CBC with diff, metabolic panel, glucose, renal function, liver function, PT/PTT, blood cultures, urinalysis and urine culture.

Measure ABG in many cases to look for evidence of hypoxemia, hypercarbia, metabolic acidosis.

CRP will be elevated in most cases; may have some prognostic significance, but not likely to change management; similar situation for pro-calcitonin and D-dimer levels.

In setting of severe sepsis and shock, elevated serum lactate levels may be further evidence of end-organ damage from hypoperfusion (and assist in facilitating aggressive management).

Noninv: Further diagnostic testing for source based on hx and physical, but can include:

- Lumbar puncture for CSF analysis, Gram stain, culture; head CT or MRI
- Chest imaging including Xray, CT; thoracentesis for effusion/empyema; sputum for Gram stain and culture

- Abdominal/pelvic imaging including Xray, US, CT; paracentesis if ascites; exploratory laparotomy

   Placement of a PA catheter (Swan-Ganz) not necessary in all cases, but may be helpful in pts not responding to initial therapies, pts at high risk for fluid overload/pulmonary edema due to CHF, pts with apparent ARDS; typically will see low SVR, normal or low PCWP (unless concomitant CHF), elevated or normal cardiac output (unless concomitant LV dysfunction).

Rx: Improved standardization of therapies due to the Surviving Sepsis Campaign international guidelines, first published in 2004 and updated in 2008 (Crit Care Med 2008;36:296).

   Mainstays of rx for sepsis include:

- Initial resuscitation, including "early, goal-directed therapy"
- Diagnosis, source control, and antimicrobial therapy
- Treatment of hypotension with fluids, vasopressors, and inotropes
- Adjunctive/supportive therapies (steroids, recombinant human activated protein C [rhAPC]), blood products, ventilatory support, sedation, glucose control, DVT and stress ulcer prophylaxis)

   Initial resuscitation should be as follows:

- As with all critically ill pts, assess ABCs; many pts may require urgent intubation for airway control and respiratory failure.
- Practice early goal-directed therapy (EGDT) for sepsis:
   - Obviously in critically ill pts, rapid eval and rx are necessary, but EGDT is a formal approach to septic pts within the first 6 hr of arrival to the hospital (usually all care provided in the ED).
   - EGDT is largely based on one well-designed study from a single center (Detroit, Michigan) (NEJM 2001;345: 1368):

- 263 pts with severe sepsis and septic shock, randomized to conventional care or EGDT, which included:
  - Placement of CVC and assessment of CVP with fluid resuscitation (500 mL of crystalloid q 30 min) to a goal CVP of 8–12 mmHg (or 12–15 mmHg in pts on mechanical ventilation)
  - Rapid assessment of MAP with addition of pressors in all pts with MAP less than 65 mmHg
  - Continuous assessment of $ScvO_2$ by the CVC and in pts with $ScvO_2$ less than 70%, addition of blood products to raise Hct greater than 30% or dobutamine infusion
  - The two study groups had no baseline differences, but within initial 6 hr the EGDT pts had higher CVP (14 vs 12), MAP (95 vs 81), and $ScvO_2$ (77% vs 66%), as well as improved APACHE-II severity scores, markers of inflammation, higher hematocrits and arterial pH, lower lactate levels.
  - EGDT pts got about 1.5L more fluid than conventional rx pts on average in the initial 6 hr (~5L total), as well as higher rates of blood and dobutamine (no difference in mechanical ventilation or pressor use).
  - EGDT pts had significantly better in-hospital mortality (30% vs 46%, NNT 6).
- Can these results be generalized to all pts with severe sepsis? Pts should be rapidly evaluated and treated with aggressive IVF and pressors. Not all centers have catheters that can measure continuous $ScvO_2$, but this can be done intermittently with blood gas analysis of blood drawn from the distal port of a central line.
- Signs of improvement with initial resuscitation can include improved tachycardia and hypotension, improved mental status, resumption of adequate urine output, reduced respiratory distress.

Guidelines for diagnosis, source control, and antimicrobial therapy:

- Diagnosis of source of sepsis based on lab, imaging, and procedural eval is crucial to adequate therapy.
- Source control includes surgical or other invasive rx, including:
  - Laparotomy for intrabdominal sepsis from bowel perforation, appendicitis, abscess, etc.
  - Thoracotomy/thoracoscopy for empyema
  - Surgery or percutaneous drainage of abscesses, ureteral obstruction
  - Drainage or surgical debridement of wound, joint, soft tissue infections
  - Removal of infected hardware or CVC
- Obtain Cx prior to any abx therapy, as abx can reduce yield of Cx by up to 50%; however, should not delay abx significantly if not able to obtain Cx (e.g., lack of vascular access, lack of personnel to perform procedure such as LP).
- Appropriate timely abx therapy is the biggest determinant of prognosis in sepsis; get the right abx into the pt asap.
  - If clear source, use appropriate abx coverage for the situation (see specific disease sections for abx recommendations).
  - If source not obvious, empiric broad-spectrum coverage can include the following:
    - Consider broad-spectrum cephalosporin, such as cefepime; broad-spectrum PCN, such as piperacillin-tazobactam; carbapenem, such as imipenem or doripenem.
    - If prior hx or high community rates of MRSA, consider addition of vancomycin or linezolid.
    - If prior hx or immunosuppression, consider addition of antifungal rx, particularly for *Candida*; however, studies supporting empiric therapy are limited (Ann IM 2008;149:83).

- Make sure to consider renal and hepatic dysfunction in dosing of abx.
- Retrospective cohort study of more than 2000 pts with septic shock; median time to effective abx therapy was 6 hr; pts who got abx within the 1st hr had survival rate of 80%, and survival fell 7.6% with each additional hour of delay to abx (Crit Care Med 2006;34:1589).
- Once diagnostic testing and culture results available, strongly consider changing broad-spectrum abx therapy to narrow-spectrum drugs.
- Duration of abx depends on source and nature of infection, as well as pt response and clinical course, but usually 7–10 d at least.

Treatment of hypotension related to sepsis involves the following:

- Initially treat with fluid resuscitation as described for EGDT above.
- Most use crystalloids for fluid resuscitation: isotonic saline (0.9% NS) or lactated ringer's (LR) solution.
- Colloid solutions are another option.
  - Volume reexpansion with less infused volume given; oncotic pressure of the colloids draw fluid from the extravascular space.
  - Options include albumin, hetastarch, dextran.
  - SAFE study: 7000 ICU pts (18% with severe sepsis) requiring fluid resuscitation; randomized to 4% albumin vs crystalloid rx; no difference in mortality, ICU LOS, or other outcomes (NEJM 2004;350:2247).
  - VISEP study: 537 pts with severe sepsis; randomized to 10% pentastarch therapy vs LR; colloid solution was associated with higher rates of acute renal failure (35% vs 22%, NNH 8) (NEJM 2008;358:125).

- Colloid solutions require less volume given (about half the rate of crystalloids), but are also more expensive.
- No evidence for IV bicarbonate therapy, but some expert opinion for use in pts with persistent hypotension and pH less than 7.10.
- Vasopressor therapy for persistent hypotension (MAP less than 65 mmHg) (Chest 2007;132:1678).
  - Consider timely addition of vasopressors if BP does not respond to adequate fluid resuscitation (CVP 8–12 mmHg); in most cases, requires central access for more than brief use, as extravasation of these agents from a peripheral line can cause skin necrosis; also, consider placement of intra-arterial catheter for BP monitoring ("A-line") as more effective than BP cuff for rapid and valid assessment of MAP.
  - Cochrane review of available studies in 2004 could not make recommendations of choice of vasopressor agents (Cochrane 2004;CD003709).
  - Consider as 1st-line agents: norepinephrine vs dopamine:
    - Norepinephrine (Levophed): Strong alpha-agonist (causing peripheral vasoconstriction) and milder beta-agonist (causing increased myocardial contractility [inotropy] and tachycardia [chronotropy]); usually start at 1–2 mcg/min and titrate up to 20-30 mcg/min (note different units than dopamine infusion; if desire weight-based dosing, use 0.02–0.04 mcg/kg/min).
    - Dopamine (Intropin): Physiologic effects are dose-dependent; at less than 5 mcg/kg/min, activates dopamine receptors (causing vasodilation in renal and mesenteric circulation); at 5–10 mcg/kg/min, activates beta-1-receptors (inotropic and chronotropic effects); at higher doses, activates alpha-1-receptors

(vasoconstriction); usually start at 5 mcg/kg/min and titrate up to 20 mcg/kg/min.

- Despite physiologic low-dose effects, the practice of using low-dose dopamine (less than 5 mcg/kg/min) for "renal protection" in crtically ill pts to maintain renal blood flow and urine output has not been proven effective; ANZICS study group of 328 critically ill pts did not show any difference in acute renal failure, need for dialysis, LOS, or mortality with low-dose dopamine vs placebo (Lancet 2000;356:2139).
- Small comparative study of 32 pts with septic shock; randomized to norepinephrine vs dopamine; norepinephrine led to achievement of hemodynamic goals (increased SVR, cardiac index, oxygen delivery and uptake) more than dopamine (94% vs 31%, NNT 2); however, this study did not measure patient-oriented outcomes (Chest 1993;103:1826).
- Prospective observational study of 97 pts with septic shock; use of norepinephrine was associated with reduced mortality (62% vs 82%) vs other vasopressors, but this was not a blinded RCT (Crit Care Med 2000;28:2758).
- SOAP II Trial: RCT of 1679 pts with shock (~60% septic); randomized to initial pressor therapy with norepinephrine vs. dopamine (if not adequate, 2nd-line therapy with norepinephrine, epinephrine, or vasopressin); no significant difference in mortality (ICU, hospital, and up to 12 months), but dopamine associated with higher rates of cardiac arrhythmias (24% vs. 12%, NNH 8), mostly atrial fibrillation (NEJM 2010;362:779).
- Choice usually falls to physician comfort of use and local practice; overall similar effects, except

norepinephrine induces less tachycardia; combination of the two drugs can be used, but given the similar receptor activations, may not be as helpful as adding another 2nd-line agent (see below).

- If require addition of 2nd-line agents, consider:
  - Epinephrine: Used more in Europe than in U.S. centers; potent alpha- and beta-agonist.
  - Phenylephrine: Alpha-agonist only; may be useful as second agent added to one of primary vasopressors, or as 1st-line agent in pts with tachycardias limiting use of beta-agonist drugs.
  - Vasopressin, aka antidiuretic hormone (ADH): Studies have shown septic pts to be ADH-deficient; physiologic effects include vascular smooth muscle contraction (V1 receptors) in addition to renal effects of increased free water resorption and increased circulating volume; can be started at 0.01 U/min, up to a max dose of 0.04 U/min, but most centers use a standard dose infusion of 0.03–0.04 U/min without titration; no studies have shown benefit to use as 1st-line monotherapy.
    - VASST trial: 778 pts with septic shock, randomized to norepinephrine alone vs norepinephrine plus vasopressin; no difference in mortality rates, except in a prespecified subset of pts with less severe shock (requiring norepinephrine doses of 5–14 mcg/kg/min) (NEJM 2008;358:877).
    - This study has led some to advocate vasopressin as 2nd-line agent to be added before maximizing doses of norepinephrine or dopamine.
    - High doses can cause digital ischemia and necrosis.
- Re inotropic therapy with dobutamine:
  - Dobutamine is not primarily used as a pressor, because its BP effects are quite variable.

- Used to increase systemic oxygen consumption in the EGDT studies described above (for pts with $ScvO_2$ less than 70%).
  - Also used to boost cardiac contractility in pts with sepsis-induced or chronic LV dysfunction, already on other pressors for BP control.
- Bottom line: Most use norepinephrine or dopamine as initial agent (NE preferred if tachycardic); use phenylephrine if tachycardia limits use of either agent; add vasopressin as 2nd-line agent if inadequate response.
- Eval and rx of resistant hypotension involves the following considerations:
  - Addition of a 2nd-line vasopressor agent (phenylephrine or vasopressin to norepinephrine/dopamine)
  - Addition of steroids if functional adrenal insufficiency (see "Adrenal Insufficiency" in Section 2.1 for full details)
  - Metabolic disturbances including severe hypocalcemia, hypophosphatemia, hypomagnesemia requiring replacement
  - Severe metabolic acidosis (pH less than 7.10), which might respond to bicarbonate therapy
  - PA catheter monitoring of cardiac output/index and addition of dobutamine, if concomitant myocardial dysfunction
  - If pt on mechanical ventilation, consider hypotensive effects of sedative meds, pos pressure ventilation and extrinsic PEEP, and possibility of tension pneumothorax

  Adjunctive sepsis therapies include:
- Steroid therapy: Controversial subject (see "Adrenal Insufficiency" in Section 2.1 for full details); if used, administer hydrocortisone 50 mg IV q 6 hr or 100 mg IV q 8 hr.
- Hyperglycemia therapy: Most centers utilize IV insulin infusion in pts with severe sepsis, although clinical evidence for improved outcomes is lacking, and may even be some

harm (see "Hyperglycemia, Inpatient" in Section 2.3 for full details).

- Activated protein C (rhAPC) therapy: Patients with severe sepsis are known to have suppressed levels of protein C; IV infusion of 24 mcg/kg/hr for 96 hr; studies have shown addition of this drug to be beneficial in pts with severe sepsis and increased risk of death by APACHE-II scoring, if no contraindications.
  - PROWESS trial: 1690 pts with severe sepsis, randomized to rhAPC vs placebo; rx improved mortality (25% vs 31%, NNT 17) with a nonsignificant trend toward increased major bleeding events (3.5% vs 2%) (NEJM 2001;344:699); subgroup analyses suggested further benefit in pts with higher risk of death by APACHE-II scores (Crit Care Med 2003;31:12).
  - ADDRESS trial: 2613 pts with severe sepsis and low risk of death (defined by APACHE-II scores of less than 25 or single organ failure only), randomized to rhAPC vs placebo; no difference in mortality rates, but rx was associated with an increased risk of serious bleeding (3.9% vs 2.2%, NNH 59) (NEJM 2005;353:1332).
  - Based on these studies, rhAPC therapy should be considered in all pts with severe sepsis and multiorgan system involvement, especially with APACHE-II scores greater than 25.
  - Multiple exclusion criteria based on PROWESS trial:
    - Age younger than 18; weight more than 135 kg
    - Pregnancy or breast-feeding
    - Increased bleeding risk including recent or planned surgery; recent head trauma, stroke, or intracranial lesions; recent GI bleeding
    - Coagulopathy including thrombocytopenia (plt less than 30K); known hypercoagulable condition; recent

use of thrombolytics, warfarin, UFH or LMWH (except for VTE prophylaxis)
- Other severe disease including AIDS (CD4 count less than 50), severe liver disease, CKD on dialysis, prior transplantation, active pancreatitis
- Treatment is quite expensive, but if used judiciously as per evidence, rx is considered cost-effective (~$25,000 per quality-adjusted year of life gained) (Crit Care Med 2003;31:1).
- Treatment of anemia: Acute anemia is common in sepsis, likely multifactorial due to blood loss and reduced RBC production.
  - Consider RBC transfusion as part of EGDT in early resuscitation sepsis, for pts with Hct less than 30% and $ScvO_2$ less than 70% (NEJM 2001;345:1368).
  - In later stages, aggressive transfusion has not shown improvement in outcomes and may be related to increased mortality; TRICC study showed that "restrictive" transfusion policy (only for Hgb less than 7 gm/dL) vs "liberal" (Hgb less than 9 gm/dL) in critically ill pts was associated with reduced in-hospital mortality (22% vs 28%, NNT 16), especially in pts younger than 55 yr and with APACHE-II scores of 20 or less (NEJM 1999;340:409).
  - Indications for transfusion include Hgb less than 7 gm/dL, concomitant ACS/STEMI with Hgb less than 10 gm/dL, active bleeding with ongoing blood loss. See Section 4.1 ("Anemia (Including Transfusion Practices)") for more details.
  - Use of erythropoietin (300 U/kg daily from ICU day 3 through day 7 or 40K units weekly) may reduce need for transfusion (Crit Care Med 1999;27:2346; JAMA 2002;288:2827), but no effect on mortality in medical pts (possibly in posttrauma) with an increased risk of thrombotic events (NEJM 2007;357:965).

- Treat coagulopathy as follows:
  - Consider FFP only in setting of active bleeding.
  - Empiric treatment of elevated INR in sepsis (not due to warfarin therapy) with FFP did not normalize INR in 99% of pts in one study (Transfusion 2006;46:1279).
  - Platelet transfusions are appropriate only w/ plt less than 50K and active bleeding, w/ plt less than 20K and high risk of bleeding, or w/ plt less than 10–15K regardless of bleeding risk; see Section 4.2 ("Thrombocytopenia") for more details.
- Mechanical ventilation: See Section 5.5 ("Pulmonary Infections") and "Acute Respiratory Distress Syndrome (ARDS)" in Section 7.3; in setting of ARDS, use low lung volume ventilation (tidal volumes of 6–8 mL/kg) and permissive hypercapnia OK.
- Nutrition: Addition of nutrition is recommended for most pts once showing signs of clinical improvement; if no preceding bowel surgery or significant ileus, prefer enteral feeds vs parenteral (TPN or PPN) (Crit Care Med 2001;29:2264; NEJM 2009;361:1088).
- VTE prophylaxis with either LMWH or UFH unless active or high risk for bleeding (then use mechanical prophylaxis with IPC or GCS); see "VTE Prophylaxis" in Section 7.1 for details.
- GI prophylaxis for stress ulcers with IV H2 blocker or PPI (or PO sucralfate); see Section 3.2 ("Gastrointestinal Bleeding") for details.

Central Venous Catheters and Associated Infections

(Surg Clin N Am 2009;89:463; Lancet 1998;351:893)

Cause: IV access is required for most hospitalized pts, usually for fluid or med administration; peripheral IVs are usually adequate for most, but central IV access is warranted in certain situations, as follows:

- Administration of multiple drugs, including continuous drips

- Poor peripheral IV access
- Prolonged IV fluid resuscitation (for initial resuscitation, large bore, short peripheral IVs are better)
- Administration of medications that might be painful or caustic if extravasated from peripheral line (e.g., vasopressors, calcium, potassium)
- Total parenteral nutrition (PPN can be given through peripheral line)
- Frequent blood draws, especially if poor peripheral venous access
- Central access for monitoring (CVP, $ScvO_2$)
- Special procedures like hemodialysis or transvenous cardiac pacing

Many hospitals are now employing peripherally inserted CVCs (i.e., PICC lines), which have lower rates of placement cmplc and can safely remain in place longer than traditional CVCs, but risks include venous thrombosis and infection; in hospitalized pts, PICC lines carry the same infection rates as other CVCs (2–5/1000 catheter days) (Chest 2005;128:489).

Tunneled catheters (e.g., Hickman catheters) are for longer-term use, such as in pts with chemotherapy; tunneling the catheter under the skin away from the entry site to the vein is associated with decreased infection rates (JAMA 1996;276:1416).

Most common organisms related to CVC infection include coagulase-negative staphylococci (CNS, *S. epidermidis*), *S. aureus* (MSSA and MRSA), *Enterococcus*, Gram-negatives (including *Klebsiella*, *Pseudomonas*, *E. coli*), *Candida albicans*.

Epidem: There are an estimated 250K catheter-related infections per year in the United States (MMWR Recomm Rep 2002;51:1).

Cost of infections: $25,000 per event, with increased ICU LOS of 2.4 days and hospital LOS 7.5 days (Crit Care Med 2006;34:2084); listed as a CMS preventable "never event," so no further reimbursement (other than primary DRGs) associated with this complication.

Pathophys: Infections within 10 days of catheter placement typically due to bacteria through the skin insertion site; after 10 days, typically due to manipulation of the hub, entrance through the catheter itself (J Clin Microbiol 1985;21:357).

Sx: Most commonly presents as fever in pt with CVC, with negative w/u for other sources; otherwise, signs of systemic infection/SIRS.

Si: May have erythema, induration, discharge from the catheter site; cardiac murmur may suggest endocarditis.

Crs: Risk factors for infected catheter include:

- CVC age
- Location of catheter (femoral risk is more than IJ, which is more than SC)
- Number of lumens (Am J Med 1992;93:277)
- Frequency of manipulation of catheter (changing drips, blood draws, dressing changes)
- Use of CVC line for TPN

Use of the catheter for abx administration reduces the risk of line infection (JAMA 2001;286:700).

Morbidity and mortality related to organism: *S. aureus* bacteremia carries mortality rate of 8% vs coagulase-neg staph rate of 0.7% (Clin Infect Dis 2001;32:1249).

Cmplc: (Crit Care Med 2007;35:1390)

Approximately 15% of CVC placement is associated with cmplc; performing more than 50 procedures lessens cmplc by 50% (Arch IM 1986;146:259); most frequent cmplc include infection (all sites, highest with femoral), venous thrombosis (highest with femoral), pneumothorax (highest with SC), vascular/arterial injury (highest with IJ), bleeding/hematoma, cardiac arrhythmias (highest with IJ and SC placement).

Placement site usually determined by provider and facility choice, but also by potential complications:

- Avoid sites of active inflammation/infection.

- In pts with high bleeding risk, avoid SC approach because of lack of compressible vessels.
- Risk for pneumothorax higher in pts with COPD and on mechanical ventilation; consider IJ rather than SC site.

Femoral site is least favorable, usually only used when other sites are inaccessible or in code situations where access can be obtained while CPR, intubation, etc., are being performed; RCT of femoral vs subclavian CVCs demonstrated higher rates of infection (20% vs 4.5%, NNH 6) and venous thrombosis (21.5% vs 2%, NNH 5) with femoral site (JAMA 2001;286:700).

Use of US guidance has helped to reduce cmplc, especially with less experienced providers, but requires IJ or femoral site (clavicle limits US imaging in SC approach), both of which carry higher rates of infection.

Catheters should be removed as soon as not necessary for pt care; routine catheter changes over a guidewire do not reduce rates of infection and are not recommended by guidelines (Crit Care Med 1997;25:1417), especially if concern for infected catheter (changing over wire will likely infect the new catheter).

Complications of catheter-related infections (especially with *S. aureus*) include septic thrombosis, endocarditis, osteomyelitis, abscess formation, septic emboli (Clin Infect Dis 1992;14:75).

Lab: Blood Cx for dx and to guide therapy; two sets are standard; can consider one set drawn from CVC, but if peripheral draw is neg, there may be concern for colonized catheter or hub rather than true source of infection.

If both Cx positive, consider colony counts (higher counts from the CVC draw) and "time to positive" Cx (quicker from CVC draw; requires a lab that has constant culture monitoring) as signs of CVC source of infection.

If catheter removed, can cut and culture the tip, but should only perform if concern for true infection (not with routine catheter removal); otherwise, if pos Cx, unclear if pt requires abx treatment.

Noninv: After CVC placement with IJ or SC site, CXR to assess proper placement (should reach the SVC/right atrial junction, should not cross midline, which suggests placement in RV) and lack of cmplc (pneumothorax, hemothorax).

In setting of infection, imaging only to r/o other sources; echocardiogram if concern for endocarditis.

Rx: Prevention of infection includes:

- Hand-washing prior to procedure
- Antiseptic scrub of site with 2% chlorhexidine (proven more effective than 70% alcohol and 10% iodine) (Lancet 1991;338:339)
- Full barrier precautions
- Choice of anatomic site (SC preferred over IJ; IJ preferred over femoral)
- Daily review for removal of CVC when no longer necessary

Evidence for CVC infection prevention includes the following studies:

- Johns Hopkins study: Prospective cohort study of surgical ICU; education and multifactorial approach to CVC line insertion and monitoring reduced central line infections from 11.3 to zero per 1000 catheter days; estimated prevention of 43 infections, 8 deaths, and $2 million in associated costs (Crit Care Med 2004;32:2014).
- Pronovost study: Multicenter trial of 108 ICUs, mostly in Michigan; similar approach as Johns Hopkins study; reduced infections from baseline 2.7 cases per 1000 catheter days to zero within 3 mo after implementation and persisted up to 18 mo (NEJM 2006;355:2725).

Use of antibiotic-impregnated catheters: Meta-analysis of 27 trials (mainly with chlorhexidine-silver sulfadiazine and monocycline-rifampicin) showed reduced risk of infection (OR 0.49) (Crit Care Med 2009;37:702); the savings in prevented infections may outweigh higher initial costs in some cases (JAMA

1999;282:554); because of the impressive effects of educational programs as described above, the CDC recommends considering impregnated catheters only if expecting prolonged use of a catheter in hospitals that have elevated infection rates despite the implementation of a CVC infection control policy (MMWR Recomm Rep 2002;51:1).

Guidelines for treatment of catheter-related infections:

- Removal of the catheter is warranted in most cases, either once infection is diagnosed or empirically in critically ill pts without other clear source.
  - In uncomplicated infections with S. *epidermidis* and other CNS, removal of the catheter does not affect cure rates, but if not removed, there is a 20% chance of recurrent infection (Inf Contr Hosp Epidem 1992;13:215).
  - In cases of essential CVCs or tunneled catheters, consider a trial of "antibiotic lock" with abx held in the catheter for a period of time to rx colonization.
- Antibiotic rx should be directed by Cx results (similar to rx of endocarditis); if empiric therapy warranted, consider broad-spectrum coverage to include Gram-positives and Gram-negatives, and MRSA coverage in most settings.
- Duration of abx typically 10–14 d; can consider 7 d in uncomplicated infections with coagulase-negative staphylococci; if associated cmplc (e.g., endocarditis, septic thrombosis), consider 4–6 wk of IV therapy.

5.4 Soft Tissue Infections

Cellulitis (Including Necrotizing Fasciitis and Gas Gangrene)

(NEJM 2004;350:904; Clin Infect Dis 2005;41:1373)

Cause: Bacterial infection with inflammation of the dermis and SQ tissues.

Erysipelas is often used interchangeably with cellulitis, but specifically defines inflammation of the upper dermis and lymphatics.

Can affect any location, but most common on the extremities, head (particularly orbital and periorbital cellulitis; facial rash from erysipelas), groin (Fournier's gangrene, spread from perianal or retroperitoneal source), buttocks.

Risk factors for cellulitis, including portals of entry, are as follows:

- IV drug abuse; i.e., "skin-popping" particularly in antecubital areas, but also can be seen in interdigital regions
- Skin lacerations, wounds, surgical sites
- Bites, including human, animal, and insect
- Interdigital and intertriginous fungal infections (always check for tinea pedis, which is a common portal of entry in lower extremity cellulitis and should be treated concomitantly to reduce risk of reinfection/relapse)
- Lymphedema

Bacterial causes include (most cases are from the first two groups):

- Group A streptococci (*S. pyogenes*); group B, C, G beta-hemolytic streptococci
- *Staphylococcus aureus,* including nosocomial and community-acquired MRSA (CA-MRSA).
- *Enterococcus*
- Gram-negative organisms, including *Pseudomonas*
- More rarely, *Vibrio vulnificus, Aeromonas hydrophila, Mycobacterium marinum*
- Bites are usually polymicrobial, often including *Pasteurella, Eikenella*
- Severe soft tissue infections such as:
  - Necrotizing fasciitis: Most are polymicrobial (59–85% in case series), with an average of 4 or more microbes present on culture (Am Fam Phys 2003;68:323)
  - Gas gangrene: Clostridial spp., including *C. perfringens*

Sx/Si: Tenderness, erythema, edema, warmth of the skin in the affected area; may be streaking of erythema in lymphatic pattern, with associated lymphadenopathy; area may be painful to touch, or in some cases, reduced sensation.

"Peau d'orange" ("orange peel") is edematous, indurated skin that has a dimpled appearance because of hair follicles held down within the edematous skin; when seen on the breast, make sure to consider and r/o inflammatory breast cancer.

Erysipelas typically has sharply demarcated edges of inflammation with a raised border.

Check for crepitus in the skin to suggest subcutaneous air, a hallmark of clostridial infection.

Infection may be associated with si/sx of sepsis: fever, tachycardia, hypotension.

Crs: In pts with recurrent or resistant infections, or other odd presentations, consider differential dx including the following (Ann IM 2005;142:47):

- Chronic inflammation related to venous insufficiency: Very common cause of "bilateral cellulitis"; although occasionally can be associated with infectious cause, especially if concomitant ulcers, most cases responsive to compression, elevation, and judicious diuretics without the need for abx
- Superficial and deep venous thrombosis: Especially in lower-extremity cellulitis with other VTE risk factors; diagnose with clinical exam (for superficial) or US (for DVT); superficial requires only symptomatic therapy (compresses, NSAIDs), DVT requires anticoagulation
- Contact or irritant dermatitis: Usually recurrent, associated with blistering, exudates; responsive to topical steroid therapy
- Allergic reactions to insect stings, immunizations
- Erythema chronicum migrans: Spreading rash associated with Lyme disease (*Borellia burgdorferi*)

- Drug rashes: Usually more widespread, involving chest, trunk, abdomen; may have associated pruritus
- Gout: Associated with underlying joint inflammation, pain
- Cutaneous lymphoma and leukemia

Many inpatients have worsening local signs of inflammation in the first 24 hr after therapy, likely due to release of bacterial toxins/antigens; after that period, worsening sx should prompt concern for resistant organisms, deep infection, or another dx.

Cmplc: Mortality generally low, except for necrotizing infections (mortality was 29% in small series of 65 pts) (Ann Surg 1995;221:558).

Differentiating uncomplicated cellulitis from deeper, more serious soft tissue infections (particularly necrotizing fasciitis and gas gangrene) can be difficult in the early setting (Clin Infect Dis 2005;41:1373); potential clues to more severe infection include:

- Pain out of proportion to physical signs, or anesthesia of the associated inflamed skin
- Associated skin changes, including bullae, hemorrhage, skin sloughing, "wooden-hard" feeling to skin
- Rapid progression of symptoms or severe sepsis and septic shock
- Laboratory abnormalities: leukocytosis more than 20K, anemia, hypocalcemia, metabolic acidosis, thrombocytopenia (Ann Surg 1995;221:558)
- Crepitus on exam or gas seen on imaging

In cases of spontaneous gas gangrene (not associated with wounds or IV drug abuse), consider immunosuppression and underlying GI malignancy.

Lab: For most inpatients, initial w/u includes CBC with diff, metabolic panel, glucose (to look for underlying diabetes); CRP and

ESR can be obtained but will not affect management in most cases, probably best reserved in pts with broader diff (to help r/o infection) or if concern for deeper infection (i.e., osteomyelitis, which often has ESR more than 70).

Consider CPK if concern for underlying rhabdomyolysis, trauma.

Blood Cx have a low yield in all pts with cellulitis; review of five studies showed positive cultures in 1–16% of pts, with no significant changes in most antimicrobial regimens (Ann EM 2005;45:548); for more severe infections, associated sepsis, immunocompromised pts, Cx should be considered.

Wound cultures also have low yield; if associated wound or bite, there may be multiple organisms on the skin surface that may or may not be the offending infectious agent; in difficult, resistant, or recurrent cases, a needle aspirate or punch bx for Cx may be helpful to determine pathogen; in one small series, a punch bx yield bacterial cause in 18% of cases, best if obtained at the wound edge (Arch IM 1989;149:293).

Consider wound Cx if associated abscess, especially if concern for MRSA.

Noninv: Most pts do not require imaging studies; consider imaging in these situations:

- Concern for underlying disease (cancer, osteomyelitis): Mammography and US if breast cellulitis, CT/MRI in other cases
- Associated abscess (based on fluctuance felt on physical exam or lack of improvement with appropriate antibiotics): US or CT
- Crepitus on exam to look for gas collection in the SQ tissues: Plain films or CT/MRI

Consider MRI if concern for necrotizing fasciitis; MRI confirmed all pts with suspected fasciitis in one small study (17 pts), based on deep fluid collections and thickening of the fascia (Am J Roentgenol 1998;170:615).

Rx: When to hospitalize for cellulitis:

- Patients with severe disease, associated sepsis, initial concern for deeper infections
- Failed outpatient therapy
- Immunocompromised patients
- Patients with associated exacerbation of chronic diseases (e.g., severe hyperglycemia in diabetics)
- Patients with lack of adequate follow-up

   Antimicrobial therapy for most cases of cellulitis:

- Most inpatients should be initially treated with IV abx.
- 1st-line therapy in uncomplicated cases without risk for MDR organisms is penicillinase-resistant PCN (e.g., nafcillin) or cephalosporin (e.g., cefazolin, ceftriaxone); fluoroquinolone is also often used and equally effective (Drugs 2002;62:967).
- Consider MRSA coverage.
  - Risk factors: (1) pts with recent wounds and hospitalization at risk for nosocomial MRSA, (2) high local rates of CA-MRSA, (3) IV drug abuse, (4) incarcerated pts, (5) younger pts involved in contact sports, (6) associated furuncles and small abscesses.
  - Initial IV therapy with vancomycin or linezolid, similar success rates (73%) in one head-to-head trial (Clin Infect Dis 2002;34:1481); tigecycline is another option (see below).
  - When able to take oral abx, choice should be based on Cx if available and local resistance patterns; many CA-MRSA strains are sensitive to trimethoprim-sulfamethoxazole, clindamycin, doxycycline, or minocycline.
  - If associated abscess, primary therapy is incision and drainage; if small abscess, I&D may be only therapy needed.
- Consideration of broad-spectrum Gram-neg coverage:
  - Appropriate for pts with h/o similar infections, immunocompromised, uncontrolled diabetes (especially with associated wounds).

- Choices include ampicillin-sulbactam, piperacillin-tazobactam, carbapenems, 3rd and 4th generation cephalosporins (ceftazidime, cefotaxime, cefepime).
- Tigecycline is another good option as it covers MRSA in addition to broad-spectrum Gram-pos and -neg coverage (but not *Pseudomonas*); does not require change in dosing for renal dysfunction.
- Treatment of bite wounds should cover multiple organisms; initial IV therapy with ampicillin-sulbactam, piperacillin-tazobactam, or carbapenems.
- Duration of abx: Usually continue IV until taking adequate PO and clinical improvement (afebrile, resolving leukocytosis and signs of inflammation) for 24 hr; in pts with uncomplicated infection and rapid clinical response, 5 d of therapy (IV and PO combined) may be adequate (study of 121 pts on monotherapy with levofloxacin) (Arch IM 2004;164:1669); otherwise 7–10 d.

  Adjunctive rx measures include:

- Analgesia
- Tetanus immunization, if associated with a wound
- In extremities, elevation and immobilization of the affected limb
- Control of peripheral edema with support stockings, or compressive dressings, in severe cases
- Treatment of concomitant fungal infections of the skin with topical therapies (clotrimazole, miconazole, terbinafine)
- I&D for associated furuncles and abscesses
- Steroids
  - Scandinavian study of 112 pts with uncomplicated cellulitis, randomized to prednisolone plus abx vs abx alone; steroid group had 1 less day of IV abx (3 vs 4 d) and faster resolution of sx (9 vs 10 d), without other side effects (Scand J Infect Dis 1997;29:377); however, use of steroids in this setting has not been generally used.

Issues re rx of necrotizing infections and gas gangrene (Am Fam Phys 2003;68:323):

- Most important is clinical suspicion for disease early in course.
- Surgical eval and debridement of necrotic tissue is the mainstay of therapy; will often require repeated surgical interventions; many require critical care and aggressive supportive measures.
- Given that most cases of fasciitis are polymicrobial, broad-spectrum abx coverage is necessary to cover Gram-pos and Gram-neg bacteria, anaerobes, and possibly MRSA as well; consider ampicillin-sulbactam, piperacillin-tazobactam, carbapenems, 3rd and 4th generation cephalosporins (ceftazidime, cefotaxime, cefepime) *plus* clindamycin or metronidazole (*plus* vancomycin or linezolid if MRSA risk).
- Confirmed clostridial infections can be managed with penicillin G and clindamycin, but may require broad-spectrum coverage until culture and sensitivities available.
- Hyperbaric oxygen therapy and IV immunoglobulin (IVIG) can be considered in some cases.

Diabetic Foot Ulcers

(NEJM 2004;351:48; Am Fam Phys 2008;78:71)

Cause: Triad of peripheral neuropathy, foot deformity, and associated trauma.

Associated infection is usually due to the loss of skin protection, rather than the cause of the ulcer; not all ulcers are infected, and should consider eval and rx of infection only when suspicion for acute infection based on hx and exam or in the setting of nonhealing ulcer with standard therapies.

Infections are typically polymicrobial, including multiple Gram-neg and Gram-pos organisms (including MRSA), anaerobes; most common pathogens are as listed for cellulitis.

Epidem: Occur in 15% of pts with DM; leading cause of diabetic-related hospitalization.

Annual incidence of 2% per year among diabetics, 5–7% if associated neuropathy.

Cost of treating one foot ulcer is approximately $28,000 (Diab Care 1999;22:382).

Sx/Si: If concern for infection, look for local (erythema, warmth, edema) and systemic (fever, sepsis) signs; other signs of infection include skin and soft tissue necrosis, foul odor, purulent wound discharge.

Look for signs of PVD (reduced or absent distal pulses; thin, shiny skin; loss of hair on the extremities).

Perform microfilament testing and check ankle jerk reflexes for peripheral neuropathy.

Sterile probe of the ulcer for bone is effective eval of osteomyelitis: PPV of 89% in one study (JAMA 1995;273:721).

Crs: Preceding event in 85% of amputations in diabetic pts; increased mortality for diabetic pts with foot ulcer vs matched diabetics (28% 3-yr mortality vs 13%) (Diab Care 1999;22:382).

Cmplc: Most concern is for underlying osteomyelitis, present in 68% of pts with foot ulcers in one series, and 64% of osteo pts had no local si/sx of inflammation (JAMA 1991;266:1246).

Lab: Initial w/u similar to cellulitis; consider osteomyelitis if ESR is more than 70 mm/hr; consider blood Cx in severe cases, but likely low yield (see "Cellulitis" earlier in Section 5.4).

Guidelines for wound cultures:

- Should not obtain routinely if no concern for infection, as all will likely grow colonized bacteria.
- If concern for infection, surface swab will probably be inadequate and likely will grow colonizers or multiple organisms.
- Consider scrubbing the affected skin and obtaining culture from either deep probe or surgical specimen (postdebridement).

Noninv: Consider assessment of PVD in all pts:

- Assessment of pulses on physical exam

- Ankle-brachial index (ABI): measure systolic BP in ankle and arm, and calculate ratio; ABI less than 0.91, consider mild to moderate ischemia; less than 0.4 indicates severe ischemia
- Noninvasive assessment of PVD, including US, MRA, CTA

Imaging for osteomyelitis is crucial in most cases, especially as there are many pts without si/sx of local infection.

- Plain films of the feet may show localized bone destruction, but limited sensitivity.
- MRI or bone scan are most sensitive (90–100%) in eval of osteomyelitis.

Rx: Surgical eval. and rx is the primary step in management:

- Debridement of necrotic tissue
- Probing and eval for osteomyelitis
- Amputation of affected bone
- Revascularization if associated PVD

Antimicrobial therapy: Reserve for true infection; do not prophylactically or chronically treat wounds, as will not likely affect long-term outcome and will lead to antimicrobial resistance.

- Due to polymicrobial infection, typically use broad-spectrum agents and anaerobic coverage.
  - In mild cases, can use 1st-line therapy of cephalosporins or fluoroquinolones *plus* clindamycin or metronidazole for anaerobic coverage.
  - In more severe cases, empiric rx with carbapenems, piperacillin-tazobactam, 3rd/4th generation cephalosporins.
  - Consider MRSA hx and risk; addition of vancomycin or linezolid, or tigecycline as monotherapy.
- Severe infections should be treated with IV therapy initially.
- Duration of therapy 10–14 d for associated cellulitis; if osteomyelitis, treatment with IV therapy for up to 6 wk (although can consider oral fluoroquinolone therapy in selected pts).

- If amputation of affected bone, can reduce duration of rx to just coverage of the wound edge after surgery (usually only 2–5 d post-op).

  Adjunctive measures include the following:

- Affected limb elevation for edema
- Removal of pressure, both at rest and with activity
- Dressing to promote wound moisture and debridement of necrotic tissue; traditionally used wet-to-dry dressings, but newer wound-filling gels may have better outcomes (but lacking large trials at this point)
- Tight control of blood sugars, both as inpatient and on hospital discharge

5.5 Pulmonary Infections

Pneumonia (Including Community-Acquired, Hospital-Acquired, and Ventilator-Associated)

(Clin Infect Dis 2007;44 Suppl 2:S27)

Cause: Definitions (Am J Respir Crit Care Med 2005;171:388):

- Community-acquired (CAP): Pneumonia that develops in pt of any age, who does not meet the criteria for other, higher-risk groups.
- Healthcare-associated (HCAP): Pneumonia in pts with prior hospitalization (more than 2 d within the past 3 mo); residing in nursing home or other long-term care facility; IV abx therapy, chemotherapy, or wound care within 1 mo; on hemodialysis.
- Hospital-acquired (HAP): Pneumonia that develops 48 hr or more after admission to the hospital.
- Ventilator-associated (VAP): Pneumonia that develops 48 hr or more after endotracheal intubation.

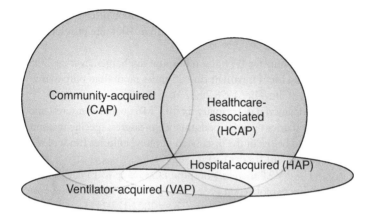

Figure 5.1 Classification of Pneumonia

Figure 5.1 illustrates the classification of pneumonia and how their causes can intersect.

Infectious causes, stratified by severity of illness (higher severity associated with less typical organisms), are as follows:

- All inpatients: *Streptococcus pneumoniae, Mycoplasma, Chlamydophila, Haemophilus influenzae, Legionella*; viruses including influenza A and B, parainfluenza, RSV, adenovirus
- Severe CAP: Above causes, plus *Staphylococcus aureus* (including MRSA), Gram-neg organisms (*Pseudomonas aeruginosa, Klebsiella pneumoniae, E. coli, Enterobacter, Acinetobacter*)
- Less common organisms to consider: *Mycobacterium tuberculosis, Chlamydia psittaci, Coxiella burnetii, Franciscella tularensis, Bordetella pertussis*, fungal pneumonias (*Histoplasma, Cryptococcus, Coccidiodes, Blastomyces*)
- HAP/VAP may be polymicrobial, and higher rates of Gram-neg organisms and MRSA

Epidem: Eighth leading cause of mortality in the United States; 5 million U.S. cases per year (more than 900K are pts older than 65 yr).

Accounts for 1.4 million hospital discharges, average LOS 5.3 days; cost of inpatient care 25 times more than outpatient therapy (Clin Ther 1998;20:820).

Pneumonia is a primary dx for CMS quality measures, and many inpatient pay-for-performance measures; specific measures are listed below in the discussion of blood cultures (under Lab) and treatment (under Rx).

HAP/VAP increases hospital LOS by up to 13 days and mortality twofold (Am J Med 1993;94:281), and increases costs by more than $40,000 per pt (Chest 2002;122:2115).

Pathophys: Interplay of microbial burden and virulence, with the host response; although adequate immune response is required to fight off infection, an inappropriately vigorous inflammatory response can lead to cell damage and death with worsening clinical status (e.g., ARDS) (for an excellent review, see NEJM 2008;358:716).

Sx: Cough (more than 90% of cases), sputum production (66%), dyspnea (66%), tachypnea, pleurisy (50%) (NEJM 2002;347:2039) are the cardinal sx; however, sx in the elderly may be nonspecific, including confusion/delirium, weakness, frequent falls, anorexia, decompensated CHF or diabetes.

Sx of sepsis occur in severe cases.

In critically ill pts, sx of HAP and VAP may be more difficult to discern; consider in pts with new-onset fever, hypoxemia, worsening sputum production.

Legionella infection is associated with diarrhea, headache, rigors.

Si: Exam is nonspecific and insensitive; lung exam for focal rales, ronchi; tactile fremitus, E-to-A changes suggest an infiltrate;

reduced breath sounds, dullness to percussion suggest an associated effusion.

Crs: Severity scoring may help to stratify pts and assist with decisions on admission vs outpatient rx and ICU vs non-ICU placement:

- Pneumonia Severity Index (PSI, also commonly called the PORT score): Checklist of multiple factors including age, comorbidities, physical exam, and lab findings; classifies pts into five categories (I is least severe, V is most severe).
  - PORT study: More than 14,000 pts with CAP; using scoring system, pts were stratified to five classes, with associated mortality rates: Classes I and II had very low mortality (less than 0.6%), suggesting possible outpatient therapy; III had intermediate mortality (2.8%), consider outpatient rx or short inpatient stay; IV and V had higher mortality (8.2%, 29%), with inpatient admission and consideration of ICU in highest risk group (NEJM 1997;336:243).
  - Online PSI calculators are available (e.g., http://pda.ahrq.gov/clinic/psi/psicalc.asp).
- British Thoracic Society (BTS) guidelines (also called the CURB-65) (Thorax 2003;58:377):
  - **C**onfusion: delirium, disorientation; **U**remia: BUN greater than 20 mg/dL; **R**espiratory rate more than 30 breaths/min; **B**lood pressure less than 90 systolic, less than 60 diastolic; **65** years or older
  - 1 point for each of the measures; 30-d mortality lowest in pts with 0–1 point (0.7%, 2.1%), intermediate with 2–3 points (9.2%, 14.5%), highest with 4–5 points (40%, 57%)
  - Provides quicker assessment than PORT score
- Severity scores are not the only consideration for admission; also look at ability to take oral meds, outpatient f/u,

compliance; pneumonia may also exacerbate another chronic illness (e.g., COPD, CHF, angina, diabetes, atrial fibrillation) requiring admission.

About 10% of pts admitted for pneumonia are admitted to the ICU.

- Strongly consider need for ICU at the time of admission.
  - Higher severity pts may lead to consideration of blood cultures and broader abx coverage.
  - Inpatient transfer to the ICU for delayed respiratory failure or sepsis is associated with increased mortality (Intensive Care Med 1995;21:24).
- Absolute requirements for ICU include mechanical ventilation and sepsis requiring pressors.
- Consider ICU placement for pts with high PSI or CURB-65 scores, immunosuppression, severe hypoxemia or hypercarbia requiring high-flow O_2 or NIPPV, or severe comorbidities.

Up to 15% of pts do not respond to initial rx, with associated higher mortality (Arch IM 2004;164:502); in the first 3 d of treatment, this may simply represent severe illness, although worsening illness in that time frame should necessitate w/u for another dx (PE, ARDS, CHF) or reconsideration of risk factors for drug-resistant organisms and broadening of abx coverage; after 3 d of no response to appropriate rx, consider the following options (Am J Respir Crit Care Med 2000;162:154):

- Resistant infection: Check cultures, if available; consider reculturing blood and sputum and broadening abx coverage to cover Gram-neg organisms, MRSA, fungal causes.
- New infection: HAP or VAP in addition to initial infectious cause, which may require broadening of coverage.
- Complication: Effusion/empyema, drug-related fever or illness; consider repeat chest imaging (CXR, CT) and thoracentesis if appropriate.

- Initial misdiagnosis: PE, ARDS, CHF, vasculitis, bronchiolitis obliterans organizing pneumonia (BOOP), pulmonary hemorrhage, acute eosinophilic pneumonia; may require further imaging, bronchoscopy to evaluate.

    Discharge decision: Consider sending pt home when these criteria are met (NEJM 2002;347:2039):

- Clinically stable for 24 hr: Afebrile, RR less than 24/min, HR less than 100/min, SBP more than 90 mmHg, O_2 saturation more than 90% on room air (or on home supplemental O_2 level)
- Able to take oral meds and maintain adequate oral intake
- Normal or baseline mental status
- Study evaluated these criteria in 680 pts admitted for CAP; 19% left the hospital without meeting more than one of the above criteria, and associated with an increased risk of death and readmission (OR 1.6); failing to satisfy more than two criteria carried even higher risk (OR 5.4) (Arch IM 2002;162:1278)

Cmplc: Acute respiratory failure, requiring NIPPV or mechanical ventilation; sepsis and septic shock.

    Parapneumonic effusion and empyema; significant effusion in the setting of pneumonia should prompt thoracentesis (especially if effusion does not easily move/layer out on CT or decubitus Xray studies); finding of empyema may necessitate chest tube placement or thoracoscopy for evaluation.

Lab: Initial lab w/u should include CBC with diff, metabolic panel, LFTs; consider ABG to quantify hypoxemia and r/o hypercarbia in select pts (i.e., those with acute respiratory failure); CRP and ESR will likely show acute inflammation, but clinical significance limited.

    Legionella infection may show hepatitis and hyponatremia as clues to dx.

Consider pro-BNP and D-dimer in select cases to help r/o other causes of dyspnea.

Considerations re tests to determine specific etiology of pneumonia:

- Particularly in ill pts requiring hospitalization, inappropriate abx therapy is associated with increased mortality (Chest 1999;115:462); however, one study suggested no difference in mortality or LOS in pts treated with specific pathogen-directed antimicrobial therapy vs appropriate empiric therapy (Thorax 2005;60:672).
- Blood cultures:
  - Yield of blood cultures in pts with pneumonia is 5–14%.
  - Most commonly isolated pathogen is *S. pneumoniae*.
  - Yield drops by 50% when abx administered prior to cultures being drawn (Am J Respir Crit Care Med 2004;169:342).
  - Patients with severe CAP have a higher yield and are more likely to lead to a change in antimicrobial therapy; this also applies to pts with immunosuppression, chronic liver disease, leukopenia, asplenia.
  - Do blood cultures change abx therapy?
    - Canadian study of 760 pts with CAP; blood Cx were positive in 5.6% (and did not correlate well with severity of illness by PSI score); Cx results changed management in 35% of pts with pos cultures, but only 2% of all pts because of low overall yield (Chest 2003;123:1142).
    - Study of 209 pts with CAP; blood Cx were positive in 13.9% (and as opposed to prior study, PSI score did correlate with pos results); Cx results changed mgt in 20% of pts with severe disease (defined as PSI Class V) (Respir Med 2001;95:78).
    - Risks of blood Cx include extra needle sticks (minimal morbidity), cost of testing, and problems related to false

positive test (usually showing Gram-positive organisms, which necessitate rx with vancomycin to cover MRSA and increased LOS to ensure pathogen vs contaminant prior to discharge).

- Blood Cx are component of CMS quality measures.
  - Originally, required blood Cx for all pts admitted with pneumonia; however, subsequent studies (as above) and clinical feedback suggested that this was not necessary in all pts.
  - Current measures:
    - If blood Cx obtained, abx should be held until after blood Cx drawn to ensure the highest yield (if significant delay for Cx, should not delay therapy, especially in critically ill pts, regardless of quality measures).
      - In pts admitted to or transferred to the ICU within 24 hr of admission for pneumonia, blood Cx should be drawn; this is based on studies showing higher yield and therapeutic value to pts with severe disease.
  - Many hospitals have decided to require blood Cx prior to abx in all pts admitted for pneumonia, so as to ensure no "drop-outs" in the quality measures; this should be an institutional decision.
  - If not required for all pts, consider blood Cx in pts with severe disease (by general appearance or severity scores), prior abx use and hospitalizations, which may suggest drug-resistant organisms.
- Sputum Gram stains and cultures:
  - Yield can be variable, even if adequate sample obtained.
    - Study of 105 pts with blood culture-positive pneumo-coccal pneumonia had sputum sample ordered; in about 40% of pts, sputum was not obtained or was inadequate for culture; however, in pts with an adequate sample,

yield of pneumococcus on Cx was 80% (Clin Infect Dis 2004;39:165).
- Study of 1669 pts with CAP; only 32% of samples were obtained and of good quality; only 14% of all sputum samples revealed a predominant organism on Gram stain, and only 16% yielded an organism on Cx; positivity of Cx did not correlate with disease severity (Arch IM 2004;164:1807).
- Can be obtained from expectorated sputum (and may be induced with some respiratory techniques); better samples obtained by endotracheal aspirates (in ventilated pts) or bronchoscopy (usually reserved for severe cases, not improving with adequate empiric therapy).
- Probably most helpful to diagnose or r/o MRSA infection.
- Antigen testing:
  - Rapid urine assays available for *S. pneumoniae* and *Legionella*.
    - Pneumococcal tests have documented specif of 90–97% and sens of 70% (Chest 2001;119:243; Clin Infect Dis 2003;36:286).
    - Legionella tests have documented specif of 99% and sens of 80% (J Med Microbiol 2001;50:509).
  - Identification of these bacteria may allow for abx narrowing, but no information on abx sensitivity; also may allow for confirmation of bacterial pneumonia in pts who have already received abx (with subsequent reduced yield on blood and sputum Cx).
  - Nasopharyngeal swabs for influenza: High specif (99%), but limited sens; may be useful in limiting abx use in low-risk pts with pos test (but high-risk, severe CAP pts may require rx for possible concomitant bacterial pneumonia).
  - Serum testing for other atypical organisms (*Mycoplasma*, *Chlamydia*) is available but with delayed results, not likely to affect clinical mgt.

Work-up for HAP/VAP generally includes repeat Cx (many times pts are pan-cultured for new fever); specifically sputum Cx in pts with VAP often obtained by endotracheal aspirate or bronchoscopic lavage (both are equivalent) (NEJM 2006;355: 2619).

Noninv: CXR required in all cases of pts hospitalized for pneumonia; in addition to confirming dx, want to r/o other comorbidities, including underlying carcinoma (with postobstructive pneumonia), parapneumonic effusion, CHF.

Study of two radiologists evaluating CXR for pneumonia showed only moderate intra-observer agreement, higher in agreeing that pneumonia was not present (94%) than was present (59%); reduced further in pts with COPD and documented pneumococcal cause (Clin Radiol 2004;59:743).

Follow-up CXR may continue to show infiltrates for up to 3–4 mo after initial infection (in pts older than 70, only 35% showed resolution within 3 wk, 84% within 12 wk) (J Am Ger Soc 2004;52:224); frequent serial imaging initially is not necessary unless concern in pts worsening despite adequate therapy; if dense, lobar infiltrate, consider f/u CXR 1–3 mo after treatment to confirm resolution and r/o underlying carcinoma.

Chest CT is more sensitive than CXR for dx of pneumonia, but not required in most cases; consider if pt having recurrent illness, possible mass on CXR, sx that suggest PE; also CT findings in the setting of normal CXR may be of questionable clinical significance (resolving pneumonia, pneumonitis) (Clin Infect Dis 1998;27:358).

Rx: Guidelines for antibiotic therapy in pneumonia:

- Determine the class of pneumonia (CAP, HCAP, HAP, VAP).
  - Has pt developed pneumonia on ventilator for more than 48 hr? If yes, then VAP.
  - Has pt developed pneumonia after hospitalized for 48 hr or more? If yes, then HAP.

- Does pt have any of the following risk factors? If yes, then HCAP.
  - Prior hospitalization (more than 2 d within the past 3 mo)
  - Residing in nursing home or other long-term care facility
  - IV abx therapy, chemotherapy, or wound care within 1 mo
  - On hemodialysis
- Otherwise, treat as CAP.
- For pts with CAP, determine severity of illness to help guide therapy (ICU vs non-ICU).
- For pts with CAP, consider the risk factors for *Pseudomonas* and MRSA infections.
  - *Pseudomonas* risk factors: Prior pseudomonal infection, chronic lung disease (including CF, bronchiectasis, severe COPD), prolonged or frequent steroid and abx use (Arch IM 2002;162:1849).
  - MRSA risk factors: ESRD, IV drug abuse, recent influenza, recent abx use (especially with fluoroquinolones) (J Antimicrob Chemother 2001;48:375).
- For pts with HAP, VAP, and HCAP, determine risk of multidrug-resistant (MDR) organisms; if pt has any of the following, consider MDR:
  - Antibiotics within the last 3 mo
  - Hospitalized for more than 5 d
  - High rates of abx resistance in community or hospital
  - Immunosuppression, including alcoholism, asplenia, long-term steroid use, chronic liver disease, chemotherapy
- Once class and risks are determined, use appropriate empiric coverage (see **Table 5.1**), usually in IV form initially.
- Administer first dose of abx as soon as dx of pneumonia is confirmed, usually in the ED prior to admission, and at least within 6–8 hr of pt arrival to the hospital.

Table 5.1 Empiric Antibiotics for Pneumonia

Patient Type	1st Abx Choice	Other Choices
CAP, non-ICU	antipneumococcal fluoroquinolone *or* beta-lactam + macrolide	beta-lactam + doxycycline
CAP, ICU (severe illness)	antipneumococcal fluoroquinolone + beta-lactam *or* beta-lactam + macrolide	antipneumococcal fluoroquinolone + aztreonam (if PCN-allergic)
CAP, at risk for *Pseudomonas*	antipseudomonal beta-lactam + antipseudomonal fluoroquinolone	antipseudomonal beta-lactam + aminoglycoside + antipneumococcal fluoroquinolone (*or* macrolide) (can substitute aztreonam for beta-lactam if PCN allergic)
CAP, at risk for MRSA	*Add* vancomycin *or* linezolid to drug choices above	
CAP, at risk for aspiration pneumonia	*Add* clindamycin to drug choices above	
HCAP/HAP/VAP, low MDR risk	Use same protocol as "CAP, non-ICU"	
HCAP/HAP/VAP, high MDR risk	antipseudomonal beta-lactam + antipseudomonal fluoroquinolone + vancomycin (or linezolid)	antipseudomonal beta-lactam + aminoglycoside + vancomycin (*or* linezolid) (can substitute aztreonam for beta-lactam if PCN allergic)

Choices within class of antibiotics:

Antipneumococcal FQ: levofloxacin, moxifloxacin, gemifloxacin

Antipseudomonal FQ: ciprofloxacin, levofloxacin

Beta-lactam: ceftriaxone, cefotaxime, ampicillin-sulbactam, ertapenem

Antipseudomonal beta-lactam: piperacillin-tazobactam, cefepime, imipenem, doripenem, meropenem

Macrolide: azithromycin, erythromycin, clarithromycin

Aminoglycoside: gentamicin, tobramycin, amikacin

Based on *Am J Respir Crit Care Med.* 2005;171:388; *Clin Infect Dis.* 2007;44 Suppl 2:S27.

- If Cx become available to guide therapy, reduce spectrum of abx coverage appropriately.
- Treat with abx therapy for a minimum of 5 d, and least 2–3 d after clinically stable.

Evidence for guidelines of empiric abx in CAP includes the following:

- Why avoid cephalosporin monotherapy?
  - Cohort studies have shown improved mortality with addition of macrolide therapy to cephalosporins in the empiric treatment of CAP (Arch IM 1999;159:2562; Chest 2001; 119:1420).
  - Effect probably due to both improved coverage of atypical organisms and double coverage of pneumococcus in areas of emerging resistance.
  - After initial rx and clinical improvement, may be appropriate to convert to monotherapy with either class of drugs to finish the course of treatment.
- Which initial choice for non-ICU CAP is the best (FQ or β-lactam/macrolide)?
  - Cohort studies have shown them to be equivalent (or at least better than cephalosporin monotherapy).
  - One RCT compared levofloxacin (500 mg IV qd, lower dose than used in most settings) to ceftriaxone (1 gm IV qd) and azithromycin (500 mg IV qd to start) in 212 pts with CAP; no difference in cure rates and outcomes (Treat Respir Med 2004;3:329).
- Why the dual drug therapy requirement in ICU pts with CAP?
  - Evidence for this is limited, but the main concern is providing adequate coverage for the sickest of pts.
  - Based on one RCT of 398 pts admitted to an ICU with severe CAP (but without shock), which showed no difference in outcomes between pts treated with FQ vs

combination of cephalosporin and macrolide, but a trend toward inferiority in FQ-treated pts (Chest 2005;128: 172).

- In addition to this (albeit limited) study, cohort studies of pts with bacteremic pneumococcal pneumonia (presumably more severe) have shown improved outcomes with multiple abx rather than monotherapy (Arch IM 2001;161:1837; Can Respir J 2004;11:589; Am J Respir Crit Care Med 2004;170:440), although the monotherapy in many of these pts was cephalosporin (not FQ) therapy.

Issues re time to first abx dose:

- Has been the subject of significant controversy in hospital and ER literature.
- Cohort studies showed improved mortality associated with abx given within 8 hr (JAMA 1997;278:2080) and improved in-hospital and 30-day mortality (and reduced LOS) for pts given first abx within 4 hr (Arch IM 2004;164:637).
- This led to development of CMS quality measure guidelines pushing for abx within 4 hr of arrival to the ED, which have since shown unintended consequences:
  - Study of 518 pts with CAP after release of 4-hr guideline (compared to prior 8-hr window) showed more pts received initial abx and blood cultures, but fewer had CXR consistent with pneumonia, or a final dx of pneumonia; no difference in mortality rates between the two time periods (Chest 2007;131:1865).
  - Many EDs with long wait times were administering abx to pts with dyspnea and then pursuing further clinical w/u, so as not to fall outside of the proscribed window for therapy.
- There is little doubt that abx should be given as soon as the dx of pneumonia is made, and should be given asap in pts with severe disease and shock (see "Sepsis and Septic Shock" in Section 5.3 for study on abx delay in sepsis).

- Current ACP/IDSA recommendations do not state a time frame, but simply that pts admitted through the ED should get abx in the ED, not delayed until admission to the floor/ICU.
- The current CMS quality measure is abx administered within 6 hr of arrival to the hospital.

    Other treatment considerations:

- Consider directed therapy in cases of known pathogen: e.g., antifungal therapy if proven aspergillosis, antiviral therapy for proven influenza (especially if severe disease or less than 48 hr of sx).
- Switch to oral abx once pt shows improvement with reduced fever, leukocytosis, delirium, stabilizing vital signs (for most pts, this will be within 3 days of admission).
- Duration of therapy for CAP should be up to 5 days and at least 2–3 days after achieving clinical stability (see Crs, above); high-dose levofloxacin and azithromycin rx have been proven effective for 5-day therapy; most other regimens suggest 7–10 days; consider longer therapy in pts with fungal, pseudo-monal, or staphylococcal pneumonia (can be from 2–6 wk depending on cause and source) or infection that spreads outside the lungs (e.g., meningitis, osteomyelitis, endocarditis).
- Duration of therapy for HAP/VAP is usually 7 days, as long as the following criteria are met prior to stopping abx (Crit Care Med 2001;29:1109):
    - Afebrile
    - WBC less than 10K
    - Improved radiographic findings (not resolved)
    - Improved respiratory secretions
    - Infection not associated with *Pseudomonas* (generally rx for 14–21 days)
- Treat concomitant sepsis and respiratory failure as appropriate; many pts require supplemental oxygen and IV hydration.
- Consider DVT prophylaxis in all pts.

- Consider GI/stress ulcer prophylaxis in appropriate pts, especially ventilated pts, critically ill, NPO, high-dose steroids.

Prevention of CAP:

- Smoking cessation counseling: This is a CMS "core measure" for quality for pts admitted with pneumonia who have smoked within the past 6 mo; many hospitals have developed inpatient smoking cessation counseling programs, including referrals for behavioral therapy, nicotine replacement.
- Pneumococcal vaccination: Consider for all pts older than 65 and those with high-risk diseases (lung disease, heart disease, cirrhosis, cancer).
- Influenza vaccination: Consider for all pts older than 50, those at risk for influenza-related cmplc, household contacts of high-risk pts, healthcare workers.
  - Pneumococcal and influenza vaccination screening (and offering vaccination to those eligible) is a CMS "core measure" for quality.

Prevention of HAP/VAP (Am J Respir Crit Care Med 2005;171:388):

- Staff hand-washing and respiratory precautions as appropriate
- Endotracheal and orogastric tubes instead of nasotracheal/nasogastric (Am J Respir Crit Care Med 1999;159:695)
- Possible prophylactic abx at the time of intubation
  - Small study of 50 pts intubated for head injury or stroke (and expected mechanical vent for more than 3 days); randomized to cefuroxime 1500 mg IV q 12 hr for 2 doses vs placebo; rx group had reduced incidence of pneumonia (24% vs 50%, NNT 4), did not affect mortality, but was associated with decreased ICU and total LOS (Am J Respir Crit Care Med 1997;155:1729).
- Elevation of the head of the bed in ventilated pts (Am J Respir Crit Care Med 1995;152:1387)
  - Elevate head of bed (HOB) more than 30–45°.

- RCT of supine vs semi-recumbent positioning of ventilated pts showed elevated HOB associated with reduced nosocomial pneumonia (34% vs 8%, NNT 4) (Lancet 1999;354:1851); however, goal elevation can be hard to meet at times and less elevation (less than 30°) not associated with any improved outcomes vs supine position (Crit Care Med 2006;34:396).
  - Risk of VAP increased with enteral feeds, so especially important to elevate HOB with any feeding.
- Limiting sedation and paralysis
- Selective decontamination of the digestive tract (SDD)
  - RCT of 546 surgical ICU pts; randomized to ciprofloxacin IV for 4 days and topical gentamicin/polymyxin vs placebo; SDD led to fewer infections including pneumonia (2% vs 10%, NNT 12), but no effect on mortality, except in the subgroup of pts with midrange APACHE-II scores (20–29) (7% vs 14%, NNT 15) (Am J Respir Crit Care Med 2002;166:1029).
  - RCT of 934 med/surg ICU pts; randomized to cefotaxime IV for 4 days and topical tobramycin/polymyxin/amphotericin vs placebo; SDD reduced hospital mortality (24% vs 31%, NNT 14) (Lancet 2003;362:1011).
  - Dutch study of 5939 ICU pts with expected LOS more than 3 days; randomized to three protocols: SDD (cefotaxime IV for 4 days and topical tobramycin/colistin/amphotericin), selective oral decontamination (topical only), placebo; after adjustment for multiple variables, both interventions reduced 28-day mortality vs placebo (oral only by 3.5% [NNT 29] and SDD by 2.9% [NNT 34]) (NEJM 2009;360:20).
  - Despite these results, many still have concerns, particularly about the use of prophylactic IV abx and emerging resistance; many ICUs have developed protocols for oral hygiene.

- GI prophylaxis (particularly with H2 blockers) (Ann IM 1994;120:653) and early enteral feedings (JPEN 2002;26:174) may be associated with increased risk of VAP, but guidelines suggest continued use because of lack of definitive proof of harm and known benefits.

5.6 Systemic Fungal Infections

Antifungal Medications

(Med Lett Drugs Ther 1997;39:86)

Azoles

(NEJM 1994;330:263)

- All can cause N/V, rashes, hepatotoxicity; all impair cytochrome p450 enzymes and so impair metabolism of many drugs (Med Lett Drugs Ther 1996;38:72) including macrolides, nonsedating antihistamines, benzodiazepines.
- Amphotericin B, 1 mg test dose, then 0.25–1.5 mg/kg IV qd, or perhaps less toxic continuous infusion over 24 hr (BMJ 2001;322:579); used for *Candida, Mucor, Cryptococcus*, histoplasmosis, blastomycosis, and extracutaneous sporotrichosis; adverse effects include RTA and renal failure (especially more than 4 gm cumulative dose), chills (rx with meperidine 25 mg IV or prevent with hydrocortisone, ASA, APAP, or antihistamines), hypokalemia, anemia, phlebitis, hypotension, pulmonary toxicity (NEJM 1981;304:1185).
- Fluconazole (Diflucan): 100–400 mg IV (or PO) qd; vs *Candida, Cryptococcus* (Ann IM 1990;113:183); none of the H2 blocker interference or testosterone problems of ketoconazole; adverse effects include alopecia (12–20%) after 2 mo rx (Ann IM 1995;123:354), toxic interactions with nonsedating antihistamines like terfenadine (JAMA 1996;275:1339).
- Itraconazole (Sporanox) 200–400 mg IV qd; may be less toxic than ketoconazole; used vs histo, blasto, invasive aspergillosis;

80–90% effective, but amphotericin still better if life threatening infection; adverse effects include toxic interactions with nonsedating antihistamines (JAMA 1996;275:1339), some benzodiazepines, and statins.

- Voriconazole (Vfend) (Med Lett Drugs Ther 2002;44:63; NEJM 2002;346:225) 6 mg/kg IV q 12 hr for 2 doses, then 4 mg/kg IV q 12 hr; for invasive aspergillosis (NEJM 2002;347:408), candidiasis.
- Oral meds include fluconazole, voriconazole, ketoconazole (Nizoral), miconazole (topical, Monistat).

Echinocandins

- Caspofungin (Cancidas) 70 mg IV load, then 50 mg IV qd; as good or better than amphotericin in safety and for monilial species (NEJM 2002;347:2020).
- Micafungin (Mycamine) (Med Lett Drugs Ther 2005;47:51) 50–150 mg IV qd; used for candidal esophagitis.

Fluorinated pyrimidines

- Flucytosine (5-fluorocystine) 50–150 mg/kg/d PO divided qid; with amphotericin for *Cryptococcus*, blastomycosis, and *Candida*; renal excretion; adverse effects include enterocolitis, dose-dependent leukopenia; emerging resistance prevents using alone.

Aspergillosis

(Am J Respir Crit Care Med 2006;173:707)

Cause: *Aspergillus* species; early studies showed mainly A. *fumigatus*, but more recent reports of multiple pathogenic species (A. *flavus*, *terreus, niger, versicolor*) (Clin Infect Dis 2002;34:909).

Epidem: Ubiquitous; environmental (e.g., from construction, air conditioners, bird guano); a pathogen primarily in the immunocompromised, especially AIDS (NEJM 1991;324:654).

Pathophys: Fungus ball (aspergilloma), allergic (Ann IM 1982;96:286), and invasive types; invasive type is associated with severe and persistent leukopenias and AIDS, as well as chronic lung disease, steroid use, and liver disease (Clin Infect Dis 2007; 45:205).

Enters through nose in immunocompromised host if nose first sterilized by abx (Ann IM 1979;90:4), or through skin ulcers or IV sites (NEJM 1987;317:1105).

Sx/Si: Hemoptysis with aspergilloma; asthma with allergic type.

Consider in pts with risk factors (immunosuppression, COPD, steroids) who have persistent febrile illness and pulmonary infiltrates, despite adequate abx therapy.

Crs: Invasive type has a 50% survival if start rx within 4 d of infiltrate appearing; much worse if delayed therapy (Ann IM 1977;86:539).

Cmplc: Disseminated aspergillosis can affect all organ systems (including endocarditis, eyes, sinusitis, GI tract, skin).

Lab: Gram stain shows mycelia in sputum 33% of time; blood Cx occasionally positive if systemic infection; nasal Cx 40% false neg, 10% false pos (Ann IM 1979;90:4).

In allergic type, eosinophilia and RIA-specific IgG and IgE, skin test positive (Ann IM 1977;86:405).

Re serum galactomannan assay:

- Component of *Aspergillus* cell wall released during fungal growth.
- Meta-analysis of 27 studies showed pooled sens of 71% and specif of 89% for invasive disease (Clin Infect Dis 2006;42:1417).
- False positive tests have been reported with piperacillin-tazobactam and ampicillin-sulbactam use, because both abx contain galactomannan (and both are used for broad-spectrum coverage of bacterial pneumonia) (J Clin Microbiol 2004;42:4744; J Clin Microbiol 2004;42:5362).

Noninv: CXR abnormal in almost all pts, but findings can include diffuse infiltrates, nodules/masses, and cavitary lesions.

Rx: Allergic type: Treat with steroids, itraconazole 200 mg PO qd–bid for at least 16 wk (NEJM 2000;342:756).

Systemic invasive types:

- 1st-line rx: voriconazole; RCT of 277 pts randomized to voriconazole (6 mg/kg IV q 12 hr for 2 doses, then 4 mg/kg IV bid for 7 d, then 200 mg PO bid) vs amphotericin B; vori showed better response (53% vs 32%, NNT 5) and mortality (29% vs 42%, NNT 8) (NEJM 2002;347:408).
- 2nd-line rx: amphotericin B (1 mg/kg qd until improved, then double-dose qod, then q 1–2 wk for 3–12 mo); itraconazole, caspofungin.
- Duration of rx usually months, until resolution of clinical sx and radiologic findings.

Blastomycosis

(NEJM 1986;314:529; NEJM 1986;314:575)

Cause: *Blastomyces dermatitidis*

Epidem: Airborne in rotten wood dust; North America, especially around the Great Lakes, and southeastern United States.

Pathophys: Lung involvement is most common (91%), but also can cause osteomyelitis (4%), prostatitis and other GU disease (2%), cutaneous involvement (18%) (Semin Respir Infect 1997;12:219).

Sx/Si: 3–12 wk incubation period; asx (50%), cough (45%), headache (32%), chest pain (30%), weight loss (28%), fever (25%).

Crs: Usually self-limited, 3–4 wk (NEJM 1974;290:540).

Cmplc: R/o South American blastomycosis, caused by paracoccidiomycosis (*Paracoccidioides brasiliensis*), which is transmitted by thorn pricks and causes skin disease that looks like leprosy; rx with sulfonamides.

Lab: Diphasic yeast form in tissue; *P. braziliensis* has multiple budding in yeast form.

Antigen testing available, sens 93%, spec 79%, but significant cross-reactivity with other invasive fungal diseases (J Clin Microbiol 2004;42:4873).

Skin test of doubtful usefulness, pos in fewer than 40% of proven cases (Am Rev Respir Dis 1988;138:1081; NEJM 1986;314:529).

Noninv: CXR; will be abnormal if pulmonic.

Rx: For severe infections (disseminated, CNS, severe lung disease), primary rx is amphotericin B; in milder forms of disease, itraconazole.

Coccidiomycosis (San Joaquin Valley Fever)

(NEJM 1995;332:1077)

Cause: *Coccidioides immitis*

Epidem: Airborne spread (inhalation) of mycelial stage infective spores; endospore spread in body.

Prevalent in American Southwest, especially Arizona, Texas, and California (e.g., San Joaquin Valley, Stockton to Bakersfield); worst in wet season, especially in pts exposed to dirt in spring and late fall.

Increased prevalence (possibly reactivation) in diabetics and pts on steroid rx, in AIDS and other immunocompromised pts.

Sx: Hemoptysis; granulomatous reactions of face and neck; pneumonitis (NEJM 1970;283:325), flu-like syndrome with generalized pruritus macular/papular rash; acute polyarthritis.

Si: Erythema nodosum, pleural effusion

Crs: Mortality 1% in Caucasians, 20% in Asians and Mexicans with disseminated disease; recurrence up to 10 yr after amphotericin rx (NEJM 1969;281:950).

Cmplc: Hypercalcemia (NEJM 1977;297:431); extrapulmonary lesions, onset more than 1 yr after primary pulmonary infection (e.g., bones, joints, skin, meninges).

Lab: Mycelial form (white, fluffy, distinctive) dangerous to lab personnel; diphasic but no yeast forms in tissue.

Urine Cx frequently pos if concentrated by lab, even when do not suspect disseminated disease; prostate secretions Cx also often pos in same circumstances (Ann IM 1976;85:34).

Complement fixation ab titer more than 1:16 suggests disseminated active disease; decreases with successful rx.

Noninv: Nodular pneumonitis; primary pneumonias; coin lesions; thin-walled cavities, r/o rheumatoid nodules and pneumatoceles.

Rx: Treat acute severe disease (NEJM 1987;317:334) as follows:

- Amphotericin 0.5 mg/kg IV biw to total of 30 mg/kg if sick, if complement fixation test is increased, or if steroids; 20% relapse (NEJM 1970;283:325); intrathecal for meningitis, many cmplc, especially with reservoir (NEJM 1973;288:186).
- Ketoconazole PO is at least static in many moderate pulmonary/skin infections (Ann IM 1982;96:436; Ann IM 1982;96:440); vs meningitis (Ann IM 1983;98:160).
- Fluconazole 400 mg qd PO for years effectively suppresses meningitis (Ann IM 1993;119:28) and treats more than 50% of nonmeningeal infections (Ann IM 2000;133:676).
- Itraconazole 200 mg PO bid, cures 63% of nonmeningeal infections (Ann IM 2000;133:676).

Meningitis after acute rx must have lifelong suppression (Ann IM 1996;124:305).

Cryptococcosis

(Rev Infect Dis 1991;13:1163; Ann IM 1981;94:611)

Cause: *Cryptococcus neoformans*

Epidem: Ubiquitous fungus; airborne; birds are probable vectors, especially pigeons, grows well in bird guano.

Worldwide; increased incidence in pts with lymphomas, AIDS, steroids.

Pathophys: Meningitis, pneumonitis (Am Rev Respir Dis 1966;94:236).

Sx/Si: Sx/si of meningitis, but may have acute or chronic, indolent course.

Crs: Without rx, nearly 100% mortality in 1 yr; with rx, 70% survival, 18% relapse in 29 mo (Ann IM 1969;71:1079); for a review of good and bad prognosis test results, see Ann IM 1974;80: 176.

Cmplc: Renal papillary necrosis (NEJM 1968;279:60); resistant prostatitis despite rx (Ann IM 1989;111:125)

Lab: Smear of sputum, CSF, urine; India ink preparation (drop of ink to CSF) reveals large clear (large capsules) organisms but 35% can have CNS crypto and neg India ink prep (Ann IM 1969;71:1079).

    Cultures have higher yield in HIV pts because of immunosuppression; in non-HIV, may need large volumes of CSF (15 mL) to find.

    Antigen by latex fixation or comp-fix is the only clinically useful test; for antibody, by indirect fluorescent antibody (IFA); 92% of pts positive for one or the other in CSF and/or serum (NEJM 1977;297:1440); pts with pos antigen levels do more poorly; false positive IFA in 2% normals, 6% blastos, 12% histos. No false positive antigen tests; hence rx a positive antigen but not a positive IFA (Ann IM 1968;69:1117).

Noninv: CT scan for mass lesions as described in the discussion of meningitis in Section 5.8.

Rx: IDSA guidelines for rx (Clin Infect Dis 2000;30:710):

- Isolated pulmonary disease: Watchful waiting in selected immunocompetent pts w/ mild disease, but for most fluconazole 200–400 mg qd for 3–6 mo; itraconazole or amphotericin B as alternatives.
- Cryptococcal meningitis (or other CNS disease): Amphotericin B 0.7–1 mg/kg/d *plus* flucytosine 100 mg/kg/d for 6–10 wk (or in select pts 2 wk may be enough for this initial IV therapy), then fluconazole 400 mg/d for 6–12 mo.

Histoplasmosis

Cause: *Histoplasma capsulatum*

Epidem: Most prevalent fungal disease in the United States; 500,000 new cases per year (Clin Infect Dis 2006;42:822).

 Bats and bird droppings are vectors via airborne spores; most common in Ohio and Mississippi River valleys in North America, but found worldwide.

 Exposures include chicken farms, caves, excavation and construction sites.

Pathophys: Intracellular; three clinical syndromes: acute primary (pulmonary), chronic cavitary (pulmonary), and progressive disseminated (Ann IM 1972;76:557).

Sx: Pulmonary, acute immune complex-type polyarthritis

Si: May present with chorioretinitis, focal, macular choroid inflammation, and hemorrhage without vitreous reaction (present with all other types of chorioretinitis).

 Other signs: hepatomegaly; erythema nodosa.

Crs: Usually benign; fewer than 5% of exposures result in symptomatic disease (Eur J Clin Microbiol Infect Dis 1989;8:480).

 In endemic areas, must r/o histo in pts with concern for sarcoidosis, because of similar appearance and worsening course with steroid or immunosuppressive rx (NEJM 2000;342:37).

Cmplc: Complications include the following:

- Fibrosing syndromes of mediastinum and/or retroperitoneum
- Endocarditis
- Adrenal insufficiency in 50% of disseminated form (Ann IM 1971;75:511)
- Chronic meningitis, like *Cryptococcus*
- Ulcerative enteritis, especially of distal ileum and colon

Lab: Silver stain; cannot see with H&E stain or Giemsa stain. Cx most likely pos in chronic pulmonary syndrome; in disseminated forms, culture of liver, marrow, nodes are pos in about 20% of cases (Ann IM 1982;97:680); slow grower, takes more than 2 wk; filamentous strands of hyphal sporangia; distinctive chlamydospores when grown at room temperature.

Labs may show anemia, thrombocytopenia.

Complement fixation ab titer pos in 96% of pts with active, disseminated disease (Ann IM 1982;97:680); immunodiffusion ab titer positive in 87%; RIA for antigen positive in urine (90%) and blood (50%) in disseminated disease (NEJM 1986;314:83) and more accurate than ab titers, which can initially be neg for 4–8 wk after exposure (Ann IM 1991;115:936).

Noninv: "Buckshot" calcifications in lungs, spleen; can have varied pulmonary findings from discrete nodules to mediastinal and hilar masses to cavitary lesions.

Rx: Most pts with mild or asx disease require no specific therapy.

Amphotericin B and itraconazole are primary antifungals, but fluconazole, voriconazole also have activity.

Pneumocystis Pneumonia (PCP)

(NEJM 2004;350:2487)

Cause: Formerly *Pneumocystis carinii*, now *P. jirovecii* (changed because PCP first described in rats is a different organism from the infectious agent in humans), reclassified as a fungus from protozoan status in 1988.

Epidem: Opportunistic; airborne from other people harboring (e.g., epidemics in tumor clinic) (Ann IM 1975;82:772).

In pts with depressed immunologic responses including hypogammaglobulinemia, premature infants, hematopoietic malignancy, immunosuppression, AIDS (vast majority of pts with pneumocystis have AIDS and CD4 count less than 200/mm^3), elderly (NEJM 1991;324:246).

Pathophys: Diffuse interstitial pneumonitis

Sx: Dyspnea, nonproductive cough

Si: Fever, normal chest exam or rales, tachypnea, tachycardia; thrush often concomitantly

Crs: Die in weeks without rx (50%), but with treatment mortality is about 3%; those who require ventilator have a 25% survival to hospital discharge (JAMA 1995;273:230); mortality is lower in pts with AIDS than those without, especially in cancer pts (Clin Infect Dis 2002;34:1098).

Cmplc: Osteomyelitis rarely (NEJM 1992;326:999); r/o other opportunistic infections.

Lab: Hypertonic saline-induced sputum (Ann IM 1988;109:7; Ann IM 1996;124:585), stain with Giemsa (72% sens), toluidine blue (80% sens), or with indirect immunofluorescence (92% sens) (NEJM 1988;318:589); does not grow in culture.

> If further testing required, consider bronchoscopic biopsy, lavage, brushings.

> Often elevated serum LDH, but nonspecific (Chest 1995;108:415).

> If HIV status unknown, test for HIV and check CD4 and viral loads.

Noninv: CXR shows diffuse interstitial infiltrate, starts perihilar, 98% bilateral.

> Gallium scan shows hot lungs even with neg plain films, but 50% false positives including sarcoid pts (NEJM 1988;318:1439).

Rx: (Med Lett Drugs Ther 1995;37:87; NEJM 1992;327:1853; Ann IM 1988;109:280)

> Treatment of acute disease includes:

- Trimethoprim-sulfamethoxazole (TMP-SMX) 15–20 mg/kg/d divided q 6–8 hr PO/IV is primary rx (Ann IM 1986;105:37; Med Lett Drugs Ther 1981;23:102); watch for allergic rash, marrow suppression, renal failure; alternatives include pentamidine IV, atovaquone PO, or primaquine and clindamycin PO.

- Supportive rx with ICU care and supplemental O_2 as needed; in non-HIV pts, may require more traditional abx coverage until CAP/HAP ruled out.
- Adjunctive steroid therapy in HIV-infected pts, starting with prednisone 40 mg bid and taper over 3 wk or IV methylprednisolone (NEJM 1990;323:1500; NEJM 1990;323:1451; NEJM 1990;323:1444); in non-HIV pts, more controversial, but recommended if significant hypoxemia and severe disease.
- Duration of therapy 14–21 d, with the latter especially in HIV pts.

Prevention (NEJM 1995;332:693; Ann IM 1995;122:755):

- Prophylaxis of HIV pts with CD4 count less than 200/mm^3, and consider in the following non-HIV pts:
  - Transplant pts, including stem cell (MMWR Recomm Rep 2000;49:1) and solid organ (J Natl Compr Canc Netw 2008;6:122)
  - Pts on long-term prednisone more than 20 mg qd (or equivalent) (Arch IM 1995;155:1125), especially if on other immunosuppressive drugs
  - Pts with other acquired or congenital leukopenias
  - Efficacy shown in meta-analysis of 12 trials (more than 1200 pts) of pts with hematologic cancer or transplant; prophylaxis led to 91% reduction in PCP infection (NNT 15) and PCP-related mortality (Mayo Clin Proc 2007;82:1052)
- Primary drug is TMP-SMX 1 double-strength tablet qd (or 3/wk) or 1 single-strength tablet qd (Arch IM 1996;156:177; NEJM 1987;316:1627); alternatives include atovaquone (NEJM 1998;339:1889), dapsone (Am J Med 1993;95:573), pentamidine aerosol (Med Lett Drugs Ther 1989;31:91; Ann IM 1990;113:677) or IV, primaquine and clindamycin.

Systemic Candidiasis

Cause: Previously *Candida albicans* in many cases, but increasing rates of other species like *tropicalis* (Ann IM 1979;91:539), *krusei*, *parapsilosis*, and *glabrata*, which are often fluconazole resistant.

Epidem: Associated with ICU care, indwelling catheters, immunosuppression, abx, TPN, acid suppressants

Pathophys: Normal flora, opportunistic invasion

Sx: In a debilitated pt, rapid deterioration to severe sepsis and shock; suppurative peripheral thrombophlebitis (Ann IM 1982;96:431).

Si: Fever, papular/pustular rash like gonococcus

Crs: 36% mortality (NEJM 1994;331:1325)

Cmplc: Systemic type: myocarditis, endophthalmitis ("a culture of fungus growing on retina") (NEJM 1972;286:675), hepatosplenic abscess (Ann IM 1988;108:88)

Lab: Positive blood Cx for *Candida* should always be treated as a true infectious agent, not colonizer (as opposed to urine, respiratory, skin culture).

Candida PCR in pts with high suspicion and neg cultures (J Clin Microbiol 2002;40:2483; Clin Infect Dis 2008;46:890).

Rx: (Med Lett Drugs Ther 1990;32:58; Med Lett Drugs Ther 1988;30:30)

1st line is amphotericin B or fluconazole (NEJM 1994;331:1325); consider caspofungin in *C. glabrata*, *krusei* (NEJM 2002;347:2020); rx for a minimum of 14 d.

Removal of infected/colonized catheters is crucial to cure. Empiric rx for candidemia:

- Consider in pts with neutropenic fever after more than 4 d of fever with no response to abx, but limited evidence to suggest use empirically in all ICU pts.
- Meta-analysis of 626 surgical ICU pts using fluconazole as empiric therapy; rx did reduce overall fungal infections, but not

candidemia (which was only diagnosed in ~2% of pts), and no effect on mortality (Crit Care Med 2005;33:1928).

- RCT of empiric fluconazole in 270 ICU pts with fever, broad-spectrum abx, APACHE-II more than 16; randomized to fluconazole 800 IV qd vs placebo; no difference in outcomes including resolution of fever and invasive candidiasis, but overall fewer than 10% of pts had documented candidemia (Ann IM 2008;149:83).

5.7 Urinary Tract Infections

Complicated Urinary Tract Infections and Pyelonephritis

(Am Fam Phys 2005;71:933)

Cause: UTIs encompasses lower urinary tract (urethra, prostate, bladder, ureter) and upper urinary tract (renal parenchyma and pelvis) infections; most lower UTIs are seen and treated as outpatients, unless inpatient-acquired (usually due to catheterization) or complicated UTI; many cases of pyelonephritis also evaluated and treated as outpatients, but higher percentage require admission than lower tract infections.

Microbial causes include:

- *E. coli* is most common; about 70% of acute cystitis and about 80% of acute pyelonephritis
- Remaining common organisms: *Staph. saprophyticus*; *Proteus*; *Klebsiella*; enterococci
- Complicated and catheter-related UTIs more closely mirror nosocomial infections, with higher rates of drug-resistant Gram-neg organisms, including *Pseudomonas*, staph including MRSA, polymicrobial infections, and *Candida*

Complicated UTIs include (Urol Clin N Am 2008;35:13):

- UTIs in immunosuppressed pts (including diabetics), at risk for drug-resistant organisms.

- Associated urinary tract obstruction:
  - Prostatic hypertrophy in males, causing bladder outlet obstruction; distended bladder, bilateral hydronephrosis, large prostate on rectal exam
  - Lower tract obstruction in females usually due to pelvic tumor (e.g., colorectal, uterine, ovarian)
  - Upper tract obstruction usually from nephrolithiasis, rarely tumor
- Catheter-associated UTI: Risk of UTI with indwelling catheter is about 5% per day; with indwelling catheter almost all pts have bacterial colonization of the urinary tract within 2–3 weeks.
- UTIs in men: Controversial; may be more likely due to obstruction (prostate), hematogenous spread, or resistant organisms, because anatomically, men at lower risk for ascending infection due to longer urethra and prostatic secretions (Urol 1976;7:169).
- Patients with CKD: Complicated due to acute renal failure with infection; reduced abx delivery to the tissue.
- Pregnancy: Associated with high rates of asymptomatic bacteriuria (usually screened for and rx early in pregnancy).

Epidem: Yearly incidence of pyelonephritis in United States: 250K cases, 100K hospitalizations.

Women have a higher risk for hospitalization (5 times higher than men), but lower mortality (50% lower).

Pathophys: 95% of cases from ascending bacteria (usually from the GI tract); 5% from hematogenous spread from other sources

Sx/Si: Lower UTI sx include urethral burning, irritation; pelvic discomfort; polyuria, urinary urgency.

Upper UTI sx include flank pain (with costovertebral angle tenderness), fevers, chills, N/V.

Sx in complicated UTIs, especially in the elderly, can be harder to distinguish; may present as sepsis, altered mental status/delirium, change in behavior/mood, irritability, weakness/fatigue.

Strongly consider sx in setting of possible catheter-related UTI, because all pts with chronic catheters will have pos urine Cx; do not order Cx unless plan to treat; avoid routine Cx or for inappropriate sx (change in urine appearance, urinary odor, etc.).

Crs: Many pts with pyelonephritis remain febrile for up to 72 hr, even after appropriate abx; if continued illness after 72 hr, consider:

- Inappropriate abx regimen or microbial resistance
- Cmplc, including perinephric abscess, ureteral obstruction
- Alternate dx: lower lobe pneumonia, intra-abdominal infection, herpes zoster (which can present with flank pain and constitutional sx, even before onset of vesicular rash), pelvic inflammatory disease

Cmplc: In pregnancy, UTIs can lead to preterm labor and low birth weight.

Emphysematous pyelonephritis (J Urol 2007;178:880): Seen in immunosuppressed and diabetics; usually presents with severe sepsis and shock; gas in the urinary tract/renal parenchyma (despite gas, most common cause is still *E. coli*, not anaerobic organisms); mortality can be very high (~40%), and many pts require surgical intervention, including early nephrostomy placement and possible nephrectomy.

Perinephric abscess (Urol Clin N Am 1999;26:753): Usually from direct extension from pyelonephritis, but can also arise from hematogenous spread; requires eval for ureteral/renal obstruction; CT is the best study; relieve obstruction with nephrostomy; may require complete I&D for large abscesses.

Infected stones with urease-producing organisms (Urol Clin N Am 1999;26:753): Urease produces a high urinary pH, which does not allow magnesium to become soluble, and then mixes with ammonia to form a $Mg\text{-}NH_3\text{-}phos$ stone; most common

INFECTIOUS DISEASE

5.7   *Urinary Tract Infections*   **333**

with *Proteus* infections; requires directed abx therapy and stone removal.

Lab: Initial w/u usually includes CBC with diff, metabolic panel, urinalysis with Gram stain and Cx.

U/A should reveal pos tests for leukocyte esterase and nitrites; micro should reveal pyuria, may also show hematuria, white cell casts; confirmatory urine Cx requires more than 10K CFUs.

Blood Cx are often drawn in pts hospitalized for complicated UTI and pyelonephritis, but rarely change management.

- Urine Cx often pos and guides abx management; usually pos Cx in 90% of pts with pyelonephritis (unless obtained after abx started).
- Retrospective analysis of 307 pts with pyelonephritis; pos blood Cx in 18%, but more than 33% were considered contaminants and only one Cx (0.2%) revealed an organism not grown on urine Cx (Am J Emerg Med 1997;15:137); results corroborated in another study of 583 women (Clin Infect Dis 2003;37:1127).
- Consider blood Cx only if critical illness/sepsis or high suspicion for resistant organisms, including immunosuppressed pts.

Noninv: Most cases do not require any imaging studies.

In pts not responding to standard antibiotic therapy, consider CT, U/S or IVP to rule out ureteral obstruction, perinephric abscess, emphysematous changes.

Rx: Most uncomplicated UTIs can be treated as outpatients with close observation (case-control study of 200 women in San Francisco showed 90% response in both outpatients and inpatients, with 7.5 times higher costs in hospitalized pts) (Am J Med 1988;85:793), but consider hospitalization if:

- Sepsis, severe illness
- Persistent vomiting, unable to take PO meds
- Associated urinary tract obstruction, requiring specific therapy

- Not responding to prior outpatient therapy
- Patients at risk for resistant organisms (immunosuppressed, severe DM, posttransplant)
- Inadequate f/u or social support

  Guidelines for rx of asymptomatic bacteriuria:

- Do not check urine Cx unless planning to treat.
- Rx with abx only in pts at risk for progression to acute disease.
  - Pregnancy, immunosuppression, pts with planned urinary tract instrumentation
- Very high rates associated with indwelling catheters—remove catheter if possible.

  Guidelines for rx of uncomplicated UTIs and pyelonephritis:

- Oral/IV fluoroquinolone: ciprofloxacin, levofloxacin, moxi-floxacin all good choices; oral bioavailability is about 100%, so oral just as good, unless pt not able to take PO.
- Other appropriate choices: Extended-spectrum cephalosporin (e.g., ceftriaxone), ampicillin-sulbactam, aztreonam (alternative to FQ, if PCN allergic); can also use ampicillin and gentamicin, but given aminoglycoside toxicity, not considered a 1st-line option.
- In pregnant pts, avoid FQs and aminoglycosides.
- Trimethoprim-sulfamethoxazole (TMP-SMX, Bactrim) has been a common empiric abx choice for uncomplicated lower UTIs, but increasing community resistance (up to 20%) (Ann IM 2001;135:41) has led to concern about use empirically; in hospitalized pts, use urine Cx and local resistance patterns to guide management.
- Switch to PO as soon as able; 7–10 d course is feasible in most healthy pts with uncomplicated disease.

  Guidelines for rx of complicated UTIs:

- Consider source: Remove infected catheters; relieve obstruction (urolithiasis with cystoscopy, lithotripsy; BPH with TURP, prostatectomy).

- If risk for nosocomial or MDR organisms, consider empirical broad-spectrum coverage: cefepime, piperacillin-tazobactam, carbapenems; vancomycin or linezolid if MRSA-risk.
- Depending on microbe and cause of infection, may require prolonged therapy, 4–6 wk; typically, true catheter-related infections (as opposed to colonization) require 14–21 d of abx.
- Recurrent UTIs may require abx prophylaxis, but suggest consultation and close f/u, as also will likely select for further resistant organisms.

Guidelines for rx of candidal UTI (Pharmacotherapy 1993;13:110):

- Usually related to urinary catheter, and most cases represent asymptomatic candiduria, which should not require rx (except removal of catheter if able).
- More rarely, may be related to systemic candidiasis; consider risk factors (immunosuppression, critical illness, multiple prolonged abx), blood Cx to look for candidemia, Cx of other sources (resp tract, GI tract).
- If felt to represent true infection, rx with oral or IV fluconazole; alternative includes IV rx or bladder irrigation with amphotericin B.

Consider a f/u urine Cx in 2–4 wk posthospitalization to ensure eradication.

To prevent catheter-related UTI in hospital inpatients, avoid initial placement of Foley catheter unless absolutely necessary, and then review necessity daily to allow removal as soon as possible (Arch IM 1999;159:800).

5.8 Central Nervous System Infections

Meningitis

(NEJM 2006;354:44; Clin Infect Dis 2004;39:1267)

Cause: Microbial causes in adults:

- Bacterial: *Neisseria meningitides* (meningococcus) and *Strep. pneumoniae* (pneumococcus) account for 80% of cases; also *Haemophilus influenzae* type b (although reduced significantly with childhood vaccination), *Strep. agalactiae*; in pts older than 50, severe alcoholism, and immunosuppression, also consider Gram negatives and *Listeria*; in pts with recent neurosurgical procedures, consider *Staph. aureus*, including MRSA.
- Viral (BMJ 2008;336:36): Enteroviruses (Coxsackie A and B, echoviruses, polioviruses), herpes simplex virus (HSV-1, HSV-2), varicella (VZV), HIV, Epstein-Barr virus (EBV), mumps (used to be most common cause of viral meningitis prior to widespread vaccination), West Nile, tick-borne.
- Rare causes can include fungal (*Cryptococcus*), atypicals (mycobacteria).

Epidem: Adult incidence: 4–6 per 100,000 people

Sx/Si: Classic triad of fever, neck stiffness, and delirium/altered mental status; found in only 44% of 696 cases in one study, but when headache added, 95% of pts had at least two of the classic sx (NEJM 2004;351:1849).

Also photophobia, focal neuro sx (see Cmplc below).

Look for signs of meningococcemia with petechial rash; vesicular or maculopapular rash may suggest viral cause.

Classic signs are Kernig's (resistance to extension of the knee when the hip is flexed at right angle) and Brudzinski's (flexion of the hips with attempts at neck flexion), which both suggest meningeal inflammation; specif is adequate (~95%), but sens in eval of bacterial meningitis is low (~5%) (Clin Infect Dis 2003;36:125).

Altered mental status based on Glasgow Coma Score (GCS) of less than 14:

- GCS allows score of altered mental status based on three criteria, with scores ranging from 3 to 15; may be difficult or impossible to score in pts on ventilator or having received sedatives or paralytics for intubation.

- Eye opening (up to 4 points):
  - Spontaneous (4), to verbal stimulus (3), to pain (2), no eye opening (1)
- Verbal response (up to 5 points):
  - Oriented (5), confused (4), inappropriate words (3), in-comprehensible sounds (2), no response (1)
- Motor response (up to 6 points):
  - Follows commands (6), localizes to pain (5), withdraws to pain (4), flexor response (3), extensor response (2), no response (1)

Crs: If worsening mental status with treatment, consider encephalitis and elevated ICP.

Overall mortality rate about 20% (NEJM 2004;351:1849), but higher with pneumococcal disease (30%); risk factors for poor outcome include:

- Older pts
- Concomitant sinusitis or otitis
- Clinical findings: tachycardia, lack of rash (suggests pneumo-coccal disease), low initial GCS score
- Lab findings: positive blood Cx, elevated ESR, thrombocy-topenia, low CSF white cell count (may indicate inability to mount adequate immune response)

Cmplc: Associated neurologic abnormalities (NEJM 2004;351:1849):

- Seizures in 5%
- Hearing loss in up to 14% of pts, due to CN VIII palsy
- Focal neuro deficits in 33% of pts; other CN palsies in 2–7% (ocular [III, VI], facial [VII]), aphasia 23%, hemiparesis 7%
- Long-term cognitive impairment in 27% (J Infect Dis 2002;186:1047)

Consider subdural empyema in pts with deterioration despite adequate therapy, especially if evidence of sinusitis or mastoiditis (Clin Infect Dis 1995;20:372).

Lab: Initial lab w/u should include CBC with diff, metabolic panel (including glucose), PT/PTT (to r/o underlying coagulopathy prior to LP).

Blood Cx should be obtained in all pts (positive in 67% of pts with bacterial cause), as may have some yield if LP unsuccessful or unable to be done.

Many cases have mild to moderate hyponatremia, due to SIADH, cerebral salt wasting, and fluid resuscitation.

Noninv: Lumbar puncture is the definitive test (JAMA 2006;296: 2012).

- Should be performed in all pts when concern for meningitis, preferably before administration of abx, unless significant delay in abx therapy.
- Most dangerous risk of procedure is brainstem herniation, due to removal of CSF in pts with elevated intracranial pressure from a CNS mass lesion; consider CT prior to LP in select pts (see "Which patients require a head CT prior to LP?" below).
- Most common adverse effects are headache (60%) and backache (40%) (Acta Neurol Scand 1998;98:445); rare events include hemorrhage (especially in pts with coagulopathy) and infection.
- Guidelines for performing the procedure:
  - Place pt in the lateral recumbent position with knees flexed to the chest to allow maximal opening of the interspinous distance (can also using a sitting position if pt not able to lie down).
  - Use the pt's posterior superior iliac crest as the guide to find the L4–L5 interspace; can go one level higher or lower if needed, but avoid anything higher than that

because of risk of puncturing the conus medullaris of the spinal cord.

- Use sterile drapes and procedures; cleanse skin with chlorhexidine.
- Some use atraumatic needles (blunt tip) to reduce risk of postprocedure headache (Neurol 2000;55:909).
- In most settings, obtain the following:
  - Opening pressure of CSF with use of a manometer (place the 0 level of manometer at the level of the needle): normally will be 6–18 cm H_2O, in bacterial meningitis, may be elevated more than 40 cm in 40% of pts (NEJM 2004;351:1849) and correlates with level of consciousness; should see some variation with respirations.
  - Collect up to four tubes of CSF (usually 1–2 mL each) for analysis: tube 1 for glucose and protein levels; tube 2 for Gram stain and culture; tube 3 for cell count and differential; tube 4 to hold for other studies (can consider in certain circumstances: bacterial antigen testing, enteroviral tests, VDRL, Lyme titer, HSV PCR, fungal culture, AFB smear and culture, lactate level).
  - Replace the stylet in the needle prior to removal from the epidural space to reduce risk of postprocedure headache (16% of pts had post-LP headache without stylet reinsertion vs 5% with reinsertion in one study of 600 pts, NNT 9) (J Neurol 1998;245:589).

  Guidelines for interpretation of CSF results:

- Other than a pos CSF culture, no single test absolutely rules in or rules out bacterial meningitis; treat empirically based on clinical suspicion and use LP results to help guide.
- Positive Gram stain has specif of 97% for bacterial cause; sens is 60–90% for negative staining.
- CSF WBC greater than 500/mm^3 suggests bacterial meningitis (Eur J Clin Microbiol Infect Dis 1988;7:374); average about

7500/mm^3, range is 100–10,000/mm^3; usually predominance of neutrophils.

- Reduced glucose levels suggest bacterial meningitis; absolute CSF glucose less than 40 mg/dL or CSF-blood glucose ratio of 0.4 or less (98% specific for bacterial meningitis) (Clin Infect Dis 2004;39:1267).
- Protein levels often elevated, more than 50 mg/dL, but non-specific (can be seen with viral meningitis, other inflammatory and neurologic diseases).
- CSF culture can be negative in 10–30%; may be due to viral disease, difficult-to-grow organism, prior abx.
- Bacterial antigen testing (most test for *S. pneumoniae*, *N. meningiditis*, *H. influenzae*, *S. agalactiae*) not necessary for all pts, but consider in those pts who have already received abx (and therefore may have neg CSF culture) and those with neg Gram stain and Cx results.
- Viral antigen testing (PCR for enteroviruses) is available in some settings, with consideration of discontinuation of abx therapy if positive, but no large clinical trials to assist decision.

  Which patients require a head CT prior to LP?

- Most pts should not get a head CT prior to LP because of the delay in dx and subsequent abx therapy (as well as the added cost of unnecessary imaging).
- Main concern is to find pts at risk for intracranial mass lesion causing elevated ICP, which in turn may cause brainstem herniation when CSF removed by the procedure.
- Studies to guide decision:
  - Study of 113 pts with need for LP; 15% had new finding of intracranial lesion on CT (2.7% were considered danger-ous enough to preclude LP); three risk factors increased the risk for finding a new lesion: altered mental status, focal neurologic deficits, papilledema; these findings with overall clinical impression (undefined in the study) were able to

provide an adequate screen for pts who require a pre-LP CT scan (Arch IM 1999;159:2681).

- Study of 301 Yale ED pts with need for LP; 24% had a new intracranial CT finding, 5% with evidence of mass effect; the following findings were associated with an increased risk for intracranial lesion:
  - Patient factors: age older than 60, immunosuppression, h/o CNS disease, seizure within the past week
  - Exam findings: altered mental status, unable to answer two questions correctly, unable to follow two commands, presence of gaze or facial palsy, abnormal visual field exam, abnormal speech, arm or leg drift
  - Absence of all of these features reduced risk of abnormal CT to 3% (NPV 97%); use of this screen prospectively would have reduced need for CT by 41% (NEJM 2001;345:1727)
- Bottom line is that the risk of an intracranial lesion should be considered in all pts prior to LP, and should use the above factors (mainly altered mental status, focal neuro deficits, recent seizure activity, and immunosuppression) and overall clinical impression to guide the need for CT imaging; if decide to proceed with CT imaging, should perform asap, draw stat blood cultures, and give empiric abx (and steroids) prior to the CT with immediate LP once CT results available.

Rx: Antibiotic therapy for bacterial meningitis:

- Empiric rx should be started as soon as dx is suspected and LP is performed (or even prior to LP if delay for imaging or procedural assistance); delay in abx more than 6 hr is associated with increased mortality in pts with acute bacterial meningitis (and delays are associated with facility transfers, wait times for CT prior to LP, and absence of classic sx) (QJM 2005;98:291).

- Empiric abx therapy guidelines:
  - For most adult pts, use a 3rd generation cephalosporin (e.g., ceftriaxone 2 gm IV q 12 hr or cefotaxime 2 gm IV q 6 hr) *and* vancomycin 15–20 mg/kg IV q 12 hr.
    - Vancomycin added for coverage of resistant pneumococcus, not MRSA, in this category of pts; due to some concern for vancomycin failure, it is not recommended as monotherapy (Antimicrob Agents Chemother 1991;35:2467).
  - For older adults, immunosuppressed, or severe alcoholics, add ampicillin 2 gm IV q 4 hr for *Listeria* coverage.
  - For pts at risk for nosocomial (MDR organism) infection and postneurosurgical pts, use broad-spectrum agent (e.g., cefepime 2 gm IV q 8 hr or meropenem 2 gm IV q 8 hr) *and* vancomycin.
    - Meropenem and imipenem have both been proven effective in small studies, but less risk of seizures with meropenem.
  - If concern for possible HSV encephalitis (see "Encephalitis" later in Section 5.8; risk factors include known HSV lesions or h/o recurrent disease, temporal lobe hemorrhage or MRI findings, lymphocytic predominance in CSF), add acyclovir 10 mg/kg IV q 8 hr.
- Once Cx and sens available, consider changing to directed therapy.
- Duration of rx is 10–14 d for most common organisms (or culture-neg, with continued suspicion for bacterial cause); consider 21 d of therapy for *Listeria* and Gram-negatives (Clin Infect Dis 2004;39:1267); unlike other infections, IV therapy is recommended for the full course to ensure high CSF concentrations of abx, but can consider home IV rx in pts showing improvement after 6–7 d, with no significant neuro deficits, stable home environment, and adequate compliance and follow-up (Clin Infect Dis 1999;29:1394).

Adjunctive therapy for meningitis:

- Supportive care; many pts need ICU-level mgt; may require ICP monitoring if worsening mental status/coma.
- Respiratory precautions for pts with suspected meningococcal meningitis.
- Steroids should be considered in all cases of suspected bacterial meningitis.
    - RCT of 301 pts with acute meningitis; randomized to dexamethasone 10 mg IV before or at the time of first abx dose, then q 6 hr for 4 d vs placebo; rx was associated with a significant reduction in "unfavorable outcome" (death or anything more than mild persistent disability) (15% vs 25%, NNT 10) and mortality (7% vs 15%, NNT 13), with most benefit seen in pts with pneumococcal meningitis, and no increased side effects (NEJM 2002; 347:1549).
    - Meta-analysis of five trials (including one above) corroborated results of reduction in mortality and poor neuro outcome from adjunctive steroid use (Lancet Infect Dis 2004;4:139).
    - Suggest all pts with suspected bacterial meningitis receive dexamethasone 10 mg IV prior to first abx dose and then q 6 hr for 4 d.
    - In pts with concomitant septic shock, no evidence to suggest either dexamethasone or hydrocortisone dosing (see "Sepsis and Septic Shock" in Section 5.3) is superior; but given significant results of the meningitis studies, dexamethasone is probably preferred over hydrocortisone.
- If associated seizures, may require anticonvulsant therapy, but no evidence for prophylactic use.
- Chemoprophylaxis for close contacts of pts with meningococcus with either rifampin 600 mg bid for 4 doses or ciprofloxacin 500 mg for 1 dose.

Encephalitis

(Clin Infect Dis 2008;47:303)

Cause: Inflammatory disease of the brain tissue associated with neurologic dysfunction.

Microbial causes of encephalitis are as follows:

- Viral: likely accounts for the vast majority of cases, but difficult to determine percentage, as most not able to be tested; major classes of encephalitis viruses include:
  - Adenovirus
  - Flavivirus: West Nile, Japanese encephalitis, tick-borne encephalitis, Powassan
  - Herpes virus: HSV-1 and HSV-2, varicella, HHV-6, CMV, EBV
  - Togavirus: rubella, equine encephalitis
  - Paramyxovirus: measles, mumps
  - Others: polio, HIV, rabies, influenza
- Bacterial: *Bartonella* (cat scratch disease), *Listeria*, *Mycoplasma*
- Mycobacteria
- Rickettsial: ehrlichiosis, *Coxiella burnetii* (Q fever), *R. rickettsii* (Rocky Mountain spotted fever)
- Spirochetes: *Borrelia burgdorferi* (Lyme), *Treponema pallidum* (syphilis)
- Fungal: *Coccidioides*, *Cryptococcus neoformans*, *Histoplasma*
- Protozoal: *Acanthamoeba*, *Naegleria*, *Plasmodium falciparum* (malaria), *Toxoplasma*, *Trypanosoma*

Consider noninfectious causes in the differential dx:

- Encephalopathies: metabolic (hyponatremia, hypoglycemia), hepatic, intoxication/overdose, related to critical illness/sepsis
- Tumors, with mass effect or paraneoplastic syndrome
- Seizures and status epilepticus
- Stroke
- CNS vasculitis

- Acute disseminated encephalomyelitis (ADEM): immuno-logic response up to 2 wk after immunization or infection

  Actual causative agent not determined in most cases; the California Encephalitis Project evaluated 334 pts from 1998–2000 with a wide array of tests to determine cause; 62% had no cause found, 9% were found to have a viral encephalitis, 3% bacterial, 10% were determined to have noninfectious cause (Clin Infect Dis 2003;36:731).

Epidem: Important aspects of hx to help determine causative agent: recent travel, employment and hobbies, ill contacts, pets or other animal contact, raw meat or milk ingestion, sexual history, vaccination status.

Sx/Si: Significant overlap with sx of meningitis (including headache, fever, delirium, seizures); mental status changes may be more protean, including cognitive dysfunction, personality changes.

Crs: High mortality with HSV encephalitis, even with prompt rx; Swedish study of 236 pts showed 1-yr mortality of 14%, and more than 20% persistent neuro deficits or seizures (Clin Infect Dis 2007;45:875).

Cmplc: Specific complications depend on the offending agent.

Lab: Multiple tests available for specific causes, but "shotgun" approach probably not helpful; focus on specific agents suggested by history and physical (consult IDSA guidelines for more information) (Clin Infect Dis 2008;47:303); widespread testing may lead to "red herrings" (prior exposures that are not the causative agent), significantly increase cost of care, and may not change management.

  Initial w/u should include CBC with diff, metabolic panel, renal and liver function tests, blood Cx (and consider Cx of urine, resp tract, wounds in specific settings).

  Consider specific testing for common pathogens with serologies: CMV, EBV, HIV, *Mycoplasma*, Lyme titers.

Noninv: Lumbar puncture required in most cases to r/o bacterial meningitis and to obtain CSF for directed testing; CSF in encephalitis (as opposed to meningitis) more likely to show lower WBC (less than 250/mm^3), elevated protein, normal glucose.

For imaging, MRI is preferred over CT (Curr Opin Neurol 2004;17:475); look for temporal lobe involvement with HSV (J Neurol Sci 1998;157:148); thalamic, basal ganglia, midbrain lesions with flaviviruses.

EEG may be helpful to r/o status epilepticus and may show temporal lobe findings with HSV.

Brain bx can be considered in difficult cases, but may be low yield for the risk.

Rx: For most causative agents, only supportive rx is available.

Based on clinical presentation, many pts will receive empiric abx for bacterial meningitis until CSF cultures negative.

All pts should receive acyclovir rx for possible HSV encephalitis, until r/o by clinical testing or lack of response to therapy; typical dose is 10 mg/kg IV q 8 hr; other than acyclovir, consider specific therapies for these causative agents:

- Rickettsial diseases and ehrlichiosis: doxycycline
- Varicella: acyclovir or ganciclovir (AIDS 1994;8:1115)
- CMV: ganciclovir and/or foscarnet (AIDS 2000;14:517)
- EBV: possibly acyclovir, but no benefit in meta-analysis of mononucleosis rx (Scand J Infect Dis 1999;31:543)
- Rabies: postexposure prophylaxis with immunoglobulin and vaccine, but no rx for acute disease without prophylaxis
- ADEM: methylprednisolone 1 gm IV qd for 3–5 d, plasmapheresis if unresponsive (J Neurol Neurosurg 2004;75 Suppl 1:i22)

Chapter 6

Neurology

6.1 Stroke and Related Disorders

Transient Ischemic Attack (TIA)

(NEJM 2002;347:1687)

Cause: Carotid or aortic arch (NEJM 1992;326:221) plaque and/or platelet emboli, cardiac emboli, vascular spasm, hypercoagulable states, and idiopathic

Pathophys: Most similar to ischemic stroke (see "Ischemic Stroke" later in Section 6.1 for details); occasionally is vasospastic (consider rx with CCB) (NEJM 1993;329:396).

Sx: Lateralized neuro sx, usually lasting less than 5–10 min but by revised definition (NEJM 2002;347:1713) always less than 1 hr, with no evidence of CVA by imaging; however, emergent MRI may change this: about 50% of TIA pts have MRI evidence of ischemia, aka transient symptoms associated with infarction (TSI).

Anterior circulation sx: amaurosis fugax (transient monocular blindness) (Stroke 1990;21:201); middle cerebral artery pattern (weakness of arm > face > leg paresis), anterior cerebral artery pattern (leg > arm > face paresis).

Posterior circulation sx: bilateral blindness, diplopia, numbness in face and mouth, slurred speech, quadriplegia.

Si: Carotid bruit, but correlates poorly with symptomatic disease (Ann IM 1994;120:633); in elderly, asx bruit present in 10% and does not correlate with CVA rate in or out of affected carotid distribution; 60% disappear over 3 yr (Ann IM 1990;112:340).

Crs: Risk of subsequent stroke after TIA by time period: 2 d (3.5%); 30 d (8.0%); 90 d (9.2%) (Arch IM 2007;167:2417); about 40% will eventually die of MI due to coexistent CAD.

ABCD scoring can help assess acute risk of recurrent CVA (Lancet 2005;366:29):

- **A**ge: older than 60 (1 point)
- **B**lood pressure: higher than 140/90 (1 point)
- **C**linical features: unilateral weakness (2 points), isolated speech deficit (1 point), other sx (0 points)
- **D**uration: more than 60 min (2 points), 10–59 min (1 point), less than 10 min (0 points)
- Risk of early stroke using ABCD score: 3 or less (0%), 4 (1–9%), 5 (12%), 6 (24–31%)

Cmplc: Differential dx includes:

- Tumor, can mimic exactly (Arch Neurol 1983;40:633)
- Carotid or vertebral dissections
- Post zoster cerebral vasculitis if recent zoster (NEJM 2002; 347:1500)
- Metabolic causes: hypoglycemia, hyponatremia, uremia, hepatic encephalopathy
- Intoxication
- Seizure with postictal (Todd's) paralysis
- Atypical migraine
- Conversion disorder

Lab: See "Ischemic Stroke" later in Section 6.1.

Noninv: See "Ischemic Stroke" later in Section 6.1.

Rx: To determine whether to hospitalize, consider if recurrent stroke risk is low by ABCD score and able to have close outpatient f/u and studies; if so, discharge from ED in some pts; but most pts benefit from short stay admission for facilitated w/u and monitoring for recurrent sx.

See "Secondary prevention for ischemic stroke" below.

Ischemic Stroke

(NEJM 2000;343:710; Stroke 2007;38:1655)

Cause: Common risk factors include heart disease/CAD/prior MI, atrial fibrillation, valvular disease, endocarditis, hypertension, smoking, diabetes/metabolic syndrome, dyslipidemia, pregnancy, drug abuse (cocaine, amphetamines), coagulopathy due to bleeding disorders/anticoagulant use.

Epidem: 700K CVAs per yr in the United States, 200K are recurrent; 80–90% ischemic; slightly more common in men (1.25:1); more common in African American, Hispanic, and Native American populations.

Pathophys: Three main categories, as follows:

- Thrombosis: Includes in situ arterial obstruction with underlying arteriosclerosis, or more rarely dissection or fibromuscular dysplasia; large vessel (carotids, circle of Willis, etc.) vs small vessel (penetrating arteries, aka "lacunar stroke"); typically has stuttering course of sx.
- Embolism: Includes arterial obstruction from another source; usually abrupt onset and if improves, does so rapidly.
  - Cardiac: atrial fibrillation or other source of atrial thrombus, heart valves (endocarditis, marantic, etc.), ventricular wall source due to prior MI or dilated cardiomyopathy, recent CABG
  - Aortic arch
  - Arterial: carotids or other large vessel
  - "Paradoxical embolus": DVT with passage to left heart circulation via patent foramen ovale (or other congenital heart defect)
- Systemic hypoperfusion: Characterized by loss of flow to watershed, border regions of the brain due to shock/hypotension, associated with overall circulatory collapse and multiorgan involvement; sx usually less focal, cortical blindness, stupor, proximal weakness.

Sx/Si: Anterior circulation sx: amaurosis fugax (Stroke 1990;21:201), middle cerebral artery pattern (weakness of arm > face > leg paresis), anterior cerebral artery pattern (leg > arm > face paresis)

Posterior circulation sx: bilateral blindness, diplopia, numbness in face and mouth, slurred speech, quadriplegia.

Crs: See "Transient Ischemic Attack" earlier in Section 6.1 for differential dx.

Cmplc: VTE: prophylaxis with LMWH better than UFH; meta-analysis of three trials, LMWH with reduced incidence of all VTE (NNT 15), proximal VTE (NNT 25), and PE (NNT 138) (Chest 2008;133:149).

Lab: Initial eval with CBC, electrolytes, glucose, LFTs, PT/PTT; in special circumstances, consider ESR, toxicology screen and alcohol level, urine/serum HCG, hypercoagulability studies.

Noninv: Noncontrast head CT: Initial screen to r/o bleed; in most cases, will not see signs of ischemic stroke unless prior CVA, massive stroke, or delayed time to eval; early signs of ischemic stroke on CT (less than 6 hr) associated with poor prognosis; generally no signs on CT for 24 hr.

MRI: Will show ischemia immediately, but not used in many emergency settings; use in nonacute setting to diagnose CVA if dx unclear, determine extent of stroke, r/o other causes.

Echocardiogram: Indicated for pts with new dx of atrial fibrillation, prior MI/cardiomyopathy that might increase risk for cardiac source, pts at risk for endocarditis (fever, leukocytosis, prosthetic valve, new cardiac murmur), young pts with cryptogenic stroke to r/o PFO; transesophageal (TEE) is more sensitive than transthoracic (TTE) but may not change management in most cases.

Carotid dopplers: Eval in all cases of new TIA/stroke for stenosis; recommendations are based on pts with appropriate sx (i.e., clear TIA/stroke sx, not vertigo or syncope).

Imaging of intracranial vessels: CT angiography, MR angiography, transcranial doppler US; not warranted in all cases (as may not change management strategies) but consider in pts younger than 50 without clear source, recurrent strokes with similar sx, posterior circulation strokes, prior to CEA.

Electroencephalogram (EEG): Consider with comorbid seizures or if dx in doubt (i.e., Todd's paralysis).

Rx: Treatment involves immediate acute rx as well as secondary prevention.

Acute treatment of ischemic stroke

- Considerations for thrombolytic therapy:
  - Must be given within 3 hr of symptom onset (not by-stander or family awareness of sx), possibly expand up to 4.5 hr (NEJM 2008;359:1317).
  - Most pts are not candidates: About 20% of pts with acute stroke present in 3 hr treatment window, and less than 10% have no contraindications to thrombolytic rx.
  - NINDS study: Two-part RCT of about 300 pts with acute stroke sx within 3 hr of arrival, with multiple exclusion criteria randomized to thrombolysis with IV t-PA vs placebo; rx was not associated with any significant difference in outcomes within 24 hr, but did show improved complete or near-complete recovery at 3 mo post-CVA (38% vs 21% in placebo, NNT 6); no difference in mortality; predictors of success include quicker time to rx, younger pts, lack of hypertension, lack of hyperglycemia, less severe sx (NEJM 1995;333:1581).
  - Major risk is intracranial hemorrhage, 6% in study population; try to obtain informed consent in all pts (but do not withhold rx in appropriate pts if not able to get consent).
  - Alteplase (t-PA) 0.9 mg/kg dose up to 90 mg; 10% as IV bolus, then remainder as infusion over 60 min.
  - Multiple exclusion criteria:
    - Active bleeding or trauma; prior stroke/head trauma within 3 mon; any prior ICH

- Surgery within 14 d; GI bleed within 21 d; acute MI or MI within 3 mon
- LP within 7 d; arterial puncture at noncompressible site within 7 d
- Rapidly improving or minor sx; seizure with postictal sx; sx of SAH, even if normal CT
- BP higher than 185/110
- Pregnancy
- Platelets less than 100K; glucose less than 50, more than 400; INR more than 1.7 or elevated PTT
- Hemorrhage on CT; "major" infarct on CT
- For many hospitals, optimizing thrombolytic rx requires multidisciplinary stroke team (ER, neurology, hospitalists, radiology, pharmacy, laboratory, nursing); goal is to get CT results within 45 min, thrombolytics infused within 60 min of arrival to ER.
- Catheter-based therapy, intra-arterial thrombolysis; studied in large centers, may be an option in pts with longer duration of sx (up to 12 hr).
- BP management: Severe hypertension is common due to autoregulation (poststroke cerebral blood flow is BP-dependent); overly aggressive BP control leads to increased mortality (Stroke 2007;38:1655).
  - BP lower than 220/120: Monitor closely but do not treat in the acute phase, unless comorbid myocardial ischemia or heart failure, arterial/aortic dissection
  - BP higher than 220/120: Rx with intermittent doses of IV labetalol, IV nitroglycerin or nitroprusside (see the discussion of hypertensive emergencies in Chapter 1).
- Antithrombotic therapy guidelines:
  - ASA rx (325 mg qd) within 48 hr unless contraindication.
  - International Stroke Trial (IST): RCT of more than 19K pts across multiple sites, with new ischemic stroke;

randomized to ASA 300 mg qd or SQ heparin; ASA-treated pts showed significant reduction in composite outcome of death or nonfatal recurrent stroke at 14 d (11.3% vs 12.4%, NNT 91) (Lancet 1997;349:1569).

- Chinese Acute Stroke Trial (CAST): RCT of more than 21K pts in China with new ischemic stroke; randomized to ASA 160 mg qd vs placebo; ASA-treated pts showed significant reduction in recurrent ischemic stroke within 4 wk (1.6% vs 2.1%, NNT 200) and death or nonfatal stroke at 4 wk (5.3% vs 5.9%, NNT 167) (Lancet 1997;349:1641).

- No available evidence for clopidogrel or dipyridamole-ASA (Aggrenox) in setting of acute stroke, but can consider clopidogrel in pts with ASA allergy (see "Secondary prevention of ischemic stroke" below).

- Heparin therapy guidelines:
  - Avoid UFH or full-dose LMWH in most cases, despite previous widespread use.
  - No evidence to support use in any setting of acute stroke, except for expert opinion in cases of carotid or vertebral dissection, large vessel arterial occlusion, cardiac embolus; mixed recommendations for use with progressive stroke sx (hard to define and classify).
  - IST study (noted above in discussion of ASA under antithrombotic rx guidelines) showed the heparin group associated with fewer recurrent ischemic strokes at 14 d (2.9% vs 3.8%, NNT 111), but offset by increased number of hemorrhagic strokes (1.2% vs 0.4%, NNH 125), so overall mortality was not affected (also higher rates of non-ICH bleeding events) (Lancet 1997;349:1569).
  - In setting of new dx of AF with acute stroke, data are limited and conflicting. If proven cardiac clot, use IV UFH; however, not seen in most cases. Likely the effect of reducing short-term stroke risk is offset by conversion to

hemorrhage (similar to results seen in all ischemic strokes). So two options for most pts:

- ASA therapy in the acute setting, with addition of warfarin (no bridging heparin) once stable (usually 4–10 d, depending on size and extent of CVA); discontinue ASA once warfarin therapy at goal
- Immediate IV UFH with bridge to long-term warfarin therapy once stable; appropriate option if plan for immediate cardioversion of atrial fibrillation (see "Atrial Fibrillation" in Section 1.3 for details); avoid in cases of "large" strokes (more than 50 cc) or high risk for bleeding (short- and long-term)

Secondary prevention of ischemic stroke

These are recommendations for approach to rx after acute phase of stroke, when preparing pt for hospital discharge and outpatient f/u.

Risk factor modification:

- Blood pressure control: goal BP lower than 130/80
  - SHEP study: Systolic HTN in pts older than 60; rx with a combination of meds (thiazide, beta-blocker, reserpine) to achieve target BP goals led to a significant reduction in both ischemic and hemorrhagic strokes at 4 yr (JAMA 2000;284:465).
  - Caution with aggressive BP lowering pts older than 80; may have some benefit in stroke reduction but also higher incidence of orthostasis and other med side effects.
  - Diuretics and/or ACE inhibitors as 1st-line agents; main concern is BP lowering, not specific drug; ARB did not decrease recurrent stroke, independent of BP effect (2nd arm of PROFESS study) (NEJM 2008;359:1225).
- Smoking cessation
- Tight diabetes control: goal HbA1c less than 7.0
- Lipid control: goal LDL lower than 70 mg/dL; meta-analysis of 121K pts, statins reduced all-cause mortality by 12% (NNT

89) and stroke by 16% (NNT 174) with no increase in hemorrhagic stroke (Am J Med 2008;121:24)
- Other lifestyle modifications: weight loss, increased activity, moderate alcohol use; consider folate, B6, B12 (MVI doses OK) but limited to no evidence

Carotid stenosis therapy:

- Based on results of NASCET (NEJM 1991;325:445; Stroke 1991;22:711; NEJM 1998;339:1415) and ECST (Lancet 1991;337:1235; Lancet 1998;351:1379)
- If ASCVD but no significant stenosis, risk factor modification only
- 100% stenosis: medical mgt only (i.e., risk factor modification and antithrombotic rx)
- 70–99% stenosis: CEA within 2 wk if good long-term survival and center with low risk of complications (less than 6%)
- 50–69% stenosis: CEA in males with same criteria as 70–99%, medical mgt in females
- Less than 50% stenosis: medical mgt for all
- In some cases, consider carotid stenting vs CEA: older pts with higher surgical risks (NEJM 2004;351:1493; NEJM 2006;355:1660; NEJM 2008;358:1572)

Antiplatelet therapy:

- Aspirin: 81–325 mg qd
  - Meta-analysis of 287 studies (more than 135K pts); antiplatelet rx (most studies with ASA) demonstrated significant reduction in "serious vascular events" (MI, stroke, vascular death) at 2 yr (NNT 27) (BMJ 2002;324:71).
  - Higher doses have more bleeding risks with no extra clinical benefit (i.e., in pt with stroke on chronic ASA rx, change regimen rather than increasing dose).
  - May see development of clinical testing for ASA-"nonresponders" who should initially receive other drugs for secondary prevention.

- Clopidogrel: 75 mg qd
  - Has replaced ticlopidine in this class because of lack of risk of neutropenia.
  - CAPRIE study: RCT of more than 19K pts with recent ischemic stroke; randomized to clopidogrel 75 mg qd vs ASA 325 mg qd; small but significant reduction in composite end point of stroke, MI, vascular death in clopidogrel pts (5.3% vs 5.8%, NNT 200) (Lancet 1996;348:1329).
  - Consider as main alternative therapy in ASA-allergic pts.
  - Avoid ASA plus clopidogrel as combo therapy because increased risk of bleeding.
    - MATCH trial: 7600 pts rx with clopidogrel and ASA vs clopidogrel alone for recent stroke; no difference in study outcome of recurrent stroke/MI/death, but significantly more life-threatening bleeding events with combination rx (2.6% vs 1.3%, NNH 77) (Lancet 2004; 364:331).
    - CHARISMA trial: RCT of 15K pts with known vascular disease or multiple risk factors; randomized to clopidogrel and ASA vs ASA alone; no difference in primary study outcome of recurrent stroke/MI/death (except in subset of pts with known atherosclerosis, NNT 100) or increased bleeding risk with combo (NEJM 2006;354:1706).
- ASA-ERDP (extended-release dipyridamole) (Aggrenox): 25/200 tablet bid
  - ESPS-2 trial: RCT of 6600 pts with recent stroke or TIA; randomized to ASA 50 mg qd (too low dose?), dipyridamole 400 mg qd, combination, or placebo; ASA and ASA-ERDP reduced stroke risk at 2 yr vs placebo (NNT 37 for ASA, NNT 18 for ASA-ERDP), but ASA-ERDP also had further benefit over ASA alone in stroke reduction at 2 yr (9.5% vs 12.5%, NNT 33) (J Neurol Sci 1996;143:1).

- ESPRIT trial: RCT of 2600 pts with recent stroke or TIA; randomized to ASA 75 mg qd vs ASA-ERDP; addition of ERDP provided significant benefit in primary outcome of stroke/MI/major bleeding/vascular death at 3.5 yr (16% vs 13%, NNT 33) (Lancet 2006;367:1665).
- PROFESS trial: RCT of more than 20K pts age 55 and older with h/o recent CVA; randomized to ASA-ERDP vs clopidogrel; at 2.5 yrs of f/u, no difference in recurrent stroke (~9% in both groups), higher rate of ICH in ASA-ERDP group (NNH 250) (NEJM 2008;359:1238).
- Headache seems to be most common and limiting side effect.
- Warfarin: variable dosing, goal INR 2–3
  - Only in the setting of AF, where warfarin is the preferred choice (see "Atrial Fibrillation" in Section 1.3 for details)
  - In non-AF settings, no clinical benefit with increased risks
    - WASID trial: RCT of 569 pts with recent TIA/stroke and known large vessel intracranial stenosis (not AF); randomized to ASA 1300 mg qd (high dose?) vs warfarin with INR goal 2–3; trial stopped early at average 1.8 yr, due to increased risks of death (4.3% vs 9.7%, NNH 18), major hemorrhage (3.2% vs 8.3%, NNH 20), and sudden cardiac death/MI (2.9% vs 7.3%, NNH 23) with warfarin (NEJM 2005;352:1305).
    - WARSS trial: RCT of 2200 pts with recent TIA/stroke; randomized to ASA 325 mg qd vs warfarin with goal INR 1.4–2.8 (too low?); no difference in outcomes of recurrent stroke, MI, or major bleeding (NEJM 2001; 345:1444).
- Final recommendations:
  - Ischemic stroke with AF: Treat with warfarin, unless very high bleeding risks, then either ASA (or possibly ASA and clopidogrel; see ACTIVE trial in Section 1.3).

NEUROLOGY

- Ischemic stroke, no AF: Three choices:
  - ASA: cheapest, most evidence to support its use, well tolerated
  - ASA-ERDP: expensive, may have additional benefit over ASA
  - Clopidogrel: expensive, may have additional benefit over ASA, probably similar effect as ASA-ERDP
- Recurrent ischemic stroke with prior ASA use: Best option is clopidogrel or ASA-ERDP.
- ASA-allergic: Clopidogrel is only choice.

6.2 Epilepsy and Seizure Disorders

(NEJM 2008;359:166)

Cause: Unknown/idiopathic in more than 60%; other causes of chronic seizures (listed by prevalence) include stroke, head trauma, alcohol, neurodegenerative disease, encephalopathy, brain tumors, infections.

Acute seizures can also be precipitated by acute renal and liver failure, hypoglycemia and hyperglycemia, hyponatremia, drug overdose and withdrawal, meningitis/encephalitis.

CVA is more common cause in elderly pts, but most cases (25–40%) are still of unknown cause (Epilepsy Res 2006;68 Suppl 1:S39).

Epidem: U.S. prevalence of epilepsy 6–8 per 1000 people; bimodal distribution with higher rates in young children and pts older than 60.

Pathophys: Generalized, tonic/clonic: Involve both hemispheres; more likely in idiopathic epilepsy.

Partial (focal) seizures: May not include altered consciousness and affect only limited areas; more likely with a specific focus of disease in the CNS.

Absence seizures: More common in children; brief, frequent staring episodes with amnesia; often misdiagnosed as ADD.

Sx: Altered consciousness, abnormal behavior, involuntary motor activity; urinary incontinence

Si: Neuro exam between episodes is usually normal after resolution of postictal sx, unless other underlying CNS abnormality.

Crs: Consider weaning antiepileptic drugs if more than 2 yr seizure-free, but recurrence risk reported to be 12–66%.

Cmplc: Differential dx includes:

- Anxiety, panic disorder, hyperventilation
- Atypical migraines
- Psychogenic, aka "pseudo-seizures"
- Syncope
- Transient global amnesia
- TIA

Comorbid depression and suicide rates higher, especially in first 6 mo after dx (Lancet Neurol 2007;6:693).

Lab: No definitive labs for dx, but consider CBC, electrolytes, renal and liver function tests, toxicology screen for initial eval.

Albumin levels if pt to get phenytoin or valproate (hypo-albuminemia will lead to increase active drug concentrations).

Elevated serum prolactin level (2 times normal value) within 20 min of seizure episode may help to differentiate true generalized or partial seizure from pseudo-seizure (Neurol 2005;65:668); study of 200 ED pts showed PPV of 74%, NPV 54% (J Neurol 2004;251:736).

Noninv: EEG, brain imaging both recommended.

EEG in all cases of first episode unprovoked seizure.

- Helpful in dx if pos for epileptiform activity (i.e., spikes and sharp waves); some abnormality in about 50% of pts after first seizure (Neurol 2007;69:1996).
- However, normal EEG does not r/o epilepsy.

- Additional information may be obtained by sleep-deprived EEG and continuous video EEG monitoring.

    CT scan is appropriate for emergency eval of seizures, with findings that affect mgt in 9–17% of cases (Neurol 2007;69:1772).

    MRI is more sensitive to find structural lesions; consider as part of routine work-up.

Rx: Considerations re whether to treat first unprovoked seizure with antiepileptic meds:

- Risk of recurrent seizure within 2 yr is 25% in pts with normal EEG and no known cause of seizure; more than 40% in pts with abnormal EEG or obvious cause (Epilepsia 2008;49 Suppl 1:13).
- Antiepileptic drug therapy overall reduces risk of recurrent seizure by 30–60%, but overall outcome 3–5 yr after seizure was similar whether drug started after first or second episode (Lancet 2005;365:2007).
- Strongly consider initiating drug therapy in obvious first seizure episode; consider watchful waiting if dx uncertain or other confounding factors (age, comorbidities, social circumstances/lack of f/u care).

    Drug therapy (adapted from NEJM 2008;359:166): See **Table 6.1** for a summary of 1st-line and 2nd-line antiepileptic drugs.

    Limited trials of drugs head-to-head: SANAD study of 716 pts showed valproate to be more effective than lamotrigine or topiramate as 1st-line drug for generalized epilepsy; lamotrigine had higher failure rate; topiramate had higher discontinuation due to side effects (Lancet 2007;369:1016).

    Phenytoin often used as initial drug therapy due to IV loading as part of rx of initial seizure activity; has limited effectiveness as 1st-line drug, so consider switch to another drug for long-term therapy in newly diagnosed pts (Epilepsia 1997;38 Suppl 9:S21).

Failure of initial drug therapy increases risk for multidrug failure, but 67% of pts become seizure-free after second or third drug trial (NEJM 2000;342:314).

Status epilepticus (NEJM 1998;338:970): Can be continuous (defined as more than 20 min, but begin treating within 5 min) or repeated seizures (two or more without regaining consciousness); many begin as tonic-clonic, but with repeated episodes, sx may be less noticeable (twitching, jerking, nystagmus); mortality about 20% and sz for 30–45 min can cause cerebral injury, particularly in hippocampus.

Management of status epilepticus includes these considerations:

- ABCs: Airway control in setting of ongoing seizures may be difficult; high-flow O_2 vs immediate intubation and mechanical ventilation; if intubate, use a short-acting paralyzing agent (succinylcholine unless concern for acute hyperkalemia or chronic neurologic disease that might precipitate severe hyperkalemia; if so, use nondepolarizing agent) and benzos should be first choice for sedation (as will be used for seizures as well).
- 1st-line rx: benzodiazepines; lorazepam (0.1 mg/kg IV, usually 4–8 mg as first dose) or diazepam (10–20 mg IV)
  - Stops 80% of status if given within 30 min of onset of seizure activity (Neurol 1993;43:483).
  - Study (NEJM 1998;339:792) compared lorazepam, phenytoin, phenobarbital, and diazepam plus phenytoin in pts with status epilepticus; all were equally effective, but lorazepam better than phenytoin when given with 20 min of seizure onset.

Table 6.1 Antiepileptic Drug Therapy

Drug Name	Daily Dose	Common Side Effects	Other Considerations
		1st-line antiepileptic drugs (for generalized or partial seizures)	
Lamotrigine (Lamictal)	Start at 25 mg; adjust to 100–200 mg	Dizziness, visual disturbances, headache	Rare significant rash, organ failure
Levetiracetam (Keppra)	Start at 250–500 mg; adjust to 1000–2000 mg	Fatigue, anxiety	Reduced dose in renal failure
Topiramate (Topamax)	Start at 25–50 mg; adjust to 100–200 mg	Drowsiness, weight loss	Rare significant metabolic acidosis; avoid if h/o kidney stones
Valproate (Depakote)	Start at 250–500 mg; adjust to 750–2000 mg	Drowsiness, ataxia, weight gain, tremor	Avoid if bleeding risk due to risk of thrombocytopenia; rare liver failure and avoid if h/o hepatic disease due to elevated ammonia levels; possible relation to polycystic ovarian syndrome
Zonisamide (Zonegran)	Start at 50 mg; adjust to 100–200 mg	Drowsiness, ataxia, weight loss, headache	Avoid if h/o kidney stones; rare aplastic anemia

2nd-line antiepileptic drugs (especially for partial seizures)		
Carbamazepine (Tegretol)	Start at 200 mg; adjust to 400–600 mg	Dizziness, visual disturbances, sedation, weight gain	Avoid in pts with marrow disorders (risk of agranulocytosis, aplastic anemia); hyponatremia; rare sick-sinus syndrome and heart block
Gabapentin (Neurontin)	Start at 300–600 mg; adjust to 900 mg	Sedation, fatigue, weight gain	Reduced dose in renal failure
Oxcarbazepine (Trileptal)	Start at 300–600 mg; adjust to 900–1200 mg	Dizziness, ataxia, nausea, confusion	Hyponatremia, rash
Phenytoin (Dilantin)	IV loading dose of 15–20 mg/kg; adjust to 200–300 mg	Dizziness, ataxia, diplopia, confusion	Bradycardias with conduction blocks; rare liver failure; lupus-like syndrome; increased risk of osteopenia
Phenobarbital	Start at 30 mg; adjust to 60–120 mg	Dizziness, ataxia, diplopia, confusion	Rare hepatic failure, rash
Pregabalin (Lyrica)	Start at 75–150 mg; adjust to 150–300 mg	Dizziness, ataxia, diplopia, weight gain, edema	Reduced dose in renal failure
Tiagabine (Gabitril)	Start at 4 mg; adjust to 16–36 mg	Fatigue, dizziness, ataxia	

- Lorazepam preferred to diazepam because of a longer duration of antiseizure effect (12 or more hr vs 30 min); both are otherwise equally effective in initial seizure control and side effects.
- If no IV access, can use im midazolam (0.15–0.3 mg/kg; 20 mg im OK for average size pt) or rectal diazepam, either as premade gel or IV solution (10–20 mg).
- Common side effects include respiratory depression, hypotension, sedation; should be prepared for intubation in all circumstances
- 2nd-line rx: phenytoin (20 mg/kg IV infused at 50 mg/min; "standard" 1000 mg loading dose will underdose most pts) or fosphenytoin (20 mg/kg "phenytoin equilavents" IV at 150 mg/min) within 5–10 min of 1st-line treatment with benzos, if no effect; consider a second 5–10 mg/kg dose within 20 min if no effect
  - Longer therapeutic effect than benzos and often used as immediate 2nd-line agent in status.
  - Can reduce dose in pts who have recent known serum levels greater than 10 mg/dL; however, do not wait for serum levels if will delay therapy for active status.
  - Phenytoin may not be best 1st-line choice for chronic seizure control (see above), so may need to consider another agent once status aborted.
  - Fosphenytoin not considered more effective than phenytoin, but less cardiotoxicity because of lack of propylene glycol in infusion and can be given faster.
  - Common acute side effects include hypotension (in up to 50% of pts); bradycardia; ventricular ectopy.
- 3rd-line rx: phenobarbital (20 mg/kg IV at 75 mg/min) or induced anesthesia
  - Considered 3rd-line rx after benzos and phenytoin.
  - Main concern is further respiratory depression and hypotension, especially after 1st-line drug therapy.

- Many skip this step and move right to continuous IV infusions of propofol (1–2 mg/kg load, then 2–10 mg/kg/hr) or midazolam (0.2 mg/kg load, then 0.75–10 mcg/kg/min); intubation and mechanical ventilation required for this step; usually continue for 12–24 hr at minimum, and continuous EEG monitoring and neurologic consultation strongly recommended.

6.3 Guillain-Barre Syndrome

(Am Fam Phys 2004;69:2405; Lancet Neurol 2008;7:939)

Cause: Rapidly progressing peripheral polyradiculopathy.

Recent prior infectious disease in about 67% of pts; *Campylobacter jejuni* is most common preceding illness, with 26% of GBS pts pos for recent *C. jejuni* infection (by culture or serology) compared to 2% of matched controls in one study (NEJM 1995;333:1374); other bacterial precipitants include *Mycoplasma* and *Haemophilus*; viral precipitants include CMV, HIV, EBV, VZV.

Influenza vaccination is also a cause (1–2 cases per million vaccinations), although risk is much less than cmplc of severe influenza disease.

Epidem: Worldwide incidence of 1–3 per 100K people per yr; increases with age, with peaks in young adults (due to increased risk of precedent illnesses) and elderly (likely due to relative immunosuppression).

Pathophys: Five subtypes of disease; most common is acute inflammatory demyelinating polyradiculopathy (AIDP).

Sx: Primary sx are proximal muscle weakness (legs more than arms) and parasthesias (usually not below wrists and ankles); pain usually in proximal muscles, and cramping.

Si: First physical finding is loss of deep tendon reflexes; cranial nerve involvement can affect facial muscles, diplopia and loss of extraocular movements, swallowing dysfunction; eval ability to stand, lift arms, lift head, and cough to assess for signs of worsening disease and pending respiratory compromise.

Crs: Acute, progressive phase within 24–48 hr; nadir of clinical sx at 1 wk in 73%; 30% will require mechanical ventilation.

Recovery is more variable; 80–85% have full function within 6–12 mo; 7–15% have permanent neurologic disability, including foot drop, muscle wasting, ataxia, dysesthesias; overall mortality less than 5% (closer to 20% in ventilator-dependent pts) and usually related to delayed dx and lack of initial appropriate care or cmplc (see below).

Predictors for poor recovery include advanced age, rapidly progressing disease, prolonged mechanical ventilation due to neurologic disease or comorbid lung disease (Neurol 2000;54:2311); rate of relapse is low, 3–5% (Neurol 2001;56:758).

Cmplc: Usually related to secondary illness, including sepsis due to hospital-acquired infection or IVIG rx, ARDS or nosocomial pneumonia in setting of mechanical ventilation, VTE due to prolonged immobilization; autonomic dysfunction can lead to hypotension/hypertension, GI ileus, urinary retention.

Differential dx includes:

- Spinal cord compression (from tumor, epidural abscess, hematoma)
- Transverse myelitis; polio
- Botulism from food or wound (consider with IVDA)
- Tick-borne paralysis
- New-onset myasthenia gravis
- Heavy metal intoxication

Lab: Elevated protein in CSF without pleocytosis, aka "albumin cytologic dissociation" (if elevated WBC, consider acute poliomyelitis, Lyme disease, cancer, HIV, West Nile virus, sarcoid); protein levels often normal within 1st wk of disease, but increased in more than 90% of pts by end of 2nd wk (Ann Neurol 1995;37 Suppl 1:S14).

Noninv: EMG studies in selected cases if dx is uncertain; consider imaging of brain (CT or MRI), spinal cord (MRI) if concern for spinal cord compression as alternative cause of sx.

Rx: Initial therapy is supportive care: Airway and ventilatory mgt; VTE prophylaxis; pain mgt (consider alternative pain modulators like carbamazepine and gabapentin in severe cases).

Serial lung function testing in acute phase to assess need for intubation; forced vital capacity (FVC) should be more than 20 mL/kg, max inspiratory pressure more than 30 cm H_2O, max expiratory pressure more than 40 cm H_2O (Arch Neurol 2001; 58:893).

Disease-specific therapies include the following:

- Steroids, once used regularly, are of no benefit alone or in combination with other therapies (Neurol 2003;61:736).
- IVIG therapy: 400 mg/kg IV qd for 5 d; multiple immune mechanisms for disease modulation, stimulating native immune cell function, binding circulating antibodies, etc.; watch for fluid overload in pts with CHF, renal and liver disease; mild side effects of fever, headache, nausea.
- Plasmapheresis: Removes circulating immune factors; controversy re number of exchanges needed; increased risk of subsequent infections/sepsis due to immunosuppressant effects.
- Head-to-head study showed no superiority to either primary therapy (NEJM 1992;326:1123).

6.4 Parkinson's Disease

(Clin Geriatr Med 2006;22:735; NEJM 2005;353:1021)

Cause: True cause of idiopathic PD is unknown, but need to r/o other disorders including these:

- Drug-induced parkinsonism: Due to dopamine antagonism by meds; most common with older typical antipsychotics, but also found with newer atypical antipsychotics, antiemetics, older antihypertensive meds (reserpine and methyldopa); rarer cases with amiodarone, valproic acid, and lithium; improves with withdrawal of rx, but may have long latency.

- Parkinsonian syndromes (aka "Parkinson's-plus"): Other primary CNS disorders that affect the basal ganglia in a similar fashion; consider in cases with bilateral onset of tremor, lack of tremor, early autonomic instability and falls, urinary retention (not due to meds), early cognitive impairment, and significant disability; also consider when pts have lack of response to 1st-line therapies.
- Essential tremor: More common in elderly than PD; differentiate by lack of other classic PD sx other than tremor; essential tremor is usually postural or with activity, rather than classic resting tremor of PD.

Epidem: Prevalence of 250 per 100K; 95% present after age 60; more prevalent in men and European descent; smokers have a lower risk of disease (unclear if neuroprotective or if there is a link between tobacco addiction and resistance to neurodegenerative disease); genetic predisposition, especially in early-onset cases.

Drug-induced parkinsonism was cause in 20% of pts in Mayo study (Neurol 1999;52:1214).

Pathophys: Deficiency/loss of dopamine in the basal ganglia of the CNS; progressive disease; characteristic cytoplasmic inclusion body in the neuronal cells (Lewy body).

Sx: Many complain of weakness but don't have true strength deficit on exam (usually sx due to slowing from bradykinesia).

Si: Four main features of disease, as follows:

- Tremor: Resting, present in limbs; usually begins unilaterally; earliest sx for most pts and present in 80% of cases.
- Rigidity: Resistant to passive movement; can be either uniform throughout the range of motion (plastic or "lead-pipe") or catching, tremulous ("cogwheeling").

- Bradykinesia: Generalized slowing of movement.
- Impaired postural stability: Difficulty maintaining proper posture with standing/walking; leads to falls.

Other signs include micrographia (small handwriting), reduced volume and clarity of speech, hypomimia (less facial expression), staring due to decreased blinking.

Crs: Chronic, progressive; treatment is to improve functional status, does not affect pathologic progression of disease.

Cmplc: Avoid abrupt discontinuation of levodopa in hospitalized pts; can precipitate NMS-like syndrome, abrupt worsening of movement disorders, delirium, and coma; small study in United Kingdom showed 74% of PD pts admitted to hospital had discontinuation or change in therapy and 61% had adverse consequence due to change (Parkinsonism Related Disord 2007;13:539).

Most common reasons for hospitalization in pts with PD include infections, cardiovascular disease, falls and impaired mobility; also delirium and psychiatric complications; LOS and discharge to nursing home is significantly higher than matched non-PD pts (Mov Disord 2005;20:1104).

Avoid dopamine antagonists, usually antipsychotics given for delirium/psych sx, antiemetics, and metoclopramide.

Constipation is a common problem; usually requires daily rx.

Noninv: Consider MRI imaging in certain cases to r/o other CNS diseases.

Rx: Some controversy re initiation of treatment; should be started when sx affect pt's QOL (as above, does not modulate disease progression); concerns re potential long-term neurotoxicity of levodopa were reduced by ELLDOPA study (NEJM 2004;351: 2498), which showed best outcomes at 40-mo f/u in pts treated with highest doses of levodopa.

Treatment options include:

- Levodopa: Direct dopamine replacement; dopamine itself does not cross blood–brain barrier (BBB), so precursor levodopa used instead; formulated with carbidopa, which does not cross BBB and blocks peripheral metabolism of levodopa and minimizes the nausea associated with peripheral dopamine receptor activation; short half-life requires frequent daily dosing; less expensive than dopamine agonists (considered the other option for 1st-line therapy).

- Start dosing with Sinemet 25/100 tid; adjust dose every 2–3 wk to minimum effective dose; max dose is 3 pills tid; should be tapered gradually and never discontinued abruptly (see cmplc above); extended-release forms available (but still given tid) and not proven to have significantly improved efficacy.
- Common side effects include nausea, anorexia, orthostasis (especially if on BP meds), hallucinations, dyskinesia.
- If not effective, reconsider dx (essential tremor, parkinsonian syndromes).
- Dopamine agonists: Older ergot agents (e.g., pergolide) not used much due to side effects, including pulmonary and cardiac fibrosis; newer meds include pramiprexole (Mirapex) and ropinirole (Requip); start with low doses and titrate slowly; similar side effects to levodopa, with sedation much more common and significant, can also cause edema.
- Anticholinergics: Including benztropine (Cogentin) and trihexphenidyl (Artane); useful for tremor in setting of minimal other sx; avoid in elderly due to cognitive impairment and other anticholinergic sx (urinary retention, constipation, blurred vision, dry eyes).
- Amantadine: Can be used in mild cases, but not 1st-line therapy.
- Surgical therapies: Thalamotomy and thalamic stimulation for tremor; pallidotomy and deep-brain stimulation for other severe sx unresponsive to medical therapy.

Chapter 7

Pulmonary

7.1 Venous Thromboembolism (VTE)

Pulmonary Embolism (PE)

(NEJM 2008;358:1037; NEJM 2008;359:2804)

Cause: Acute obstruction of a branch (or branches) of the pulmonary artery, usually from venous clot originating in the lower extremities (DVT); less common sources include upper extremity DVT, right atrial or ventricular clot, right-sided endocarditis lesions.

Causes of thrombosis represented by Virchow's triad of (1) stasis, (2) venous injury, and (3) hypercoagulability.

Risk factors for VTE (one risk factor present in 80% of adult pts, multiple in 40%) include:

- Age: Risk increases in linear fashion with age after 40.
- Illness: Risk increases with hospitalization for acute illness or surgery; trauma; spinal cord injury; cancer.
- Smoking, obesity: Risk increases if pt smokes or is obese.
- Inactivity: Risk increases with bed rest, reduced mobility, prolonged air or ground travel.
- Hormones: Risk is associated with pregnancy, oral contraceptive, and postmenopausal hormone use.
- Catheterization: Risk increases with central venous catheterization, especially femoral CVC.
- Thrombophilias: Risk increases with deficiencies of Factor V Leiden (FVL, with activated protein C resistance), antithrombin III (AT-III), proteins C and S, plasminogen; prothrombin

gene mutation; hyperhomocysteinemia; antiphospholipid antibody syndrome; polycythemia vera.

- Family hx of VTE likely related to underlying thrombophilia.

Epidem: About 1 case per 1000 people in the United States (Arch IM 1998;158:585), but may be underrecognized as cause of sudden death, especially with decrease in autopsy rates.

Causes 300K U.S. deaths per year; accounts for 15% of all inpatient deaths, 20–30% of all pregnancy-related deaths.

Pathophys: Arterial obstruction leads to release of inflammatory substances from blood vessels and platelets; ventilation-perfusion mismatch occurs; increase in RV afterload leads to RV wall stress, causing dilation and ischemia of RV.

Sx: Classic sx include dyspnea, pleuritic chest pain, cough; occasionally hemoptysis; combination of sx may not be present in many pts, but 97% have at least one of the following: dyspnea, tachypnea, pleuritic chest pain (Chest 1991;100:598).

Massive PE can present as syncope, cardiac arrest.

Si: Tachypnea, tachycardia; hypoxemia by O_2 saturation monitoring; pleural rub may be present with subsegmental PE, causing focal infarction.

Massive PE can present with hypotension, shock; elevated JVP, accentuated P_2 heart sound (delayed closure of pulmonic valve), RV heave.

Look for signs of DVT (see "Deep Venous Thrombosis" later in Section 7.1).

Crs: Average 2-wk mortality of 11%; 3-mo mortality 15–18%; most mortality occurs at or near time of dx; risk factors for PE mortality include age older than 70, cancer, CHF, COPD, hypotension (Lancet 1999;353:1386).

High index of suspicion based on sx and then quick determination of pretest probability is crucial in assessment of VTE (Am J Med 2004;117:676).

- Wells's criteria for PE (Ann IM 2001;135:98):
  - 1 point each for hemoptysis; underlying cancer
  - 1.5 points each for prior VTE; recent bed rest or surgery; tachycardia (HR more than 100)
  - 3 points each for DVT si/sx; clinical suspicion of PE as most likely dx
  - More than 6 is high probability for PE; 2–6 is intermediate; less than 2 is low
  - Online calculators available (e.g., www.mdcalc.com/wells -criteria-for-pulmonary-embolism-pe)
- Geneva score for PE (Ann IM 2006;144:165):
  - 1 point for age older than 65
  - 2 points each for recent surgery; lower extremity fracture; cancer; hemoptysis
  - 3 points each for prior VTE; unilateral leg pain; HR 75–94 bpm
  - 4 points for unilateral leg edema or tenderness
  - 5 points for HR greater than 95 bpm
  - More than 10 is high probability; 4–10 is intermediate; less than 4 is low
- Common dx error is to disregard pretest probability based on results of f/u testing; for example, avoid using a low D-dimer result to r/o VTE despite an intermediate or high pretest probability (always get a dx imaging study); do not use a low probability V/Q scan or negative LE doppler as lone study to r/o VTE if intermediate or high pretest probability (see Lab and Noninv below).

Long-term recurrence rates, probably 3–4% per yr after discontinuation of anticoagulation; study of 355 pts s/p 3 mo of rx for VTE showed 2-yr recurrence of 17%, 5-yr recurrence of 25%, and 8-yr recurrence of 30% (Ann IM 1996;125:1).

Screen for underlying cancer? In addition to initial tests (labs and CXR) and recommended screenings (mammography, colonoscopy, etc., for appropriate populations), consider abd/

PULMONARY

pelvis CT in idiopathic VTE pts (Ann IM 2008;149:323); yield of finding cancer may be high (10–12%) (Thromb Haemost 1997;78:1316), but no evidence of mortality benefit.

Cmplc: Heparin-induced thrombocytopenia (HIT) in 1–3% (from UFH or LMWH therapy; usually presents with drop in plts by 50% within 5–14 d of therapy unless prior exposure). See "Heparin-Induced Thrombocytopenia" in Section 4.2 for details.

Chronic thromboembolic pulmonary hypertension (CTPH) in 1% at 6 mo, 3% at 1 yr after acute PE (NEJM 2004;350:2257); 10–15% of pts have pos APA (Chest 2004;126:401S).

Lab: Initial labs to include CBC with plt; metabolic panel; renal and liver function tests; PT/PTT; consider D-dimer, TnI, BNP.

Consider hypercoagulability profile (FVL, proteins C and S, AT-III, homocysteine, antiphospholipid ab, prothrombin gene studies) in young pts or recurrent disease; panel testing must be done prior to anticoagulation (affects proteins C and S, and AT-III levels); not necessary in all cases, especially first episode and with transient risk factors (recent surgery, bed rest), as may not change long-term management.

Consider screening for HIT if presence of thrombocytopenia in pts on heparin rx prior to thrombosis; see "Heparin-Induced Thrombocytopenia" in Section 4.2 for details.

Once dx made, will require regular inpatient monitoring of PTT (if choose UFH), PT/INR, platelets.

Consider initial ABGs in most cases to determine degree of hypoxia (although PaO_2 is more than 80 mmHg in 25% of pts with PE) (Chest 1991;100:598); most common findings are hypoxia (with high arterial-alveolar O_2 gradient) and respiratory alkalosis from hyperventilation.

Considerations re D-dimer testing:

- D-dimer is a by-product of fibrin degradation and a sign of activation of the coagulation cascade.

- Most useful as a test to r/o the presence of VTE (PE or DVT) in pts with low pre-test risk for VTE (see discussion of risk models under Crs above); less useful in elderly (Am J Med 2000;109:357), hospitalized pts (Clin Chem 2003;49:1483) and those with cancer (Ann IM 1999;131:417) or other chronic diseases, due to high false positive rates.
- Most labs now use the highly sensitive ELISA tests (98% sens), which have been used in multiple clinical trials.
- In pts with low pretest probability of PE, a neg D-dimer can effectively r/o VTE as cause of sx (DVT or PE), with 6-mo risk of VTE less than 1% (Ann IM 2006;144:812; JAMA 2006;295:172); in all other pts, need to pursue further dx testing; a pos D-dimer, especially in hospitalized pts, is of no value in diagnosing PE.

Troponin (Chest 2003;123:1947) elevation is not dx for PE, but may be present in 47%; predicts higher RV pressure, hypokinesis, and cardiogenic shock (Am Hrt J 2003;145:751); predictor of PE mortality (Arch IM 2005;165:1777); BNP levels may have similar role (Eur Respir J 2003;22:649).

Noninv: EKG part of initial evaluation; nonspecific for PE, but used to r/o ACS as cause of presenting sx; EKG signs of PE (Chest 1991;100:598):

- Normal EKG (most common result)
- Sinus tachycardia (most common abnormal finding)
- Incomplete or complete RBBB; right axis deviation
- Atrial fibrillation (may develop from acute right-sided volume overload)
- $S_1Q_3T_3$ pattern (large S wave in lead I, significant Q wave with inverted T wave in lead III); suggests pulmonary hypertension and RV insufficiency

Review of imaging tests for PE (BMJ 2005;331:259):

- Chest Xray: Many pts have normal or nonspecific CXR (including atelectasis), but done to r/o other causes of initial sx and potential contraindications to anticoagulation (always consider risk for dissecting thoracic aneurysm with widened mediastinum on CXR); nonspecific signs of PE on CXR:

- Hampton's hump: peripheral wedge-shaped opacity, due to pulmonary infarction
- Westermark's sign: focal oligemia (lack of blood flow and lung markings in a peripheral site) suggesting arterial obstruction
- Palla's sign: enlarged right descending pulmonary artery

- CT scan:
  - CT angiography has become the primary dx imaging for PE, based on improved specif and sens (NPV better than 99%) (JAMA 2005;293:2012), widespread availability, and ease of testing.
  - Contraindications are primarily due to contrast dye administration, namely acute and chronic renal failure, and dye allergy.
  - Advent of spiral CT with faster scanning and increased number of "cuts" has allowed for detection of even small, subsegmental PEs.
  - Meta-analysis of 23 studies (~4600 pts) showed the 3-mo rate of VTE after a neg CT study was 1.4% and rate of fatal PE was 0.5%, similar to "gold standard" pulmonary angiography (Ann IM 2004;141:866).
  - Based on current evidence, most dx eval for PE begins and ends with CT; if high pretest probability for PE with neg scan, consider LE doppler US as an additional test to r/o PE.

- Ventilation-perfusion (V/Q) scan:
  - Has largely been supplanted by CT scanning as primary test for PE.
  - Still an appropriate 1st-line test in younger pts, without h/o lung disease; also used in pts who cannot tolerate contrast dye.

- "Normal" diagnostic scans (present only about 33% of time) (JAMA 2007;298:2743) r/o PE; "high probability" scans rule in PE; all other readings, including "low" or "intermediate" probability, still have risk of underlying PE and should be considered nondiagnostic based on PIOPED studies (JAMA 1990;263:2753); PIOPED study did suggest than PE can be ruled out with a "low" probability V/Q scan with low pretest probability based on clinical scoring (however, in current age of D-dimer testing, those pts would not require V/Q scan with a neg D-dimer assay).
- Overall, definitive dx made with V/Q scans in 28% of pts in PIOPED I study (JAMA 1990;263:2753) and 74% of pts in PIOPED II study (Radiol 2008;246:941); higher percentage of outpatients/ED pts in PIOPED II suggests reduced dx capacity for inpatient eval of PE.
- Pulmonary angiography:
  - Represents the "gold standard" for PE dx; not performed in many centers.
  - Due to improved dx with CT scanning, pulmonary angiography is now reserved for cases where interventional therapies are used for treatment of PE.
- Lower extremity doppler US:
  - While not a direct test for PE, can be useful in pts unable to tolerate contrast dye (renal failure, allergy) and high likelihood of nondiagnostic V/Q scan.
  - Presence of DVT (may be found in up to 80% of PE pts at autopsy, lower rates with usual testing) with si/sx of PE is enough evidence to initiate rx.
  - Not required testing in all PE pts, as finding DVT will not change mgt, unless pt has large PE and low pulmonary reserves (finding of large residual DVT may suggest benefit to IVC filter placement).

PULMONARY

- Echocardiography:
  - Not a direct test for PE, but often performed to evaluate for underlying cardiac function and evidence of RV failure (high pulmonary pressures, RV hypokinesis, tricuspid regurgitation) to suggest massive or submassive PE.
  - Not required in all cases of PE, but consider acutely if associated hypotension or shock; may also be helpful test acutely if not able to get CT due to contraindications.

Rx: (Chest 2004;126:401S; Ann IM 2007;146:211)

Overview of treatment for PE

- Most pts require hospitalization, at least initially, for monitoring and initiation of anticoagulation; see "Deep Venous Thrombosis" later in Section 7.1 for discussion of outpatient therapy.
- Cardiac monitoring for all pts; may require IV hydration and resuscitation if evidence of hypotension with RV failure.
- Eval for massive PE and consideration of thrombolytic therapy.
- Anticoagulation recommendations for DVT and PE are the same, because they are within the same clinical spectrum; most pts studied in the anticoagulation trials have DVT, please refer to DVT guidelines later in Section 7.1 for details.
  - Start anticoagulation with heparin immediately; if delay in dx imaging, start pts with moderate to high probability of PE on anticoagulation prior to imaging.
  - Initiate long-term anticoagulation on day 1 (unless pt not able to take oral warfarin).

Treatment for massive PE

- Requires high degree of suspicion on presentation and rapid dx w/u (CT scan, bedside echo).
- May require initial rapid IV fluid administration with isotonic saline (to improve RV filling), and vasopressor therapy if persistent hypotension.

- May require intubation and mechanical ventilation if associated respiratory failure with severe hypoxemia or hypercarbia.
- Thrombolytic therapy (Chest 2009;135:1321):
  - Consider strongly in cases of massive PE associated with cardiogenic shock or persistent hypotension.
  - Meta-analysis of five trials of thrombolytics in pts with PE and hemodynamic compromise showed reduced mortality with thrombolysis vs treatment with heparin alone (9% vs 19%, NNT 10) (Circ 2004;110:744).
  - Some also argue for treatment in pts with submassive PE, with echo evidence of RV dilation and hypokinesis, elevated TnI and BNP, but evidence is mixed.
  - Alteplase (t-PA) 100 mg IV infusion over 2 hr is FDA-approved regimen; hold heparin initially after thrombolysis.
  - Contraindications are similar to those for thrombolysis in AMI and acute stroke (NEJM 2008;359:2804; Chest 2009;135:1321):
    - Absolute: any h/o hemorrhagic stroke; ischemic stroke within 2 mo; trauma, surgery, head injury within 3 wk; cerebral neoplasm or AVM; active bleeding or coagulopathy (including meds, liver disease)
    - Relative: age older than 75 yr; pregnancy; resistant HTN with SBP higher than 180; noncompressible venipuncture (or CVC placement)
  - Risks of thrombolysis include intracranial hemorrhage (1–3%) (Lancet 1999;353:1386), other massive bleeding (~10%).
- Surgical embolectomy should be considered in pts with contraindication for thrombolytics and if available on-site; catheter-based thrombolysis with pulmonary angiography available at some centers (Radiol 2005;236:852).
- IVC filter placement may have mortality benefit in massive PE (see "Deep Venous Thrombosis" below for further discussion of IVC filters), but requires larger study (Circ 2006;113:577).

PULMONARY

Deep Venous Thrombosis (DVT)

(Ann IM 2008;149:ITC3; Lancet 2005;365:1163)

Cause: In situ venous thrombosis; most common in lower extremity, but can occur anywhere.

Risk factors for VTE are listed under "Pulmonary Embolism" earlier in Section 7.1.

Epidem: See "Pulmonary Embolism" earlier in Section 7.1.

Sx: Leg pain, warmth, unilateral swelling

Si: May feel palpable cord (thrombosed vein) in few pts.

Homan's sign is calf pain with dorsiflexion of the foot; of little dx value (Arch Surg 1976;111:34).

Crs: Wells criteria for assessing pretest probability for DVT (Lancet 1997;350:1795):

- 1 point each for active cancer, paralysis/immobilization, major surgery (or bed rest more than 3 d), localized tenderness, swollen leg, calf asymmetry of more than 3 cm, pitting edema, superficial venous distension
- Subtract 2 points if clinically feel another dx more likely than DVT
- 3 points or more is high probability for DVT; 1–2 points is intermediate; 0 points is low
- Review of 15 studies of the Wells score for DVT (Am J Med 2004;117:676) showed the following:
  - Score of 0 has NPV of 96% to r/o DVT, and neg D-dimer result increased NPV to 99%.
  - High probability score had PPV of only 75%, so further testing (US) needed to confirm dx.
- Online calculators available (e.g., www.mdcalc.com/wells -criteria-for-dvt).

Cmplc: Pulmonary embolism in up to 50% (many may be asx).

Postthrombotic syndrome in 30% with persistent sx of pain, edema (Ann IM 1996;125:1).

HIT in 1–3% (from UFH or LMWH therapy; usually presents with drop in plts by 50% within 5–14 d of therapy unless prior exposure). See "Heparin-Induced Thrombocytopenia" in Section 4.2 for details.

Lab: Initial lab w/u includes CBC with plt; metabolic panel; renal and liver function tests; PT/PTT; consider D-dimer, especially if low suspicion for DVT to r/o disease (see D-dimer discussion under "Pulmonary Embolism" earlier in Section 7.1).

Consider screening for HIT if presence of thrombocytopenia in pts on heparin rx prior to thrombosis; see "Heparin-Induced Thrombocytopenia" in Section 4.2 for details.

Noninv: (JAMA 2006;295:199)

Initial test is doppler US for venous flow and compressibility; sens 97–100%, specif 98–99% for proximal DVT (lower for calf DVTs); in study of 1700 pts with neg US for DVT, 0.7% had confirmed VTE within 6 mo (BMJ 1998;316:17).

Contrast venography is "gold standard," but rarely used; CT venography is gaining use in some centers (especially combined with CT angiography for PE), but added contrast and radiation exposure may not be worth the benefit.

Rx: (Chest 2004;126:401S; Ann IM 2007;146:211)

Overview of treatment for DVT

- Does the pt require hospitalization?
  - With the advent of LMWH, some pts can treat themselves at home (or go to outpatient offices or ED for injection therapy).
  - Patient self-treatment at home requires stable clinical sx, pt compliance with med regimen, adequate f/u.
  - Can consider short admission for initiation of therapies and monitoring, with discharge planning for full heparin course at home until INR adequate.
- Start anticoagulation with heparin immediately; if delay in dx imaging, start pts who have moderate to high probability of

DVT on anticoagulation prior to imaging; see initial antico-agulation guidelines below for details.

- Initiate long-term anticoagulation on day 1 (unless pt not able to take oral warfarin); see long-term anticoagulation guide-lines below.
- Bed rest is not recommended for most pts; does not reduce in-cidence of PE once pt on anticoagulation (Thromb Haemost 2001;85:42), and may increase duration of DVT sx (J Vasc Surg 2000;32:861).
- Consider addition of compression stockings initially and long-term to prevent postthrombotic syndrome.
- Unlike PE, there is little role for thrombolysis in DVT; expert opinion to consider for pts with massive DVT with risk of limb gangrene due to venous occlusion (Chest 2004;126: 401S).
- Special considerations:
  - Upper extremity DVT: Many associated with CVC place-ment; if idiopathic, high rates of thrombophilia (consider hypercoagulability panel prior to rx); does carry risk of PE; if present, remove catheter and otherwise rx similar to lower extremity DVT.
  - Superficial thrombophlebitis forms in the superficial venous system, many times due to IV placement (or idiopathic); carries no risk of embolism; rx with removal of IV, NSAIDs, and warm compresses; in severe cases with persistent sx and pain, can use short-term anticoagulation until resolution.
  - Calf-vein DVTs: Distal DVTs carry little to no risk of embolism, but main risk is propagation to proximal veins (with subsequent risk of embolism), but still less than 5% within 1–2 wk; controversy re immediate anticoagulation vs close monitoring for resolution (or therapy if extends to proximal veins); should base decision re therapy on individual pt circumstances and risk factors.

Initial anticoagulation for VTE

- Unfractionated heparin has been the mainstay of therapy since initial study in 1960 showing high mortality in pts with VTE not treated with anticoagulation (Lancet 1960;1: 1309).
- IV UFH had been the primary therapy for many years, until advent of LMWH.
  - Continuous IV infusion of UFH is preferred; although there is evidence for intermittent SQ dosing (Ann IM 1992;116:279; Cochrane 2009;CD006771), not used much in the era of LMWH (and no large head-to-head studies to show equivalency).
  - Typical regimen is 80 U/kg (up to 5K U) IV bolus, then continuous infusion of 80 U/kg/hr; recheck PTT in 6 hr and adjust to maintain PTT 1.5 to 2 times normal.
  - Most hospitals have protocols for weight-based heparin dosing and adjustment.
- LMWH is now the preferred initial anticoagulation for VTE.
  - Benefit of not requiring continuous infusion, reduced fluid administration, once to twice daily dosing, and no need for routine monitoring of PTT.
  - Meta-analysis of 13 studies comparing UFH and LMWH showed no difference in recurrent VTE or bleeding events, but reduced mortality associated with LMWH (RR 0.76), mainly driven by pts with cancer; on either rx, risk of recurrent VTE within 3 mo is 3–4%, risk of major bleeding event is 1–2% (Arch IM 2000;160:181).
  - LMWH is the preferred treatment initially and long-term for pts with VTE related to cancer (see discussion of long-term anticoagulation therapy below).
  - Typical dosing regimens include:
    - Enoxaparin 1 mg/kg SQ q 12 hr (or 1.5 mg/kg SQ q 24 hr)

- Tinzaparin 175 U/kg SQ qd
- Dalteparin 200 U/kg SQ qd
- Daily dosing of enoxaparin is as effective as bid dosing for DVT, unproven in PE (Ann IM 2001;134:191)
- Other considerations:
  - Requires renal dosing for CrCl less than 30 (enoxaparin 1 mg/kg SQ qd), and some avoid entirely (use UFH instead).
  - LMWH has lower rate of HIT than UFH, but still contraindicated if prior hx of HIT (use fondaparinux, argatroban, or lepirudin initially).
  - No monitoring is necessary (PT/PTT), but in pts with very high or low body weight, consider Factor Xa levels to direct therapy if used long term (not necessary or helpful in short-term use, less than 2 wk).
  - No specific reversal agent for bleeding.
  - Safe for use in pregnancy.
- Alternative to UFH and LMWH is fondaparinux, a direct Factor Xa inhibitor (NEJM 2003;349:1695; Am J Cardiovasc Drugs 2005;5:335).
  - Weight-based dosing: 5 mg SQ qd for pts less than 50 kg; 7.5 mg SQ qd for pts 50–100 kg; 10 mg SQ qd for pts more than 100 kg.
  - Avoid in pts with renal dysfunction (CrCl less than 30).
  - No specific reversal agent for bleeding.
  - No risk of HIT; does not require any plt monitoring and can be used in pts with prior h/o HIT.
- Initial anticoagulation (with UFH, LMWH, or fondaparinux) should be continued at least 5–7 d, or until INR on warfarin therapy is in therapeutic range of 2–3; if pt achieves INR greater than 2 before 5 d, consider overlap of therapy for 48 hr because of initial procoagulant effects of warfarin (on protein C and S) and PT measured by Factor VII activity (and may still be incomplete control of Factors II, IX, X).

Long-term anticoagulation for VTE

- Warfarin is the preferred long-term anticoagulant for most pts with VTE; can be safely started on the first day of admission (as long as pt is clinically stable and taking PO).
- Loading dose is typically 5–10 mg qd to start.
  - 5 mg qd loading dose is probably better than 10 mg; higher dose may have initial hypercoagulable effect by inhibiting protein C (Ann IM 1997;126:133), and may not achieve goal INR any quicker than 5 mg dose (research shows mixed results) (Arch IM 1999;159:46; Ann IM 2003;138:714).
  - Would consider 10 mg loading dose in larger pts (but no direct evidence to support) or in pts with previous use of warfarin requiring daily doses in excess of 5 mg.
- Goal INR is 2.5 (range 2–3) as used in most clinical studies of VTE.
  - ELATE trial: Low-intensity regimen (INR 1.5–1.9) tested in RCT of 738 pts who completed 3 mo of standard warfarin rx for VTE; randomized to goal INR 2–3 vs goal INR 1.5–1.9; low-intensity regimen had higher rate of VTE recurrence (4.3% vs 1.6%, NNH 37), with no difference in bleeding episodes (2% in both groups) (NEJM 2003;349:631).
  - High-intensity regimen (INR 3–4) tested in RCT of 114 pts with prior VTE and antiphospholipid ab; randomized to goal INR 2–3 vs goal INR 3–4; high-intensity regimen had a nonsignificant trend toward more recurrent VTE and no difference in bleeding rates (NEJM 2003;349:1133).
- LMWH therapy should be considered as the primary long-term anticoagulant for the following pts:
  - Patients with VTE related to cancer
    - CLOT study: 672 pts with cancer and VTE; randomized to dalteparin 200 U/kg SQ qd for 5–7 d, then standard

dose warfarin for 6 mo vs dalteparin alone for 6 mo; LMWH therapy alone was associated with decreased risk of recurrent VTE (17% vs 9%, NNT 12), with no difference in bleeding or mortality (high mortality rates due to cancer, ~40% in each group) (NEJM 2003;349:146).

- Pregnant pts, until delivery, as warfarin is teratogenic; hold LMWH 1 d prior to planned induction or C-section
- Patients with difficult-to control INR on warfarin; no clinical evidence to support this use, but may be easier to administer and keep a consistent level of anticoagulation
- Newer oral agents, including dabigatran (NEJM 2009;361:2342) and rivaroxaban (NEJM 2008;358:2765), may have a more significant role in the future for VTE rx and prophylaxis, based on fixed-dose oral administration, without the need for close lab monitoring.
- Considerations re duration of therapy
    - Duration depends on initial cause (if any) and risk factors for recurrence.
    - Short-term treatment of VTE (less than 6 to 12 wk) is not recommended.
        - Duration of Anticoagulation trial group: 902 pts with first episode of VTE; randomized to 6 wk of standard dose warfarin rx vs 6 mo; after 2 yr of f/u, 6-mo therapy was associated with less recurrent VTE (9% vs 18%, NNT 11) with no difference in mortality or bleeding (NEJM 1995;332:1661).
    - See **Table 7.1** for ACCP recommendations of therapy.
    - Indefinite therapy should be considered in following pts:
        - Patients with recurrent VTE
            - Duration of Anticoagulation trial group: 227 pts with a second episode of VTE; randomized to 6 months of standard warfarin rx vs indefinite therapy; after 4 years of f/u, indefinite therapy was associated with less VTE recurrence (3% vs 21%,

NNT 5), but with a nonsignificant trend toward
more bleeding (9% vs 3%) and no difference in
mortality (NEJM 1997;336:393).
- Patients with VTE and underlying cancer (at least until
  cancer is considered cured)
- Patients with VTE and underlying thrombophilia
  (especially APA syndrome)
- Prior to discontinuation of therapy, could consider repeat
  venous doppler to confirm resolution of clot or D-dimer
  level (persistently high level corresponds with increased
  risk of recurrence) (Ann IM 2008;149:481).
- See **Table 7.1** for overview.

Table 7.1 Type and Duration of Anticoagulant Therapy for VTE

Group	Preferred Anticoagulant	Length of Therapy
First VTE episode, transient or reversible risk factor (including trauma, surgery)	Warfarin	3 mo
First VTE episode, idiopathic	Warfarin	6–12 mo
First VTE episode, with cancer	LMWH, then warfarin	LMWH for at least 3–6 mo, then consider switch to warfarin for indefinite use, based on individual patient factors
First VTE episode, with known APA syndrome or multiple thrombophilias	Warfarin	12 mo, then consider indefinite therapy based on individual patient factors
First VTE episode, with known single thrombophilia (other than APA)	Warfarin	6–12 mo, then consider indefinite therapy based on individual patient factors
Recurrent VTE	Warfarin	Indefinite
Any VTE, with pregnancy	LMWH	Through pregnancy and 6–8 wk postpartum (can consider warfarin rx post-partum)

Based on 2004 ACCP recommendations in *Chest.* 2004;126:401S.

PULMONARY

Consideration for IVC filter placement

- Primary indication is DVT with inability to anticoagulate (usually due to active bleeding).
- Also consider if recurrent DVT or PE despite adequate anticoagulation; large DVT with compromised pulmonary status that would suggest high mortality with PE.
- Newer filters are removable; consider if able to anticoagulate at later time or DVT resolved and risks reduced (i.e., remission of cancer, removal of other prior risk factors).
- IVC filters have not been proven to improve mortality (NEJM 1998;338:409).

VTE Prophylaxis in Hospitalized Patients

(Chest 2008;133:381S; NEJM 2007;356:1438)

Cause: Almost all inpatients have one risk factor for VTE; 40% have three or more; see "Pulmonary Embolism" earlier in Section 7.1 for list of risk factors.

Epidem: Worcester DVT study: Incidence of DVT as inpatients or posthospitalization was 48/100K; PE was 23/100K (Arch IM 1991;151:933).

ACCP guidelines (Chest 2008;133:381S) suggest the following rates of DVT (including asx) in inpatients:

- Medical: 10–20% for all pts; stroke 20–50%; critical care 10–80%
- Surgical: general 15–40%; orthopedic (joints) 40–60%

VTE is third most common inpatient cmplc (behind obstetrical trauma and decubitus ulcers), causing an average of 5 d excess LOS, $21,000 excess charges, and 6.5% excess mortality (JAMA 2003;290:1868).

Cmplc: Bleeding risks associated with VTE prophylaxis generally low for short-term use and most studies show no increased bleeding vs placebo; contraindications to prophylaxis include:

- Active bleeding, thrombocytopenia (plt less than 50K), coagulopathy, severe cirrhosis
- Recent severe trauma, craniotomy, intraocular surgery, GI/GU hemorrhage
- Intracranial neoplasm or AVM; prior intracerebral hemorrhage
- Post-op bleeding concerns
- Hypertensive emergency
- Epidural catheter in place (avoid in most cases)

Heparin-induced thrombocytopenia is low-risk (less than 1%) with short-term use, but still consider monitoring platelets with more than 4 d of UFH, LMWH; if prior HIT, avoid UFH and LMWH; fondaparinux has no risk of HIT, and may be used safely.

Lab: Consider plt monitoring for HIT (for pts on UFH or LMWH); no need for PT/PTT (unless if long-term prophylaxis with LMWH in pts of low or high body weight, consider Factor Xa levels to guide therapy).

Noninv: No role for asx screening for DVT in most medical and surgical inpatients.

Rx: Approach to VTE prophylaxis (see **Table 7.2**):

- Assess risk for VTE in all hospitalized pts:
  - Although complex risk models are available, current guidelines suggest simple assessment based on pt factors and clinical scenario.
  - Low risk pts (VTE risk less than 10%) include:
    - Minor surgery or short-stay medical pts, with full mobility
    - Consider ambulation only for VTE prophylaxis

PULMONARY

Table 7.2 VTE Prophylaxis Recommendations

Category	OOB only	SCDs	LMWH	UFH bid	UFH tid	Fondaparinux	Warfarin	Notes
Medical								
Inpatients								
Bed-confined + one additional risk factor			×	×	×	×		Encourage OOB as soon as tolerated
High bleeding risk		×						
Critical care patients								
Moderate risk, postoperative or medically ill			×	×	×			
High risk, major trauma or orthopedic surgery			×					
High bleeding risk		×						Reassess frequently for bleeding risk and addition of medical prophylaxis
Surgical								
General surgery								
Low risk, minor procedure	×							
Laparoscopic procedure only, low VTE risk	×							
Laparoscopic procedure only, additional VTE risk		×	×	×				
Moderate risk, benign disease			×	×	×	×		
High risk, cancer surgery		×	×	×	×	×		Consider 4-wk rx
Highest risk, multiple risk factors		×*	×	×	×	×		*Medical prophylaxis + SCDs; consider 4-wk rx

Procedure						Comments
Inpatient bariatric procedures			x		x	x	Consider higher doses of drugs in morbidly obese pts
High bleeding risk	x					
Vascular surgery						
No additional VTE risk factors	x					
Significant VTE risk factors		x	x	x		
High bleeding risk	x					
Gynecologic surgery						
Low risk, minor procedure	x					
Laparoscopic procedure only, low VTE risk	x					
Laparoscopic procedure only, additional VTE risk		x	x	x		
Major surgery, benign disease		x	x	x		
Major surgery, cancer or high VTE risk	x*	x	x	x		*Medical prophylaxis + SCDs; consider 4-wk rx
High bleeding risk	x					
Urologic surgery						
Low risk, minor procedure, including TURP	x					
Major surgery	x*	x	x	x		*Consider medical prophylaxis + SCDs in high-risk pts
High bleeding risk	x					
Cardiac and thoracic surgery						
Major surgery		x	x	x		
CABG surgery	x	x	x	x		Controversial; at least SCDs, but consider medical prophylaxis
High bleeding risk	x					

Table 7.2 VTE Prophylaxis Recommendations (*Continued*)

Category	OOB only	SCDs	LMWH	UFH bid	UFH tid	Fondaparinux	Warfarin	Notes
Orthopedic surgery								
Elective total hip replacement (THR)			x			x	x	Continue rx up to 35 d post-op
• THR, high bleeding risk		x						
Elective total knee replacement (TKR)		x	x			x	x	Continue rx up to 35 d post-op
• TKR, high bleeding risk		x						
Knee arthroscopy, no additional VTE risk	x							
• Knee arthroscopy, additional VTE risk			x					
Hip fracture surgery (HFS)			x	x	x	x	x	If delayed surgery, start on admit; continue rx up to 35 d post-op
• HFS, high bleeding risk		x						
Below-the-knee injuries/fractures	x							Unless bed-confined with other VTE risk factors

Neurosurgery

					Notes
Elective spine surgery only, low VTE risk	x				
Major surgery, standard VTE risk		x	x	x	
Major surgery, high VTE risk	x*	x	x	x	*Consider medical prophylaxis + SCDs in high-risk pts
High bleeding risk	x				

Major trauma/burns

					Notes
Major trauma patients	x*	x			*Consider medical prophylaxis + SCDs in high-risk pts
• Major trauma, high bleeding risk	x				In high-risk trauma pts, consider screening for asx DVT
Rehabilitating patients with low mobility		x			x Warfarin: INR goal 2–3
Spinal cord injury, no high bleeding risk	x*	x	x	x	*Consider medical prophylaxis + SCDs in high-risk pts
Burn patients		x	x	x	
• Burn patients, high bleeding risk	x				

Based on 2004 ACCP recommendations in *Chest.* 2008;133:381S.

- Moderate risk pts (10–40%) include:
  - Medical pts with significant illness or bed rest
  - Most general surgery pts
  - Consider medical prophylaxis, unless bleeding risk
- High risk pts (risk greater than 40%) include:
  - Orthopedic surgery pts, trauma, spinal cord injury
  - Most pts with ischemic strokes
  - Medical pts w/ prior VTE or multiple risk factors
  - Consider medical prophylaxis and/or SCDs, unless bleeding risk
- Considerations re special populations:
  - Critical care: Higher VTE risk and higher bleeding risks; most should receive medical prophylaxis, but requires regular assessment for risks/benefits.
  - Cancer pts: For inpatients, assess risk as for any med/surg pt, but most are moderate to high risk; do not require long-term prophylaxis for cancer or central venous access.
- Choices for VTE prophylaxis: Refer to **Table 7.2** for 2004 ACCP recommendations (Chest 2008;133:381S).
  - Early and frequent ambulation: Important for all pts, and likely reduces incidence of other inpatient cmplc (decubitus ulcers, HAP, delirium, catheter-related UTI).
  - Mechanical (i.e., graduated compression stockings [GCS] or intermittent pneumatic compression [IPC]):
    - Some studies show reduction in post-op DVT (Cochrane 2000;CD001484), but generally considered less effective than medical prophylaxis.
    - Reserve for pts with contraindication to meds or as adjunctive measures in very high-risk pts.
  - Medications:
    - Aspirin: Antiplatelet Trialist's Collaboration (BMJ 1994;308:235) and PEP trial (Lancet 2000;355:1295) showed that ASA has some evidence of benefit for VTE

prophylaxis; but based on the weight of evidence, current guidelines suggest ASA is inferior to other choices and should not be 1st-line prophylactic therapy.

- Unfractionated heparin (UFH):
  - Proven reduction in DVT, PE, fatal PE; low risk of major bleeding (0.3–2 cases/1K pt days)
    - First large study in 1975; 4121 postsurgical pts randomized to UFH prophylaxis vs placebo; heparin rx reduced clinically evident VTE (0.9% vs 2.7%, NNT 55) and findings of PE on autopsy (0.2% vs 1.1%, NNT 111); wound hematoma was more common in the heparin group, but no difference in transfusion needs or bleeding-related mortality (Lancet 1975;2:45).
    - Meta-analysis of nine studies with medical inpatients (~20K pts) showed significant reductions in all PE (NNT 345) and fatal PE (NNT 400) with UFH prophylaxis (Ann IM 2007;146:278).
  - Least expensive, less than $2 per dose in most hospital pharmacies
  - Typical dose is 5,000 U SQ bid–tid
- Low-molecular-weight heparin (LMWH):
  - Proven as or more effective than UFH in multiple studies.
    - MEDENOX trial: RCT of 1102 medical inpatients older than 40 yr; randomized to enoxaparin 40 mg SQ qd, 20 mg SQ qd, and placebo; 40 mg dose reduced the 14-day incidence of VTE, defined as DVT by US or clinical PE (5.5% vs 14.9%, NNT 11); 20 mg dose no better than placebo; no differences in mortality or adverse events (NEJM 1999;341:793).
    - PREVENT trial: RCT of 3076 medical inpatients; randomized to dalteparin 5,000 U SQ qd

vs placebo; rx reduced the risk of VTE, defined as symptomatic VTE, sudden death, or US-detected DVT at 21 d (2.8% vs 5.0%, NNT 45) (Circ 2004;110:874).

- Common choices include enoxaparin, dalteparin, tinzaparin
- Enoxaparin 40 mg SQ qd; alternative dosing 30 mg SQ bid (used in some orthopedic studies)
- Requires renal dosing: if CrCl less than 30, enoxaparin 30 mg SQ qd or avoid using LMWH entirely (choose UFH instead)

- Fondaparinux:
  - Considered as effective as UFH and LMWH in most settings:
    - ARTEMIS trial: RCT of 849 medical inpatients older than 60 yr; randomized to fondaparinux daily vs placebo; rx reduced VTE, defined as symptomatic VTE or venogram-detected DVT (5.6% vs 10.5%, NNT 20); no difference in mortality or major bleeding (0.2% in both groups) (BMJ 2006;332:325).
  - No risk of HIT
  - Avoid in pts with CrCl less than 30
  - Dose: 2.5 mg SQ qd

- Warfarin:
  - Used for longer-term prophylaxis in orthopedic pts.
  - Generally takes 48 hr to have any measurable effect and 5–7 d for effective anticoagulation; but in prophylaxis situations, bridging therapy not necessary.
  - Dosing typically starts at 5 mg qd, and adjust to goal INR 2–3.
  - If pt already on warfarin (and at goal INR) for another indication (e.g., AF), no need to add 2nd-line agent for VTE prophylaxis.

7.2 Diseases of the Airway

Chronic Obstructive Pulmonary Disease (COPD) Exacerbations

(NEJM 2002;346:988)

Cause: COPD (including emphysema and chronic bronchitis) represents a spectrum of diseases characterized by nonreversible reduction in airflow and destruction of alveolar tissue; exacerbations typically defined as an increase in sx of dyspnea, sputum production, or sputum purulence.

Primary cause of COPD is tobacco abuse (or significant secondhand exposure); other less common causes include alpha-1-antitrypsin deficiency, chemical pollutants.

Cause of COPD exacerbations:

- Infections (80%): half due to bacterial illnesses (most common isolates are *H. influenzae, Strep. pneumoniae, Moraxella catarrhalis*); half due to viral
- Irritants: cigarette smoke, smog, ozone, chemical exposures
- Medication noncompliance
- Complications/comorbid diseases (other than infection): pulmonary embolism (up to 20% of idiopathic COPD exacerbations in one review of five studies [Chest 2009;135:786]; but yet to be corroborated in larger studies); pneumothorax, ACS, CHF

Epidem: COPD exacerbations account for an estimated 500K hospitalizations in the United States per year.

Pathophys: Emphysema occurs with nonfibrotic bronchioloalveolar wall destruction, leading to enlarged air spaces and abnormal gas exchange; loss of elastic recoil leads to distal air trapping, increasing functional residual capacity (FRC), which causes further impairment of chest wall.

Chronic bronchitis is increased inflammation and obstruction of the airways with mucous and inflammatory cells.

PULMONARY

Sx: Most common presenting sx is dyspnea; diff dx of acute dyspnea (Am J Respir Crit Care Med 1999;159:321):

- Pulmonary:
    - Infections: pneumonia, viral upper and lower respiratory tract infections, fungal infections
    - Airway obstruction: asthma and COPD exacerbations; lung cancer or other chest mass; foreign body aspiration; interstitial fibrosis; tracheal or laryngeal stenosis (mechanical, infectious, iatrogenic due to prior intubation); airway trauma and thermal injury; anaphylaxis
    - Pleural causes: pleural effusion, pleural masses, pneumothorax (including tension)
    - Other: pulmonary embolism; aspiration
- Musculoskeletal:
    - Severe kyphoscoliosis, morbid obesity
- Cardiac:
    - ACS; CHF with pulmonary edema
    - Valvular disease including aortic stenosis, mitral regurgitation, mitral stenosis
    - Cardiac tamponade from pericardial effusion, constrictive pericarditis, pericardial tumor
- Neuromuscular:
    - Myasthenic crisis, Guillain-Barre syndrome, poliomyelitis (and other ascending neuropathies)
    - Central or peripheral nervous system insult: brain-stem and cervical spine disorders affecting respiratory centers and respiratory drive; phrenic nerve disruption causing diaphragm dysfunction; recurrent laryngeal nerve injury causing vocal cord paralysis
- Other: anxiety, including panic disorder, somatization; deconditioning; severe anemia

Other sx include cough, fatigue; lower extremity edema associated w/ cor pulmonale (right-sided heart failure due to pulmonary hypertension).

Si: Tachypnea, prolonged expiration, wheezing, sputum production are usually present.

Signs of severe respiratory failure include cyanosis, pursed lip-breathing (creates positive end-expiratory pressure [PEEP]), accessory muscle use, "tripoding" (leaning forward with hands on knees to increase accessory muscle recruitment).

Lethargy, somnolence, delirium suggest hypercarbia ("CO_2 narcosis").

Crs: Average pt has 2–3 exacerbations yearly (mostly in winter months) (Br J Dis Chest 1980;74:228; Am J Respir Crit Care Med 1998;157:1418); 3–16% lead to hospitalization (Med Clin N Am 2006;90:453); 25% require ICU care (JAMA 1995;274:1852).

In-hospital mortality associated with COPD exacerbation is about 10% (30% if older than 65 and requiring ICU care) (JAMA 1995;274:1852); 43% 1-yr mortality; 50% risk for readmission within 6 mo (Am J Respir Crit Care Med 1996;154:959).

Cmplc: Possible cmplc include respiratory failure requiring intubation; also secondary infections, especially VAP, *C. difficile* colitis; pneumothorax.

Severe emphysema is often complicated by malnutrition, cachexia, and wasting.

Lab: Initial eval of dyspnea should include CBC with diff, metabolic panel, renal function; consider PT/PTT if concern for coagulopathy or on warfarin therapy; consider D-dimer in eval of possible PE; consider cardiac enzymes to r/o ACS (may have mild troponin elevations associated w/ severe respiratory failure and right heart stress); consider theophylline levels if on chronic therapy.

ABGs if severe respiratory distress to assist in decision on assisted ventilation; may show respiratory alkalosis due to tachypnea, but more commonly hypoxia and respiratory acidosis with hypercarbia; important to consider degree of renal compensation in assessing hypercarbia, as some long-term COPD pts renally compensate by holding on to serum bicarbonate to buffer $PaCO_2$

rise; presence of pH around 7.30 or better (with elevated $PaCO_2$ and HCO_3) suggests renal compensation and may not require assisted ventilation.

BNP eval may be helpful with new presentation of dyspnea and uncertain if caused by CHF or COPD exacerbation; elevated BNP can suggest cardiac cause, but false positives can result from severe COPD and cor pulmonale (or also increased right-sided pressures from massive PE); see Section 1.2, "Congestive Heart Failure," for further details on BNP.

Procalcitonin levels may assist in determining need for abx; use of an algorithm based on serum levels to initiate or discontinue abx was associated w/ similar rates of adverse outcomes (composite of death, ICU admission, cmplc, or recurrent infection) with reduced abx use in pts with pneumonia (not specifically COPD) (JAMA 2009;302:1115); assays not readily available in many centers.

Consider alpha-1-antitrypsin levels in young pts, with severe COPD, associated liver disease, family history (Lancet 2005;365:2225).

Noninv: CXR is the best initial imaging test; typical appearance in COPD is hyperinflated lungs with flattened diaphragm and "hanging heart" (reduced heart silhouette due to hyperinflation of lungs); use CXR to r/o pneumonia, pneumothorax, effusion, lung masses, etc.; ER study showed 16% yield of important findings (including infiltrates, masses, pneumothorax) in pts seen for COPD exacerbation (Ann EM 1993;22:680).

Chest CT not necessary in most cases, but consider in following:

- For further eval of abnormal CXR (masses, effusion, etc.)
- To look for PE in pts with no other obvious cause of exacerbation and risks factors for VTE

Pulmonary function testing (spirometry) not usually performed acutely, but could consider in hospital setting once acute sx improved to diagnose airway obstruction or determine degree of severity; PFT findings that suggest COPD include forced expiratory volume in 1 second (FEV_1) less than 80% predicted for age and size, ratio of FEV_1 to forced vital capacity (FVC) of less than 70%, decreased diffusing capacity (all are similar in asthma, except nonreversible in COPD) (Eur Respir J 2003;22:1).

Rx: Treatment includes both general and long-term measures, as follows.

General measures for rx of acute exacerbation of COPD

- Admission decision, based on many factors:
  - Severity of sx and need for monitoring
  - Availability of home treatments (oxygen, nebulizers)
  - Home environment (including ongoing tobacco use and secondhand smoke exposure) and compliance with follow-up
- Oxygen administration:
  - All pts should have immediate eval of oxygenation with pulse oximetry, and ABG in severe cases.
  - Goal SaO_2 is greater than 90% in most cases, unless h/o hypercarbia (but still try to keep higher than 88%).
    - Hypercarbia can be exacerbated by supplemental oxygen therapy, even at low rates (e.g., via nasal cannula at 2–4 LPM); may be due to decreased respiratory drive and subsequent hypoventilation, but more likely due to worsening V/Q mismatch (Am Rev Respir Dis 1980;122:747).
    - Take care in pts with known hypercarbia to use the minimal oxygen delivery necessary to maintain adequate oxygenation; if worsening hypercarbia, will need to consider assisted ventilation.
- Assisted ventilation:
  - Initial rx directed at improving hypoxemia, usually with high-flow oxygen by nasal cannula, face mask, or

nonrebreather mask; watch closely for si/sx of worsening hypercarbia and consider serial ABGs.

- Noninvasive positive pressure ventilation (NIPPV):
  - Can be administered as CPAP with single pressure setting or BiPAP with dual pressure settings for inspiration and expiration; typically, order set back-up respiratory rate (8–12), oxygen dose (40–100%), and pressure settings (initially, inspiratory pressure of 10–12 cm H_2O and expiratory pressure of 4–6 cm H_2O, but may require further adjustment based on pt tolerance and oxygenation).
  - Benefit of therapy is to reduce work of breathing and provide stenting of small airways, improving gas exchange; can be used to improve both hypoxemia and hypercarbia.
  - Many small studies have been performed and proven benefit in COPD; for example, review of current studies (Chest 2008;133:756) showed the following:
    - Average study pt had mean pH of 7.31 and $PaCO_2$ of 68 mmHg prior to therapy; average duration of use was 8 hr per day.
    - NIPPV reduced need for intubation by 65%, reduced in-hospital mortality by 55%, reduced LOS by 1.9 d.
  - Consider in all hospitalized pts with COPD exacerbation, especially these:
    - Resistant hypoxemia despite high-flow O_2
    - Respiratory acidosis with pH less than 7.35
    - Hypercarbia, especially if symptomatic
    - Evidence of respiratory fatigue, impending respiratory failure
  - Avoid NIPPV in the following pts:
    - Respiratory arrest
    - Severely obtunded and at risk for aspiration

- Hemodynamically unstable pts with shock
- Facial anomalies, with inability to properly wear mask (beards may add difficulty but not a contraindication)
- Patients with severe anxiety and claustrophobia, unable to tolerate mask (may use benzodiazepines or morphine to treat, but watch closely for worsening respiratory distress with sedation)
- Typically, recheck ABGs after 1–2 hr on appropriate therapy; if worsening respiratory acidosis or hypercarbia, proceed with endotracheal intubation; if stable or improving, continue NIPPV and follow clinically (or with serial ABGs or end-tidal CO_2 monitoring).
- Is NIPPV underutilized? One review showed NIPPV used in only 2.6% of inpatient COPD exacerbations (Ann IM 2006;144:894).
- May also have a role in facilitating earlier weaning from ventilator (Ann IM 1998;128:721).
- Endotracheal intubation and mechanical ventilation (Crit Care Med 2008;36:1614):
  - Consider in pts with worsening respiratory failure despite other measures.
  - Goal of rx is to reduce work of breathing and respiratory muscle fatigue; support ventilation through the acute phase of illness, then wean as able.
  - Avoid hyperventilation solely to reduce hypercarbia.
    - Goal of ventilation should be to improve pH close to normal (7.35), not necessarily normalization of $PaCO_2$.
    - Aggressive hyperventilation and subsequent reduction in $PaCO_2$ can lead to posthypercapneic metabolic alkalosis (from unopposed elevated serum bicarbonate due to chronic compensation).

- Also watch for dynamic hyperinflation, as a consequence of intrinsic PEEP (or auto-PEEP).
  - Air trapping can lead to compression of "normal" lung and worsening hypoxia, as well as pt discomfort, leading to asynchrony with the ventilator.
  - Difficult to assess degree of auto-PEEP, but can dx by rising plateau pressures (as opposed to peak inspiratory pressures, which may be high just because of bronchospasm).
  - Can treat by increasing sedation and even adding paralytics; increasing time for expiration (by reducing set respiratory rate or increasing inspiratory flow times); addition of extrinsic PEEP may also help, but may have variable effects, and requires very close monitoring.
- Bronchodilator therapy:
  - Albuterol is the most commonly used.
    - Beta-2 agonist action causes smooth muscle relaxation and dilation of the airways.
    - Available in MDI and nebulized forms; but in acute exacerbation, nebulizers may assist in improved drug delivery to the airways (although limited clinical evidence) (Ann IM 2001;134:600).
  - Levalbuterol (Xopenex) is an R-isomer of albuterol; although studies indicate there may be fewer side effects (tachycardia, anxiety, tremors) associated with its use (J Asthma 2000;37:319), the high cost vs albuterol does not justify routine use, except in pts who cannot tolerate albuterol.
  - Ipratropium bromide (Atrovent) is an anticholinergic bronchodilator; similar effects to albuterol with less systemic side effects (NEJM 1988;319:486).
  - Evidence does not support superiority of any individual agent (Ann IM 2001;134:600), and combination of

albuterol and ipratropium probably has additive effects (as measured by FEV_1, not clinical sx) (Chest 1994;105:1411).

- Suggest combination of albuterol and ipratropium, given as nebulizer (Duoneb) or MDI (Combivent), initially and every 4–6 hr while hospitalized; if rescue dosing required in between, use albuterol only.
- In ventilated pts, can use nebulizers or MDIs, but need to use higher doses of MDIs, as significant amount of medication is lost in dead space of the tubing and ETT (Am J Respir Crit Care Med 1996;154:382); common regimen is Combivent 8 puffs q 4 hr.
- Antibiotic therapy:
  - Bacterial infections are a common cause of COPD exacerbation.
  - Pneumonia should be treated with abx therapy as outlined in the discussion of pneumonia in Section 5.5 (including assessment of risk for MDR organisms, which are common in COPD pts on chronic steroids and frequent antibiotic regimens).
  - Review of available studies (Chest 2008;133:756) concluded:
    - Antibiotic use in COPD exacerbations significantly reduced treatment failures (defined as addition of abx within 7 d or worsening sx within 21 d) by 46% (and by 66% in hospitalized pts) and reduced in-hospital mortality by 78%.
    - Most frequent abx used in the studies were beta-lactams and tetracyclines.
  - Most pts with severe COPD exacerbations requiring hospitalization should receive abx with the following caveats:
    - Probably most effective in those pts with obvious si/sx of pneumonia, and with increased sputum production.

- Consider blood and sputum cultures to guide therapy, but limited evidence for efficacy; probably most helpful if risk of MDR organisms and frequent abx use.
- No consensus on abx regimen; consider:
  - If definite pneumonia, use standard pneumonia guidelines.
  - Mild to moderate exacerbation and no recent abx use, consider azithromycin, doxycycline, cephalosporins, fluoroquinolones.
  - Severe exacerbation or recent abx use may require broad-spectrum therapy to cover MDR organisms and MRSA.
- Corticosteroids:
  - Theoretically, steroids reduce airway inflammation in COPD exacerbations.
  - Largest study was RCT of 271 VA pts with COPD exacerbation; randomized to three groups: (1) IV methylprednisolone 125 mg q 6 hr for 72 hr, then oral prednisone taper (starting at 60 mg) for 8 wk, (2) IV methylprednisolone, then oral prednisone taper for 2 wk, (3) placebo; steroid therapy (either course) was associated with less treatment failure at 30 d (23% vs 33%, NNT 10) and reduced LOS (1.2 d), with the main adverse effect of hyperglycemia (15% vs 4%, NNH 9); there was no difference between the short and long course of steroid therapy (NEJM 1999;340:1941).
  - Review of all available studies showed steroid rx associated with reduced rx failure by 46% and reduced LOS by 1.4 d (Chest 2008;133:756).
  - Most inpatients initially receive high dose IV methylprednisolone with doses up to 125 mg IV q 6 hr, but lower doses may be as effective (60–80 mg IV q 8 hr).
  - Once improvement shown, convert to oral prednisone and continue for 7–14 d.

- Additional oral dosing shown to benefit in one trial of ED-treated pts, who received oral prednisone vs placebo after IV steroid therapy for acute exacerbation; oral course of prednisone 40 mg qd for 10 d reduced risk of relapse (27% vs 43%, NNT 6) (NEJM 2003;348:2618).
  - Unclear if tapering dose required for short therapy (less than 2 wk); above studies have shown both modes to be effective.
  - Main side effect is hyperglycemia, which should prompt therapy; other risks include GI ulcers, weight gain, anxiety/agitation, and increased infection risks, but none shown to be significant in clinical trials.
- No evidence for benefits to chest physiotherapy or mucolytics in acute COPD exacerbations (Ann IM 2006;144:894), although still used in some settings based on individual pt factors.

Long-term COPD therapy to prevent further exacerbations

(NEJM 2004;350:2689; JAMA 2003;290:2301)

- Smoking cessation:
  - Continued tobacco use associated with more rapid decline in pulmonary function, and cessation results in improved outcomes (JAMA 1994;272:1497).
  - Direct physician counseling is helpful, but minimally effective in long-term abstinence.
  - Consider nicotine replacement (patches, gum, inhalers, nasal spray), behavioral therapy.
  - Bupropion therapy also effective, but 6-mo abstinence rates still only 16% with rx (vs 9% with placebo, NNT 14) (Lancet 2001;357:1571).
- Vaccinations:
  - Pneumococcal vaccination, one dose, may repeat after age 65 if more than 5 yr since prior dose

PULMONARY

- Influenza vaccination yearly
- Little direct evidence of benefit in pts with COPD but presumed due to larger population studies and high-risk group for infection-related morbidity and mortality
- Medications:
  - Initial long-term rx is combination of inhaled bronchodilators (albuterol and ipratropium bromide); long-acting beta-agonist therapy associated with 21% reduction in COPD exacerbations in a meta-analysis (JAMA 2003;290:2301); then add inhaled corticosteroid (Eur Respir J 2003;22:1).
  - Long-term oral corticosteroid rx likely has more risks than benefits, except in severe, end-stage disease.
  - Tiotropium, a long-acting anticholinergic, has been proven to reduce exacerbations.
    - Not necessary in acute therapy, if short-acting ipratropium used.
    - Reduces rates of exacerbation compared to placebo and short-acting ipratropium (RRR of about 20%) (JAMA 2003;290:2301).
    - Consider starting once clinically stable and ready for discharge.
    - Dosed as one inhalation daily.
  - Theophylline can be added for additional bronchodilation in pts with severe disease already on other maximized rx, but narrow therapeutic window requires regular monitoring for adverse effects; watch for drug interactions with fluoroquinolones and macrolides, antiseizure meds, benzodiazepines, beta-blockers.
- Home oxygen therapy:
  - Medicare guidelines require resting oxygen saturation 88% or less, or PaO_2 less than 55 mmHg on room air to qualify.
  - Has been shown to improve mortality in COPD (Lancet 1981;1:681), especially with 24-hr use (Ann IM 1980;93:391).

- Pulmonary rehab: Reduced total time spent in hospital in 1 year by 11 d (21 vs 10 d) (Lancet 2000;355:362).

Asthma Exacerbations

(Chest 2004;125:1081)

Cause: Hyperresponsive airways due to multiple causes:

- Infections: viral URI, bacterial pneumonia, acute sinusitis
- Irritants: allergens (airborne, dietary), pollution, ozone
- Other: anxiety, exercise, menstruation

Epidem: 1.5 million ED visits per year for asthma-related sx; up to 30% are admitted (Am J Med 2002;113:371); 4–7% require ICU care (Lancet 2001;358:629; JAMA 1990;264:366).

Acute asthma exacerbations are more common in females (Arch IM 1999;159:1237).

Pathophys: Airway obstruction due to multiple factors:

- Mucosal edema
- Increased secretions of mucus, desquamated cells
- Smooth muscle hyperplasia
- Inflammatory response of eosinophils, mast cells, and lymphocytes

Sx: Dyspnea, cough

Si: Tachypnea, wheezing, sputum production; tachycardia is common due to both disease and side effect of bronchodilator therapy

As for COPD exacerbations, signs of severe respiratory failure include cyanosis, pursed lip-breathing (PEEP), accessory muscle use, "tripoding" (leaning forward with hands on knees to increase accessory muscle recruitment).

Lethargy, somnolence, delirium suggest hypercarbia ("CO_2 narcosis"), but less common than in COPD.

Pulsus paradoxus (drop in SBP of more than 10 mmHg with inspiration) can be a sign of severe respiratory distress with asthma.

PULMONARY

Crs: Most pts have rapid improvement with acute rx and little long-term morbidity and mortality; mortality of severe cases ("status asthmaticus") requiring ICU admission can be as high as 8%, with most mortality related to pneumothorax and nosocomial infection (Chest 2001;120:1616).

Lab: If asthma exacerbation is obvious based on history and exam, initial lab work may be unnecessary.

Initial eval of dyspnea of uncertain etiology should include CBC with diff, metabolic panel, renal function; consider D-dimer in eval of possible PE; consider cardiac enzymes to r/o ACS (may have mild troponin elevations associated with severe respiratory failure and right heart stress).

Consider ABGs in assessment of severe respiratory distress; most asthmatics initially will show hypoxemia and respiratory alkalosis; hypercarbia and respiratory acidosis less common than in COPD (signs of fatigue and impending respiratory failure).

Noninv: Consider CXR for pts being admitted, mainly to r/o cmplc (pneumonia, pneumothorax, pleural effusion, pulmonary edema); one study showed 34% of pts had abnormal findings, but not all change mgt (Chest 1991;100:14).

Spirometry not necessary or helpful in acute setting; assessment of peak expiratory flow (PEF) may be helpful, but by the time hospitalization is necessary, this may not change mgt; could consider PEF measurements to assess improvement with therapies.

Rx: General measures for treatment of acute exacerbation of asthma are as follows:

- Admission decision, based on many factors:
  - Severity of sx and need for monitoring
  - Availability of home treatments (nebulizers, need for supplemental oxygen)
  - Home environment (including ongoing tobacco use and secondhand smoke exposure) and compliance with follow-up

- Oxygen administration:
  - All pts should have immediate eval of oxygenation with pulse oximetry, and ABGs in severe cases.
  - Goal SaO_2 is more than 92% in most cases; risk of high concentrations of oxygen precipitating hypercarbia are much less in asthma than COPD, but still has been reported (Chest 2003;124:1312).
  - Consider routine humidification; one small trial showed asthmatics routinely have drier expired air, and may have worsening bronchoconstriction associated with dry oxygen administration (Chest 2002;121:1806).
- Assisted ventilation:
  - Initial therapy directed at improving hypoxemia, usually with high-flow oxygen by nasal cannula, face mask, or nonrebreather mask.
  - Noninvasive positive pressure ventilation (NIPPV):
    - Less evidence for benefit in acute asthma than in COPD, but still may be beneficial.
    - See "Chronic Obstructive Pulmonary Disease Exacerbations" earlier in Section 7.2 for more details on use and indications.
  - Endotracheal intubation and mechanical ventilation:
    - Consider in pts with worsening respiratory failure despite other measures.
    - Goal of therapy is to reduce work of breathing and respiratory muscle fatigue; support ventilation through the acute phase of illness, then wean as able.
    - See "Chronic Obstructive Pulmonary Disease Exacerbations" earlier in Section 7.2 for more details on use and indications.
    - Posthypercapneic metabolic alkalosis less common in acute asthma than in COPD due to lack of chronic respiratory failure and renal compensation, but avoid hyperventilation due to risks of dynamic hyperinflation.

- Bronchodilator therapy:
  - Albuterol is the most commonly used.
    - Beta-2 agonist action causes smooth muscle relaxation and dilation of the airways.
    - Available in MDI and nebulized forms; but in acute exacerbation, nebulizers may assist in improved drug delivery to the airways (although limited clinical evidence) (Ann IM 2001;134:600).
  - Levalbuterol (Xopenex) is an R-isomer of albuterol; although studies indicate there may be fewer side effects (tachycardia, anxiety, tremors) associated with its use (J Asthma 2000;37:319), the high cost vs albuterol does not justify routine use, except in pts who cannot tolerate albuterol.
  - Ipratropium bromide (Atrovent) is an anticholinergic bronchodilator; similar effects to albuterol with less systemic side effects (NEJM 1988;319:486).
  - Evidence does not support superiority of any individual agent (Ann IM 2001;134:600), and combination of albuterol and ipratropium probably has additive effects (as measured by FEV_1, not clinical sx) (Chest 1994;105:1411).
  - Suggest combination of albuterol and ipratropium, given as nebulizer (Duoneb) or MDI (Combivent), initially and every 4–6 hr while hospitalized; if rescue dosing required in between, use albuterol only.
  - Continuous nebulizers not more effective than frequent intermittent dosing (Chest 2002;122:160).
  - In ventilated pts, can use nebulizers or MDIs, but need to use higher doses of MDIs, as significant amount of medication is lost in dead space of the tubing and ETT; common regimen is Combivent 8 puffs q 4 hr.
  - Can resume usual doses of long-acting beta-agonists once acute episode resolved.

- Corticosteroids:
  - Theoretically, steroids reduce airway inflammation in asthma exacerbations.
  - Cochrane review of eight studies concluded that steroids in acute asthma reduced the rate of relapse at 1 and 3 wk after initial episode, reduced use of rescue inhalers, with minimal side effects; no evidence for more efficacy of IV/im steroids vs oral (Cochrane 2007;CD000195).
  - If IV form used, often initial dosing of methylprednisolone at 125 mg IV, then 60–80 mg IV q 6–8 hr; oral dosing of prednisone 60 mg qd.
  - Once stable, convert to oral prednisone and continue for 7–14 d; unclear if tapering dose required for short therapy (less than 2 wk).
  - Main side effect is hyperglycemia; other risks include GI ulcers, weight gain, anxiety/agitation, and increased infection risks, but none shown to be significant in clinical trials.
  - Resume inhaled corticosteroids once acute rx completed.
- Antibiotic therapy: Routine abx in asthma exacerbations are not suggested, except in cases of concomitant pneumonia or sinusitis.
- Magnesium:
  - Acts as a smooth muscle relaxant.
  - RCT of ED pts with severe asthma exacerbation, already treated with bronchodilators and steroids, had a significant increase in FEV_1, mainly in pts with initial FEV_1 less than 25% predicted; no difference in need for hospitalization (Chest 2002;122:489).
  - Probably best reserved as an adjunctive agent for severe attacks acutely; little need for continued hospital dosing; minimal side effects.
  - Dose is 1–2 gm IV for 1 dose.

There are further considerations for asthma exacerbations in pregnant pts (NEJM 2009;360:1862; Crit Care Med 2005;33:S319):

- Often hospital physicians may be asked to help manage exacerbations in pregnant women.
  - Chronic asthma complicates 8% of pregnancies.
  - 18% of pts have at least one ED visit, and most acute episodes require hospitalization (Am J Ob Gyn 1996;175:150).
- Asthma is a risk factor for many obstetric cmplc, including preeclampsia, preterm birth, low-birth-weight infants, and perinatal death.
- The usual meds for treatment of acute asthma, including bronchodilators (beta-agonists and anticholinergics), corticosteroids, and most abx (avoid fluoroquinolones and tetracyclines), are safe for use in pregnant pts.
  - Magnesium is often used as a tocolytic and for treatment of preeclampsia.
  - Terbutaline, an IV/im beta-agonist, is used for treatment of preterm contractions and is safe to use as a bronchodilator in pregnancy (although no evidence that it is better than inhaled bronchodilators).
- Try to maintain oxygen sats at least 95% (as opposed to 92% in others) to allow sufficient maternal and placental oxygen concentrations.
- ABG analysis in healthy pregnant women often shows respiratory alkalosis, so the presence of even a mild degree of hypercarbia ($PaCO_2$ of 28–32 mmHg) may be a sign of respiratory fatigue and failure in acute asthma.
- May require frequent fetal assessment if gestation age is more than 23 wk, with fetal heart-rate monitoring, nonstress tests.
- In severe cases requiring mechanical ventilation, take care to avoid hyperventilation and alkalosis, as this may have adverse fetal effects; also avoid hypotension for the same reason.

7.3 Inflammatory Lung Disorders

Acute Respiratory Distress Syndrome (ARDS)

(NEJM 2007;357:1113; Am Fam Phys 2002;65:1823)

Cause: Acute inflammatory disease of the lungs, characterized by noncardiogenic pulmonary edema; first described in 1967 (Lancet 1967;2:319).

American-European Consensus Conference definition (Am J Respir Crit Care Med 1994;149:818) includes the following:

- Acute onset of respiratory sx, usually associated with an underlying illness (see causes of ARDS listed below)
- Bilateral infiltrates on CXR
- Severe hypoxemia
  - Defined as a PaO_2/FiO_2 ratio of 200 or less (300 or less is defined as "acute lung injury")
  - The ratio in normal situations would be (PaO_2 100 mmHg / FiO_2 0.21) = 476
- Lack of evidence of left heart failure (i.e., CHF)
  - Defined as pulmonary capillary wedge pressure (PCWP) 18 mmHg or less.
  - Although this definition requires placement of PA catheter, cases can be diagnosed without one, based on lack of other evidence of left heart failure (e.g., normal or low CVP, lack of cardiac dysfunction on echocardiography or cardiac catheterization).

Causes of ARDS include the following:

- Infection: sepsis (most common cause) (Crit Care Med 2008; 36:296), pneumonia
- Pulmonary injury: aspiration (including drowning), fat embolism, thermal injury, trauma with pulmonary contusion
- Trauma, surgery
- Drug overdose

- Acute pancreatitis
- Blood transfusions (aka TRALI) (Crit Care Med 2006;34:S114; Crit Care Med 2005;33:721)

Epidem: Based on difficulty to dx, incidence reports have been varied; probably 10–50 cases per 100K people.

Pathophys: Alveolar damage leads to increased permeability of the alveolar-capillary membrane; alveoli are flooded with fluid and inflammatory cells; diffuse inflammatory cascade leads to worsening V/Q mismatch, low lung compliance ("stiff lungs"), and severe hypoxemia; for a good review of ARDS pathophys, see Ann IM 2004;141:460.

Sx: Dyspnea, cough; usually in the setting of other critical illness

Si: Tachypnea, tachycardia; depending on underlying cause, likely to occur in the setting of SIRS sx

Crs: Overall mortality of ARDS is 40–50%, usually within 2 wk of onset; death usually due to multiorgan system failure; higher mortality rates in men and African Americans (Crit Care Med 2002;30:1679), thin (low BMI) pts (Crit Care Med 2006;34:738), immunosuppressed.

Consider differential dx, especially in pts with ARDS not related to a clear source, as follows:

- CHF, or cardiogenic pulmonary edema: Will not meet ARDS criteria based on evidence of left heart failure (either PCWP greater than 18, or evidence of LV dysfunction on echo, cardiac cath, etc.).
- Pneumonia: Infiltrates may be more focal; fever, leukocytosis, copious airway secretions; consider respiratory and blood Cx to direct therapy; should respond to appropriate abx regimen; however, ARDS may be seen with pneumonia and sepsis.
- "Imitators" of ARDS (Chest 2004;125:1530): These meet dx criteria for ARDS and may be hard to differentiate; consider

bronchoscopy in suspected cases to help guide therapy; some of these may be responsive to steroid therapy.

- Acute interstitial pneumonia (AIP, aka Hamman-Rich syndrome) (Clin Chest Med 2004;25:739): May occur with collagen vascular diseases or due to drug toxicity; pathologic samples do not help to differentiate from ARDS.
- Acute eosinophilic pneumonia (AEP) (Crit Care Med 2009;37:1470): Look for respiratory tract eosinophils, but not consistently associated with peripheral eosinophilia.
- Bronchiolitis obliterans organizing pneumonia (BOOP) (Arch IM 2001;161:158): Usually presents as nonresolving focal infiltrate (after rx for infectious pneumonia), but may also be diffuse.
- Diffuse alveolar hemorrhage (DAH) (Clin Chest Med 2004;25:583): Consider in pts with coagulopathy (anticoagulant use, thrombocytopenia, liver disease), with diffuse pulmonary infiltrates and drop in Hct; may be associated with hemoptysis, but not in all cases; bronchoscopy should reveal blood in airways.
- Acute hypersensitivity pneumonitis (HP, aka allergic alveolitis) (Clin Chest Med 2004;25:531): Associated with acute inhalation injury.

Cmplc: Most cmplc are iatrogenic: HAP/VAP, gastric "stress" ulcers, VTE, critical illness polyneuropathy from sedation and paralysis.

Ventilator-associated lung injury can include frank pneumothorax, as well as further inflammatory changes from barotrauma.

Even with survival, ARDS can have long-term pulm, neuro, and psychiatric sequelae (Chest 2007;131:554).

Lab: No routine lab work necessary in the eval and mgt of ARDS; often requires frequent monitoring of blood count, renal function, electrolytes due to cmplc of critical illness.

Noninv: CXR is primary choice for initial imaging; diffuse bilateral infiltrates (may be interstitial or alveolar) required for dx; can be very difficult to distinguish from cardiogenic pulmonary edema, even with expert reading (Radiol 1988;168:73; Chest 1999;116:1347), but clues to suggest CHF include cardiomegaly, pleural effusions, peribronchial cuffing (extravasated fluid around the airway causes it to appear more prominent), Kerley B lines (horizontal lines in upright pt showing edema tracking in from the pleura).

Chest CT can help to quantify severity, may show some sparing of the anterior lung fields; also can help to dx cmplc (pneumothorax, abscess, etc.).

Consider bronchoscopy with lavage for Cx to r/o infection, "imitators" (see Crs above).

Consider echocardiogram to evaluate LV function and r/o CHF. May be difficult to assess for ARDS in pts with sepsis-induced acute LV dysfunction, and may require invasive monitoring and treatment for both CHF and ARDS.

Considerations re PA catheter for pts with ARDS:

- Although use of PA wedge pressure to define ARDS is not necessary, many still advocate for regular use of PA (or Swan-Ganz) catheter for mgt of pts with ARDS.
- Should be used in pts with uncertain cardiac status and need for proper dx of ARDS vs cardiogenic pulmonary edema.
- Two large trials of pts with ARDS did not show PA catheter use leading to improvement in mortality or other ICU outcomes (JAMA 2003;290:2713; NEJM 2006;354:2213).
- If no PA catheter in place, can use other measures of volume status, including weight, I/O, CVP measurements by CVC, urine output, physical exam, chest imaging, etc.

Rx: Therapy for ARDS involves general measures as well as special considerations for mechanical ventilation.

General measures of treatment for ARDS

- Recognition and rx of underlying cause, especially abx for infection

- Treatment of hypoxemia with assisted ventilation
  - Some mild cases may be treated with NIPPV, but limited evidence (Respir Med 2006;100:2235); consider in pts without hypotension, delirium, severe respiratory distress, with expected improvement in 2 to 3 d (a minority of ARDS pts).
  - Endotracheal intubation and mechanical ventilation required in most cases; see mechanical ventilation guidelines below for more details.
- Assessment of nutritional status and initiation of enteral or parenteral feedings as needed
- Avoidance of cmplc of critical illness
  - VTE prophylaxis, as described in Section 7.1
  - Stress ulcer prophylaxis, as described in Section 3.2, "Gastrointestinal Bleeding"
  - Prevention of nosocomial infection
    - Prevention of VAP, as described under "Pneumonia" in Section 5.5
    - Prevention of catheter-related UTI, as described in Section 5.7
    - Prevention of CVC infection, as described under "Central Venous Catheters and Associated Infections" in Section 5.3
- Issues re use of corticosteroids in ARDS
  - Controversial subject; multiple studies of various sizes have been performed, but difficult to summarize data and reach conclusions because of variety of dosing regimens, duration of treatment, and pt populations (early vs late therapy).
  - Early, high-dose IV steroids (methylprednisolone 30 mg/kg) have no benefit to mortality or other ICU outcomes (NEJM 1987;317:1565), nor does it prevent ARDS in pts with severe sepsis (Chest 1987;92:1032; Am Rev Respir Dis 1988;138:62).

PULMONARY

- However, studies have shown mixed results on benefits of steroids in pts with nonresolving ARDS (after 7 d or more of standard therapy).
  - Small RCT of 24 pts w/ severe ARDS, not improving after 7 d of care; randomized to methylprednisolone 2 mg/kg/d for 32 d vs placebo; steroid therapy led to reduced mortality (12% vs 62%, NNT 2) and improved oxygenation and successful extubation (JAMA 1998; 280:159).
  - ARDSNet study of 180 pts w/ severe ARDS, not improving after 7 d of care; randomized to methylprednisolone vs placebo; steroid therapy did improve shock and oxygenation, but no effect on mortality (60-day mortality was 29% in both groups), and steroids actually increased mortality in pts with ARDS more than 14 d prior to addition of steroids (NEJM 2006;354: 1671).
  - Review of all RCTs and cohort studies of low- to moderate-dose steroid therapy in ARDS suggested that there may be a mortality benefit to use of steroids (Crit Care Med 2009;37:1594); different meta-analysis, containing many of the same studies, had more guarded recommendations (BMJ 2008;336:1006).
- Bottom line is that there is little convincing evidence that potential benefits of steroid use in ARDS outweigh the risks (including increased secondary infections, hyperglycemia, stress ulcers and GI bleeding, critical illness polyneuropathy); larger RCTs are needed to help determine benefit; current expert opinion does not suggest routine use (Crit Care Med 2004;32:S548).
- Patients with ARDS may receive steroids for other indications, usually septic shock (see discussion under "Adrenal Insufficiency" in Section 2.1), bronchospasm related to asthma or COPD, or for rx of other inflammatory diseases.

- Issues re fluid management in ARDS
  - Because the nature of pulmonary edema in ARDS is different from cardiogenic pulmonary edema, pts do not respond similarly to diuresis; also, diuretic rx can be difficult to manage, especially in pts with concomitant sepsis and shock.
  - A neg fluid balance (driven by good urine output) within 3 d in pts with septic shock (not specifically ARDS) is linked to better prognosis (Chest 2000;117:1749).
  - FACTT study: RCT of 1000 pts with ARDS; randomized to liberal vs conservative fluid mgt; liberal fluid mgt resulted in a pos fluid balance of about 7 L over 1 wk, conservative had a net neg fluid balance of −0.1 L over 1 wk; conservative mgt was associated with improved oxygenation and 2 fewer days on the ventilator and in ICU; no difference in mortality, shock, or need for dialysis between the two groups (NEJM 2006;354:2564).
    - Management strategy was complex; refer to study for full details.
    - Goal of conservative mgt was to maintain CVP less than 4 (or PCWP less than 8), as long as MAP was greater than 60 (without need for vasopressors).
      - If MAP is less than 60, treat with vasopressors and IVF boluses (see "Sepsis and Septic Shock" in Section 5.3 for more details).
      - If MAP is more than 60 and urine output more than 0.5 mL/kg/hr, then treat with IV furosemide if CVP is more than 4, to goal CVP less than 4.
      - If MAP is more than 60, and urine output less than 0.5 mL/kg/hr, then give IV furosemide if CVP is more than 8, or IVF bolus if CVP is less than 8.
  - Bottom line is that minimizing IV fluid in pts with ARDS may improve respiratory status; should still use IVF in the

initial phases (especially early goal-directed therapy for sepsis, as described in Section 5.3) and for shock (MAP less than 60); in all others, should try to achieve input about equal to output; may be difficult to follow the study algorithm, but avoid "maintenance" fluids and closely monitor additional fluids given with drips and intermittent meds (abx, acid suppressants, steroids, etc.).

- Other measures
  - Surfactant has been tried, due to its efficacy in newborn respiratory distress syndrome (RDS), but no effect in ARDS (NEJM 1996;334:1417).
  - Multiple anti-inflammatory drugs have been tried without benefit (Mayo Clin Proc 2006;81:205).

Mechanical ventilation of patients with ARDS

(Chest 2007;131:921)

- The majority of pts with ARDS and acute lung injury require intubation and mechanical ventilation for hypoxemic respiratory failure.
- Cornerstone of ARDS mgt is low-tidal-volume ventilation (NEJM 2007;357:1113).
  - Older therapies were directed at high tidal volumes, suspecting that this would lead to hyperinflation of the lungs and "recruitment" of normal, but atelectatic, areas; but two subsequent studies suggested that lower tidal volumes, with the need for lower driving pressures in the airway, were associated with improved outcomes:
    - Amato study: RCT of 53 pts w/ ARDS; randomized to conventional ventilation (Vt 12 mL/kg with goal to reduce $PaCO_2$ to 35–38 mmHg) vs protective ventilation (Vt 6 mL/kg, allowing $PaCO_2$ to rise with main goal to maintain airway pressures less than 20 cm H_2O); low tidal volume was associated with reduced 28-day mortality (71% vs 38%, NNT 3) and improved

weaning from ventilator (29% vs 66%, NNT 3) (NEJM 1998;338:347).

- Three other subsequent studies did not show any benefit (or harm) to low-tidal-volume ventilation (NEJM 1998;338:355; Am J Respir Crit Care Med 1998;158:1831; Crit Care Med 1999;27:1492).
- ARMA (part of the ARDS Network) study: 861 pts w/ ARDS randomized to similar arms as Amato study; low-tidal-volume ventilation was associated with re-duced mortality (40% vs 31%, NNT 11) (NEJM 2000; 342:1301).

- Approach to low-tidal-volume ventilation:
  - Based on assist-control ventilation with set volume (can use pressure control ventilation, with variable tidal volumes, but no direct evidence to support this)
  - Set initial tidal volume at 6 mL/kg (for non-ARDS pts, typically use 10 mL/kg), based on ideal body weight, not actual body weight; calculate using the following formulas:
    - Men: 50 + 0.91 (Height in cm − 152.4)
    - Women: 45.5 + 0.91 (Height in cm − 152.4)
    - See **Table 7.3** for estimated ideal body weights
  - Set initial RR at 18–22 breaths/min (for non-ARDS pts, typically use 10–14 breaths/min); somewhat higher than traditional settings due to need for maintaining adequate minute ventilation (RR × Vt) in the face of low volumes.
  - Set initial PEEP to at least 5 cm H_2O (and maybe higher depending on degree of hypoxemia and pt hemo-dynamic status).
  - Set initial FiO_2 at 100%, but wean quickly, with addi-tion of PEEP to maintain O_2 saturation at 88–92%.
  - Goal is to keep airway plateau pressure at less than 30 cm H_2O.

Table 7.3 Ideal Body Weight

Height (in)	Height (cm)	Male IBW (kg)	Female IBW (kg)
60	152	50	46
62	157	55	50
64	163	59	55
66	168	64	59
68	173	68	64
70	178	73	69
72	183	78	73
74	188	82	78
76	193	87	82

- Adjust initial settings based on pt response:
  - Airway pressures remain high (more than 30 cm H_2O): Reduce tidal volume to 4–5 mL/kg.
  - Severe respiratory acidosis (pH less than 7.20): Increase RR to improve minute ventilation; if concomitant metabolic acidosis, can consider bicarbonate infusions to keep pH in reasonable range.
  - Hypoxemia: Add additional PEEP if tolerated; adjunctive measures as described below.
- Low-tidal-volume ventilation may lead to some degree of hypoventilation, persistent respiratory acidosis and hypercapnia; this is termed "permissive hypercapnia" and has not been shown to have any unfavorable effects (except in pts with increased intracranial pressure, as may worsen cerebral edema); goal should be to keep $PaCO_2$ less than 80 mmHg, pH greater than 7.20.
- Other modes of ventilation may be considered, but lack of significant evidence of benefit; some centers are using high-frequency oscillatory ventilation, which delivers very low tidal volumes (1–5 mL/kg) at very high rates, with some success.

- Considerations re PEEP in ARDS:
  - Improves oxygenation in ARDS, likely by improving V/Q mismatch and stenting open small airways, preventing alveolar collapse and atelectasis.
  - Traditionally set at 5 cm H_2O initially, then can titrate up to as high as 20–25 cm H_2O based on degree of hypoxemia; higher settings will contribute to plateau pressure (with goal to keep less than 30 cm H_2O); also watch blood pressure closely, as increased intrathoracic pressure will reduce ventricular preload and may cause hypotension (treat with IVF boluses if needed).
  - ALVEOLI trial showed that higher PEEP levels (mean of 13, high of 24) were associated with improved oxygenation, but no difference in mortality or ventilator-free days compared to traditional low PEEP levels (mean of 8) (NEJM 2004;351:327).
- Management of refractory hypoxemia in ARDS involves the following considerations:
  - Persistent hypoxemia despite low-lung-volume mechanical ventilation is common in severe ARDS.
  - Strategies to improve oxygenation include:
    - Increase FiO_2.
    - Increase RR to improve minute ventilation.
    - Increase PEEP as tolerated based on hemodynamics and airway pressures.
    - Prone positioning: Studies have shown that placing pts on their stomachs for a period of time will improve oxygenation but not mortality (NEJM 2001;345:568; JAMA 2004;292:2379; Am J Respir Crit Care Med 2006;173:1233); likely due to temporary improvements in V/Q mismatch with ventilation of anterior lung fields that contained less dependent edema, improved drainage of airway secretions (Eur Respir J 2002;20:1017);

PULMONARY

requires physical ability to move pt and ventilator/lines, etc., without dislodging catheters.

- Nitric oxide: Has been evaluated in multiple studies (NEJM 1993;328:399; JAMA 2004;291:1603); shown to improve oxygenation short-term, but no effect on mortality or other clinical outcomes; not available in many centers, and expert opinion suggests use only in clinical trials or for rescue therapy (Crit Care Med 2004;32:S548).

- Approaches to ventilator weaning include:
  - Consider weaning once FiO_2 is 50% or less, PEEP 5 cm H_2O or less, stable respiratory secretions and airway reflex (cough), hemodynamically stable, stable mental status off sedatives.
  - Consider daily spontaneous breathing trial (SBT).
    - Patient has 30 min to 2 hr of spontaneous respiration on vent with small amount of pressure support (5–10 cm H_2O) and PEEP (5 cm H_2O), or T-tube (as described along with other weaning procedures below).
    - Assess rapid shallow breathing index (RSBI), calculated by RR (in breaths/min) divided by Vt (in liters).
      - For example: stable pt may have SBT with RR = 15/min and Vt = 0.5 L, so RSBI = 15/0.5 = 30; unstable pt may have SBT with RR = 40/min and Vt = 0.25L, so RSBI = 40/0.25 = 160.
      - RSBI of less than 100–105 suggests increased probability of successful extubation (NEJM 1991;324:1445).
    - Consider repeat ABG after SBT to evaluate degree of hypoxemia and hypercarbia.
  - Consider other weaning procedures:
    - Pressure support ventilation (PSV): Spontaneous mode that provides constant inspiratory pressure to

assist pt ventilation; for weaning, can start at higher pressures (e.g., 20 cm H_2O) and wean slowly to lower amounts of support; requires pt to breathe spontaneously as no backup rate, so must monitor pt's RR and Vt closely.

- Synchronous intermittent mandatory ventilation (SIMV): Provides a set rate of ventilator breaths (with preset Vt) and any pt breaths above that rate can be supported with pressure support; can start with higher number of "machine breaths" (e.g., 10–12/min) and slowly wean down; essentially acts as a transition between assist-control and pressure support ventilations.
- T-tube: Spontaneous breathing w/ no additional support other than supplemental blow-by oxygen.
- Daily SBT may be the best choice (NEJM 1995;332:345).
  - Study from the Spanish Lung Failure Collaborative Group: RCT of 133 pts w/ ARDS on mechanical ventilation for mean of 7 d and ready for weaning, but failed initial SBT; randomized to four weaning techniques:
    - Once daily SBT
    - Intermittent SBT 2–3 times daily
    - SIMV weaning, initial RR of 10, decreased by 2–4/min once to twice daily as tolerated
    - PSV weaning, initial pressure support of 18 cm H_2O, decreased by 2–4 twice daily as tolerated
  - Average wean time was 3 d for SBT trials (daily or intermittent), compared to 4 d for PSV, and 5 d for SIMV.

Interstitial Lung Diseases (ILDs)

(South Med J 2007;100:579; Mayo Clin Proc 2007;82:976)

Cause: Also called diffuse parenchymal lung diseases; heterogeneous category of multiple pulmonary diseases, categorized by progressive respiratory sx, due to noninfectious causes (if cause known at all); categories of diseases include the following:

- Idiopathic interstitial pneumonias
  - Includes the most common ILD, idiopathic pulmonary fibrosis (IPF) (~60% of ILD cases) (Am J Respir Crit Care Med 1994;150:967; NEJM 2001;345:517).
  - Also includes acute interstitial pneumonia (AIP), bronchiolitis obliterans organizing pneumonia (BOOP); see the discussion of ARDS earlier in Section 7.3 for some details on these illnesses, which can be very similar in appearance and presentation to ARDS.
- Collagen vascular disease–related lung disease
  - Related to underlying SLE, scleroderma, rheumatoid arthritis (RA), polymyositis
- Exposure-related lung disease
  - Drugs, including amiodarone (Chest 1988;93:1067; Chest 1988;93:1242), methotrexate (Arthritis Rheum 1997;40:1829), nitrofurantoin (Mayo Clin Proc 2005;80:1298), chemotherapy drugs
  - Radiation, toxins, chemicals
  - Pneumoconioses: asbestosis (NEJM 1989;320:1721), silicosis (Lancet 1997;349:1311)
- Hypersensitivity pneumonitis due to exposure to organic antigens ("farmer's lung")
- Sarcoidosis (NEJM 2007;357:2153)
  - Chronic granulomatous disease of uncertain origin
  - Affects multiple systems besides the lungs, including heart, skin, lymphatics, and eyes; may present as asymptomatic hilar lymphadenopathy on CXR
  - More common in African Americans, younger pts (younger than 40 yr)
- Pulmonary vasculitis (Chest 2006;129:452)
  - Often affects kidneys as well, leading to term "pulmonary-renal syndrome"

- Includes Wegener's granulomatosis (Ann IM 1992;116: 488), Churg-Strauss syndrome (Lancet 2003;361:587), microscopic polyangiitis, Goodpasture's syndrome (aka anti-GBM diseases) (NEJM 2003;348:2543; South Med J 2002;95:1411)

Epidem: Population study in New Mexico showed ILD prevalence of approximately 70 cases per 100K; incidence of new cases approximately 30 per 100K per year (Am J Respir Crit Care Med 1994;150:967); most pts older than 60 yr; more common in men (1.4:1).

Pathophys: Varying pathophys due to underlying cause; most lead to pulmonary fibrosis causing shunt and V/Q mismatch with subsequent hypoxemia.

Sx: Progressive dyspnea, cough in most pts.

Depending on cause, may have other evidence of connective tissue diseases, including arthralgias, myalgias, rash; constitutional sx including fever, anorexia, weight loss.

Right-sided heart failure (cor pulmonale) may lead to peripheral edema.

Si: Hypoxemia; common lung finding is Velcro-like inspiratory crackles.

Digital clubbing may also be seen, especially in IPF (50%) (Thorax 1980;35:171), but not specific to ILDs.

Crs: Most have slowly progressive disease, but specific types (as detailed in the discussion of ARDS earlier in Section 7.3) may present acutely

High mortality; 30–50% of pts eventually die from cmplc of the disease; significant mortality at the time of initial dx (especially with lung bx), 15–20% within 30 d (Eur Respir J 2001;17:175); pts who require ICU care have even higher mortality (92% within 2 mo) (Am J Respir Crit Care Med 2002;166:839); mean survival is 3–5 yr (CMAJ 2004;171: 153).

Risk factors for poor prognosis include age older than 50, male, severe respiratory sx, smoking hx, honeycombing pattern on HRCT, lack of response to therapy (South Med J 2007;100:579).

Course may be complicated by acute exacerbations (Am J Respir Crit Care Med 2007;176:636), with worsening sx and hypoxemia; CT may show new opacities; many cases require rx for infectious causes until can be r/o by course, cultures, etc.

Lab: Initial eval similar to that for dyspnea (as described in the discussion of COPD in Section 7.2) or pneumonia (as described in Section 5.5)

If specifically concerned for ILD as cause of pulmonary sx, consider the following labs:

- ESR, CRP: Nonspecific, but may be useful in some settings to r/o disease or follow course of rx.
- ANA, RF: Nonspecific and may be elevated in a variety of diseases; if specifically concerned for SLE, scleroderma, or other collagen vascular diseases, consider extractable nuclear antigens (anti-SS-A/Ro, anti-SS-B/La, anti-Scl-70, anticentromere, anticyclic citrullinated peptide); CPK, aldolase for myositis.
- Antineutrophilic cytoplasmic antibodies (ANCA): Specific to pulmonary vasculitis syndromes; p-ANCA suggests microscopic polyangiitis (50–75%) or Churg-Strauss (45–70%); c-ANCA suggests Wegener's granulomatosis (more than 90%) (Chest 2006;129:452); anti-PR3 and antimyeloperoxidase may also be of value.
- Anti-glomerular basement membrane (GBM) antibodies: Seen in Wegener's granulomatosis and Goodpasture's syndrome.
- Angiotensin-converting enzyme (ACE) levels: Often performed with sarcoidosis eval, but limited specif and sens make it less useful (NEJM 2007;357:2153).
- Peripheral eosinophilia may suggest eosinophilic pneumonia, Churg-Strauss syndrome, drug reactions.

- Hypercalcemia may be seen with sarcoidosis.
- Anemia of chronic disease may be present.
- U/A for proteinuria, hematuria, RBC casts; serum BUN/Cr for glomerulonephritis in vasculitis syndromes.

Noninv: CXR usually shows diffuse parenchymal lung disease with a variety of patterns, including "honeycombing," ground-glass opacities; may have associated effusions in some cases.

HRCT has become the study of choice for evaluation of ILD (Am J Respir Crit Care Med 2005;172:268), and in some cases may be able to replace bx (80% dx with clinical si/sx) (Radiol 1994;191:383).

Spirometry may be helpful in some cases; should show restrictive disease (reduction in FEV_1 and FVC; may have preserved FEV_1/FVC ratio), but may also have concomitant obstruction if smoking hx; will also have reduced diffusing capacity for carbon monoxide (DLCO).

Echocardiogram may be useful to assess degree of pulmonary hypertension, and to r/o LV dysfunction as cause for dyspnea.

Rx: Treatment for most cases of ILD are based on sparse evidence-based data and expert opinion; RCTs are very limited due to the rarity of these diseases, the severity of disease, and the difficulty in obtaining precise diagnoses.

Some cases can managed expectantly, if sx are minimal; but most hospital physicians will be seeing pts with severe disease, either as initial presentation or exacerbation, which usually warrant therapy, if available.

General measures for treatment of ILD:

- Proper dx is important to tailor appropriate rx; occasionally in end-stage disease, or pts with other severe comorbidities, rx can be undertaken based on a presumptive dx.
  - If cause not apparent based on clinical hx and HRCT, consider bronchoscopy with lavage and transbronchial bx, or surgical lung bx (e.g., video-assisted thoracoscopic surgery).

PULMONARY

- Supportive care with O_2 usually required; may need assisted ventilation with NIPPV or mechanical ventilation; if the latter, most use the low-tidal-volume approach described in the discussion of ARDS earlier in Section 7.3.
- If co-existent COPD, consider therapies as detailed in Section 7.2.
- Detailed h/o drug/med use, exposures, occupation, family hx are all crucial; stress removal of any possible offending agents.
- Antibiotics have no specific role in treatment, but are often used initially because of concern for pneumonia; if bacterial pneumonia present in pts with ILD, consider broad-spectrum therapy due to lung disease, frequent hospitalizations, and use of steroids or other immunosuppressive drugs.
- As in ARDS, watch and provide prophylaxis for specific inpatient cmplc (VTE, stress ulcers, decubiti, malnutrition, etc.).
- Anti-inflammatory therapy is the mainstay; most studies look at treatment of IPF specifically.
  - Usually steroids are the initial rx of choice (Cochrane 2003;CD002880); may be high-dose IV (methylprednisolone 125–250 mg IV q 6–8 hr) initially (in new dx or exacerbations), then slow taper to chronic dosing.
  - Consider addition of other immunosuppressive drugs, either as 1st-line or 2nd-line therapy, including azathioprine (Am Rev Respir Dis 1991;144:291), cyclophosphamide (Eur Respir J 1998;12:1409; Chest 2000;117:1619; Respir Med 2006;100:340), colchicine (Am J Respir Crit Care Med 1998;158:220), methotrexate, hydroxychloroquine, pirfenidone (Am J Respir Crit Care Med 2005;171:1040); please refer to local experts and specific disease guidelines for therapy (Am J Respir Crit Care Med 2000;161:646).
  - Anticoagulation with warfarin or LMWH may have role in exacerbations and severe disease (Chest 2005;128:1475), but yet to be proven in larger trials.

- If chronic steroids employed, watch for hyperglycemia and consider prophylaxis against gastric ulcers (H2B or PPI), osteoporosis (calcium, vit D, bisphosphonates), and *Pneumocystis* infection (see discussion of PCP in Section 5.6 for details).
- Pulmonary rehab may have some benefit.
- Consider early referral to specialty center for lung transplant eval in appropriate pts; most pts with ILD are not good candidates for lung transplant based on age (most cases occur in pts older than 65, who infrequently get transplants), other comorbid diseases, or rapid progression of illness.

Chapter 8

Renal/Urology

8.1 Acid-Base Disorders

(NEJM 1998;338:26; NEJM 1998;338:107)

Cause: Common causes of acid-base disorders in hospitalized pts, by type:

- Metabolic acidosis: low pH, low $PaCO_2$, low HCO_3; further characterized by presence or lack of anion gap (see anion gap calculation in Lab below for details)
    - Presence of anion gap (defined as more than 10–12 mEq/L; remember as mnemonic, MUDPILES:
        - **M**ethanol ingestion: accidental or intentional (for suicide or intoxication); commonly found in windshield washer fluid
        - **U**remia: renal failure, associated with buildup of organic acids
        - **D**iabetic ketoacidosis: due to accumulation of beta-hydroxybutyrate and amino-acetate; see "Diabetic Ketoacidosis" in Section 2.3 for more details; also consider alcoholic ketoacidosis in nondiabetic pts
        - **P**araldehyde ingestion
        - **I**soniazid or iron overdose
        - **L**actic acidosis: due to accumulation of lactate from reduced tissue perfusion (but can also be due to metformin toxicity) (Crit Care Med 2009;37:2191); see "Sepsis and Septic Shock" in Section 5.3 for more details

- **E**thylene glycol ingestion: accidental or intentional (for suicide or intoxication); commonly found in antifreeze; associated with acute renal failure
- **S**alicylates: ASA overdose
- Lack of anion gap; most due to bicarbonate loss, associated with hyperchloremia:
  - Lower GI fluid losses from diarrhea, ileal loop, or fistula drainage
  - Renal tubular acidosis: variety of syndromes associated with defect in renal tubular acidification (South Med J 2000;93:1042)
- Metabolic alkalosis: high pH, high $PaCO_2$, high HCO_3
  - Upper GI HCl losses, due to vomiting, NG suction
  - Renal losses (aka "contraction alkalosis") due to loop or thiazide diuretic rx
  - Mineralocorticoid excess, due to hyperaldosteronism, Cushing's syndrome, oral replacement; excessive licorice ingestion also has similar effects (NEJM 1991;325: 1223)
  - Posthypercapneic: due to mechanical hyperventilation in pts with prior compensated resp acidosis; see the discussion of COPD exacerbations in Section 7.2 for details
  - Milk-alkali syndrome: excess ingestion of milk or other calcium-containing products induces hypercalcemia; kidneys increase resorption of HCO_3, leading to alkalosis
  - Hypokalemia, hypercalcemia
- Respiratory acidosis: low pH, high $PaCO_2$, high HCO_3; degree of acidosis and HCO_3 elevation can be used to determine acute vs chronic (with renal compensation)
  - Acute: respiratory insufficiency/arrest from infection, inflammatory or obstructive lung disease, pulmonary edema; neuromuscular disease (myasthenia gravis, Guillain-Barre syndrome); overdose/intoxication

- Chronic: chronic obstructive or restrictive lung disease; OSA, obesity-hypoventilation (Pickwickian syndrome); chronic neuromuscular diseases
- Respiratory alkalosis: high pH, low $PaCO_2$, low HCO_3; degree of alkalosis and HCO_3 reduction can be used to determine acute vs chronic (with renal compensation)
  - Most cases are acute, associated with hyperventilation from anxiety, respiratory diseases (pneumonia, PE), ASA toxicity (may have mixed resp alkalosis and metabolic acidosis), sepsis, liver failure
  - More rarely, chronic cases due to high-altitude exposure, pregnancy, liver failure

Sx/Si: Mainly due to underlying disease, but severe acidosis or alkalosis may be associated with cardiovascular compromise (hypotension, decreased perfusion), neuro deterioration (delirium, coma).

Toxic alcohol ingestions are usually associated with signs of inebriation, delirium, N/V, ataxia; visual disturbances leading to blindness with methanol.

ASA toxicity is associated with tinnitus, vertigo, N/V, seizures, delirium.

Cmplc: Metabolic acidoses are commonly associated with hypokalemia and hypoglycemia (may require IV dextrose).

Lab: ABG analysis crucial to determination of acid-base disorders; above deflections in pH, $PaCO_2$, HCO_3 are generally seen, but may be variable based on chronicity of problem with compensation, and mixed acid-base disorders.

In w/u of metabolic acidosis, should initially check electrolytes, glucose, renal and liver function tests, serum lactate, serum ketones, serum osmolality; also consider:

- Anion gap calculation (see DKA discussion in Section 2.3 for details): $Na - (HCO_3 + Cl)$; normal is less than 10–12 mEq/L

- Osmolar gap calculation: Measured serum osmolality − Calculated serum osmolarity
  - Calculated osmolarity: $[(Na \times 2) + (Glucose/18) + (BUN/2.8) + (Ethanol/4.6)]$
  - Typically, osmolar gap is less than 10; if higher, consider methanol, ethylene glycol, DKA, lactate
- Toxicology eval based on concern for ingestions (ASA; APAP does not cause acidosis, but commonly co-ingested in overdoses; can test directly for ethylene glycol and methanol levels)
- Urine for calcium oxalate crystals in ethylene glycol overdose

Noninv: Imaging studies should be based on underlying causes of acid-base disorders. Delirium associated with intoxications may prompt head CT in some cases to r/o other causes (stroke, intracranial mass, hemorrhage).

Rx: Rx of respiratory acid-base disorders is based on the underlying disease and ventilatory support, as needed; please refer to specific sections for details.

General measures for treatment of metabolic acidosis

- Determine cause by hx, lab eval; rx underlying disease as appropriate.
- See "Diabetic Ketoacidosis" in Section 2.3 for specific details on rx.
- See "Sepsis and Septic Shock" in Section 5.3 for specific details on rx of lactic acidosis; usually requires aggressive IV hydration, vasopressors for persistent hypotension, possibly mechanical ventilation.
- Watch for hypoglycemia and rx with IV dextrose if needed.
- Serum bicarbonate rx is controversial, although many advocate use in severe acidosis (pH less than 7.10–7.15) due to concern for cardiovascular compromise; see discussion of DKA in Section 2.3.

- If used, continuous infusion usually preferred over bolus therapy (unless in ACLS settings); initial dosing of 1–2 mmol of $NaHCO_3$/kg.
- Commonly, use 2 ampules (50-mL ampule contains 50 mmol of $NaHCO_3$) in 1 L of 0.45% NS or 3 ampules in D_5W to make an isotonic solution (addition to 0.9% NS will create a hypertonic, hypernatremic solution).
- Follow pH and serum HCO_3 closely, as difficult to assess response to therapy; consider stopping once pH is greater than 7.25–7.30.

Specific measures for treatment of ingestion-related metabolic acidosis

- Have a high index of suspicion for ingestions based on presence of anion gap metabolic acidosis, particularly if osmolar gap (although may not be present in all cases, especially if immediate presentation for care) (Ann EM 1996;27:343).
- Supportive care; may require aggressive hydration, pressors, mechanical ventilation for resp arrest or airway protection if obtunded.
- Start specific rx if delay in results of serum testing.
- Gastric lavage and activated charcoal are often used; charcoal is not effective for alcohol intoxications, but may help if co-ingestion of other meds; consider aspiration risks before giving.
- Follow guidelines for methanol and ethylene glycol ingestions (NEJM 2009;360:2216):
  - Guidelines re fomepizole (aka 4-methylpyrazole):
    - Competitive inhibitor of alcohol dehydrogenase; prevents the creation of toxic alcohol metabolites.
    - Consider rx in all cases of pts with significant ingestion, evidence of metabolic acidosis and/or osmolar gap, or methanol/ethylene glycol levels 20 mg/dL or more.

- Dose is 15 mg/kg initially, then 10 mg/kg q 12 hr; if used more than 48 hr, increase to 15 mg/kg/dose; requires dose adjustment if receiving dialysis.
  - Consider co-factor therapy with pyridoxine, folate (or leucovorin), MVI.
  - Continue therapy until plasma toxin levels are less than 20–30 mg/dL.
- Alcohol has been also been used, as it also inhibits alcohol dehydrogenase; but difficult to dose, and fomepizole therapy does not lead to further intoxication.
- Hemodialysis (HD) may be warranted if persistent acidosis, fluid overload, renal failure (with ethylene glycol), or visual disturbances (with methanol).
- Guidelines for salicylate ingestions (Crit Care Med 2003;31: 2794):
  - Consider additional rx if serum levels are more than 35–40 mg/dL, or associated sx.
  - Increase urinary alkalinization (to increase drug clearance) with sodium bicarbonate infusion; goal urine pH 7.45–7.50.
  - HD in severe cases.
  - Watch for concomitant bleeding and coagulopathy.
  - Consider possibility of APAP ingestion with combination meds.
- Metformin toxicity with lactic acidosis: stop metformin; supportive care; dextrose for hypoglycemia; IV hydration.

Treatment of metabolic alkalosis

- Determine cause by hx, lab eval; rx underlying disease as appropriate.
- Contraction alkalosis: hold diuretic therapy; volume repletion with isotonic saline (0.9% NS); look for concomitant hypokalemia and hypomagnesemia to replete as well.

- GI losses: antiemetics; hold NG suction; volume repletion with isotonic saline (0.9% NS); addition of H2B or PPI to reduce gastric pH may minimize HCl losses.
- Posthypercapneic: see discussion of COPD exacerbations in Section 7.2; reduce minute ventilation; may consider acetazolamide therapy in severe cases resistant to ventilator adjustments.

8.2   Sodium and Potassium Disorders

Hyponatremia

(NEJM 2000;342:1581)

Cause: Defined as serum Na less than 136 mmol/L.

Common causes of hyponatremia in hospitalized pts include:

- Hypotonic/dilutional hyponatremia (majority of cases); all have low serum osmolality, and are further characterized by extracellular fluid volume (ECF)
  - Hypovolemic hyponatremia (reduced ECF)
    - Renal fluid loss: diuretics, salt-wasting nephropathy
    - GI fluid losses: diarrhea, vomiting
    - Acute blood loss
    - Sweat losses, especially in marathon runners
    - 3rd spacing of fluids in acute illness
  - Euvolemic hyponatremia (normal ECF)
    - SIADH secretion (NEJM 2007;356:2064)
      - SIADH is most common cause of hyponatremia, especially in hospitalized pts.
      - Most cases are related to secretion of ADH independent of serum osmolality; some pts will have depressed levels of ADH but at a lower than normal level of osm ("reset osmotat") (Am J Med

RENAL/UROLOGY

2006;119:S36); even rarer is ADH-receptor defect in kidneys (NEJM 2005;352:1884).
- Condition is usually related to underlying cancer, pulmonary illness, CNS lesion or neurologic illness, or many drugs (especially SSRIs, TCAs, antipsychotics, antiepileptics, NSAIDs, opiates).
- Post-op hyponatremia, especially associated with hypotonic fluid administration
- Hypothyroidism
- Adrenal insufficiency
- Hypervolemic hyponatremia (increased ECF)
  - Cirrhosis
  - CHF
  - Nephrotic syndrome, CKD
- Hypertonic hyponatremia (rare): all have high serum osmolality
  - Due to accumulation of impermeable solutes, especially seen in severe hyperglycemia (correct Na with formula: $Na_{corr} = Na_{serum} + [1.7(Glucose - 100)/100]$), mannitol infusion, excessive sorbitol use
- Psychogenic polydipsia: psychiatric illness with excessive free water intake, overwhelming the kidney's ability to excrete (kidney can usually handle up to 15L/d in normal circumstances); may also be seen in severe alcoholics (aka "beer-drinker's potomania")
- Pseudo-hyponatremia: false reduction in Na due to hypertriglyceridemia or hyperproteinemia, due to lab measurement of excessive fluid volume; no longer seen with newer lab measurements of serum electrolytes
- Cerebral salt-wasting syndrome (CSWS): excessive BNP release due to intracranial insult (usually subarachnoid hemorrhage or neurosurgical procedure) that leads to renal sodium loss, usually associated with fluid depletion, hypovolemia (Neurosurg 2004;54:1369)

Epidem: Prevalence of hyponatremia in hospitalized pts may be as high as 30–40% (Am J Med 2006;119:S30), with values less than 125 mmol/L in 3–6%; two-thirds of pts with moderate to severe hyponatremia acquired it during the hospitalization (Ann IM 1985;102:164; Clin Nephrol 1984;22:72).

Higher risk in elderly pts (especially nursing home residents), and those with low body weight.

Incidence of hyponatremia in chronic diseases (with hypervolemic hyponatremia as above): CHF 20% (JAMA 2005;294:1625); cirrhosis 35% (Arch IM 2002;162:323).

Pathophys: Sodium and water balance is driven by neg feedback loop between the brain (hypothalamus) and kidneys; osmoreceptor cells in the hypothalamus sense increased serum osmolality and release ADH (vasopressin) from the posterior pituitary gland (as well as stimulate thirst); ADH stimulates aquaporins in kidney to retain free water; subsequent decrease in osmolality leads to suppression of ADH secretion (South Med J 2006;99:353).

Hyponatremia is mainly due to excessive free water, not a lack of sodium (except in CSWS).

Sx/Si: Sx related to severity of hyponatremia and acute vs chronic course (latter usually associated with less pronounced sx); women may have sx at higher sodium levels than men (Am J Med 2006;119:S59).

Mild hyponatremia (125–135 mmol/L) may be largely asx, but in elderly may contribute to imbalance, falls (Am J Med 2006;119:S79).

Moderate hyponatremia (115–125 mmol/L) may have sx of headache, N/V, lethargy, muscle cramps, delirium.

Severe hyponatremia (usually less than 110–115 mmol/L) may have seizures, coma, respiratory arrest.

Evaluate fluid volume; si/sx of dehydration (tachycardia, orthostasis, dry mucous membranes, diminished skin turgor, poor capillary refill) to suggest hypovolemia; edema, other sx to suggest hypervolemia from cirrhosis, CHF, CKD.

Crs: Associated with higher mortality than matched nonhyponatremic pts, but may simply be a marker of more severe illness.

Cmplc: Severe hyponatremia may cause cerebral edema, with seizures, brain-stem herniation.

Overly aggressive repletion of sodium, especially in chronic cases, can lead to osmotic demyelination (aka central pontine myelinolysis, but also affects the basal ganglia and cerebellum), marked by progressive (and possibly irreversible) neuro dysfunction, seizures, coma (Ann Neurol 1982;11:128); very rare in cases of acute or mild hyponatremia (more than 125 mmol/L); sx may be acute or delayed up to 6 d after correction of sodium (Am Fam Phys 2004;69:2387).

Lab: Initial dx may be incidental finding or may be based on neuro sx; once low sodium established, consider the following:

- Renal function (BUN, Cr) to r/o underlying acute renal failure or CKD
- U/A to r/o proteinuria from nephrotic syndrome
- Serum osmolality: will be low (less than 275) in most cases, except hypertonic hyponatremia due to hyperglycemia, other solutes
- Urine osmolality: use to distinguish hypovolemia (associated with concentrated urine, high S_{osm}, 200–600 mOsm/L) from euvolemia (lower S_{osm}, especially in SIADH, 100–300 mOsm/L) and polydipsia (should have very dilute urine, less than 100 mOsm/L)
- Urine sodium: spot urine electrolytes should be low in hypovolemia, high in SIADH (more than 40 mmol/L)
- Also, check TSH to r/o hypothyroidism and consider cortisol stimulation testing to r/o adrenal insufficiency (especially if concomitant hyperkalemia; see "Adrenal Insufficiency" in Section 2.1 for details)

Make the diagnosis of SIADH based on the following criteria (NEJM 2007;356:2064):

- Hyponatremia
- Clinically euvolemic: no signs of dehydration or fluid overload
- No recent diuretic use
- Lab eval: low serum osm (less than 275 mOsm/L), inappropriately high urine osm (more than 100 mOsm/L), high urine sodium (more than 40 mmol/L)
- Normal thyroid and adrenal function
- Does not require serum ADH level; no role in dx, as spot levels may be low, normal, or high

Noninv: No routine testing necessary, but in cases of SIADH without an apparent cause, could consider chest imaging to r/o infection, tumor; CT head to r/o intracranial mass/abnormality.

If acute neuro sx, consider brain imaging with CT or MRI to look for cerebral edema and r/o other causes.

Rx: Approach to the treatment of hyponatremia:

- Diagnose and assess severity of hyponatremia based on the following:
  - Serum Na level: most cases with Na greater than 130 mmol/L do not require rx, other than monitoring
  - Symptoms, as described above: presence of severe neuro sx requires emergent eval and rx
  - Assessment of fluid volume: hypervolemia vs euvolemia vs hypovolemia
- Assess renal function, serum and urine osmolality, urine sodium, as described above.
- If determined to be hypovolemic:
  - If hemodynamically unstable, rx initially with isotonic IV fluids (i.e., 0.9% NS), regardless of serum Na, until BP, HR, urine output improved.
  - In stable, asx pts with mild to moderate hyponatremia, if hypovolemia uncertain, consider infusion of 1–2 L isotonic

saline over 24 hr and reassess sx and serum Na; urine Na less than 30 mmol/L has a high PPV for pos response to saline infusion (Am J Med 1995;99:348); pos response confirms hypovolemic hyponatremia.

- Can use the correction formulas for severe hyponatremia detailed below if needed based on severe sx, but take care not to overshoot; once fluid volume restored, pt will likely have rapid free water diuresis and resolution of hyponatremia.

- If determined to be euvolemic:
  - Eval meds for common causes of SIADH; consider holding diuretics (unless clearly mild hyponatremia related to CHF, cirrhosis).
  - In most pts with minimal or no sx and moderate hyponatremia, the primary rx is fluid restriction (500–1000 mL qd) with adequate dietary intake of protein and salt.
  - In resistant cases, consider demeclocycline (a tetracycline derivative, which induces nephrogenic diabetes insipidus) 300–600 mg bid; but can have adverse renal effects.
  - Can also consider vasopressin-receptor antagonists (see hypervolemic guidelines below).
  - In cases associated with severe hyponatremia or severe sx, consider IV sodium repletion as described below; but IV 0.9% NS in the setting of mild to moderate SIADH has no role and may actually worsen sodium levels.

- If determined to be hypervolemic:
  - Main therapy is treating the underlying cause, as appropriate; mild, asx hyponatremia in these cases does not likely require specific therapy.
  - Consider adjustments to chronic diuretic therapy.
  - Consider addition of vasopressin-receptor antagonists (Geriatrics 2007;62:20), as follows:
    - Only currently available option in the United States is conivaptan (Vaprisol); IV and PO forms have been

proven to increase serum sodium in pts with euvolemic and hypervolemic hyponatremia (with Na 115–130 mmol/L), but no studies have tested significant clinical outcomes (J Clin Endocrinol Metab 2006;91:2145).

- Oral tolvaptan studied in the SALT trials (NEJM 2006;355:2099), starting dose of 15 mg qd (increased as needed up to 60 mg) proven to improve serum sodium and increase urine output, but no other clinical outcomes tested.

- These meds may have much more promise once further studies have shown improvement in true clinical outcomes (mortality, hospitalizations, sx) rather than just improved lab values; until then, would reserve use to pts with recurrent or recalcitrant episodes; avoid use in severe hyponatremia (use hypertonic saline as described next).

- In pts with severe hyponatremia associated with neurologic sx, treat with hypertonic saline as follows:
  - Set goal for sodium correction rate (in mmol/hr); typically in cases of chronic (or unknown duration) hyponatremia, try to increase serum sodium no more than 0.3–0.5 mmol/L/hr (or about 8–12 mmol/L/d); in cases of acute hyponatremia or associated with severe neuro sx, can increase faster (1–2 mmol/L/hr, at least until sx resolve); faster rates of repletion increase the risk of CPM.
  - Use the equation proposed by Adrogue and Madias (NEJM 2000;342:1581) to calculate the change in serum sodium with 1 L of infusate:
    - Change in $Na_{serum} = ([Na_{infusate} - Na_{serum}] / [TBW + 1])$
    - TBW is total body water, calculated as weight (in kg) $\times$ 0.6 (in men); for women and elderly men, use 0.5; for elderly women, use 0.45
    - Na concentrations of commonly used hypertonic solutions: 3% NaCl 513 mmol/L; 0.9% NS 154; 0.45% NS

77; LR 130; 3% NaCl is the most commonly used in this situation
- Divide the Na correction goal (in mmol/hr) by the change in Na_{serum} per 1 L (1000 mL) of infusate to determine the total amount of fluid (in mL/hr) to give to correct the sodium.
- For example, a 50 kg 80-yo woman presents delirium and lethargy with a serum sodium of 105 mmol/L:
  - Set a goal correction rate of 0.5 mmol/hr
  - Calculate that 1 L of 3% NaCl would be expected to raise her Na_{serum} by 17 mmol ([513 − 105] / [(50 × 0.45) + 1])
  - Divide correction rate by the expected change with 1000 mL of fluid; (0.5 mmol/hr) / (17 mmol/1000 mL) = 29 mL/hr of 3% NaCl
- If potassium is added to the fluid, must add potassium concentration to the $Na_{infusate}$; e.g., 0.9% NS with 40 mEq KCl has cation concentration of 194 mmol/L (154 + 40).
- Requires frequent assessment of serum electrolytes q 4–6 hr, with readjustment of goal and rates (and possibly change in infusate) based on response.
- If pt has evidence of fluid overload, can give IV furosemide, but this will also affect the rate of sodium correction.
- Patient should be kept NPO and any other IVF fluids given (e.g., IVP with meds, abx) must be accounted for.
- Should continue hypertonic saline infusion until sx improved and serum Na usually more than 125 mmol/L.
- Watch closely for si of neuro deterioration to suggest CPM; if so, check serum Na immediately and infuse hypotonic saline to temper rate of rise (Am J Med Sci 1989;298:41).
- Other considerations:
  - Seizures may be treated with anticonvulsant therapy, including benzodiazepines (see "Epilepsy and Seizure Disorders" in Section 6.2 for details).

- Prevent iatrogenic hyponatremia by avoidance of hypotonic IV solutions (e.g., D_5W) as routine IV therapy, especially in the post-op period.

Hypernatremia

(NEJM 2000;342:1493)

Cause: Defined as serum sodium more than 145 mmol/L.

Common causes of hypernatremia in hospitalized pts include:

- Severe dehydration with loss of free water or hypotonic fluid
  - GI loss from vomiting, diarrhea, NG tube suction
  - Renal losses from diuretics, severe hyperglycemia (with osmotic diuresis), underlying acute or chronic renal disease
  - Insensible losses (sweating, tachypnea) in a pt with reduced thirst (hypodipsia) or no access to water (fall, bed-bound, intubated)
- Diabetes insipidus (DI): marked by polyuria and polydipsia, due to lack of ADH or resistance to ADH; many pts can avoid hypernatremia by increasing fluid intake, so usually requires reduced access to free water (post-op, critically ill, fall, bed-bound, etc.) to lead to hypernatremia
  - Central DI: Loss of ADH secretion, usually related to damage/trauma to the hypothalamus or pituitary gland; may be associated with surgery, stroke, infection, tumor, perinatal (Sheehan's syndrome).
  - Nephrogenic DI (Ann IM 2006;144:186): Reduced or complete resistance to ADH in the kidneys; may be related to underlying kidney disease, response to severe hypercalcemia or hypokalemia, drug-induced (lithium most commonly; demeclocycline in the rx of SIADH), or congenital.
- Iatrogenic hypernatremia: by infusion of hypertonic solutions (3% NaCl, $NaHCO_3$, enteral or parenteral feeding); seawater ingestion
- Adrenal excess: Cushing's syndrome, hyperaldosteronism

Epidem: May be present in up to 30% of hospitalized pts from nursing homes (J Am Ger Soc 1988;36:213); in one study of 103 inpatients, more than 80% developed hypernatremia after admission, usually related to ongoing fluid losses with inadequate fluid replacement (Ann IM 1996;124:197).

Pathophys: Sodium and water balance is driven by neg feedback loop between the brain (hypothalamus) and kidneys; osmoreceptor cells in the hypothalamus sense increased serum osmolality and release ADH (vasopressin) from the posterior pituitary gland (as well as stimulate thirst); ADH stimulates aquaporins in kidney to retain free water; subsequent decrease in osmolality leads to suppression of ADH secretion (South Med J 2006;99:353).

Hypernatremia is mainly a deficit of free water, not an abundance of sodium (except in cases of significant iatrogenic hypernatremia).

Sx/Si: Sx related to severity of hypernatremia and acute vs chronic course (latter usually associated with less pronounced sx).

Initial sx include increased thirst, then lethargy, weakness, hyperreflexia; if Na is more than 160 mmol/L, can have delirium, coma.

Evaluate fluid volume; si/sx of dehydration (tachycardia, orthostasis, dry mucous membranes, diminished skin turgor, poor capillary refill) to suggest hypovolemia.

Look for si/sx of DI; presence of significant polyuria despite hypernatremia suggests DI (in normal cases of dehydration, would expect oliguria).

Crs: In one study of 103 pts, mortality with hypernatremia was 40%, but electrolyte disturbance primarily contributed in about 15% (Ann IM 1996;124:197).

Cmplc: Severe hypernatremia can lead to shrinkage of the brain, causing vascular rupture with ICH, SAH.

Similar to hyponatremia, overly rapid correction of severe hypernatremia can lead to brain damage; in this case, related to cerebral edema from rapid fluid shifts into the cerebral tissue (Lancet 1967;2:1385).

Lab: Once high sodium level is established, usually does not require significant further w/u; cause usually obvious based on hx and clinical sx.

If tested, pts with purely dehydration from GI or insensible losses will have high urine osm (more than 700), low urine Na (less than 20 mmol/L); pts with renal free water loss will have high urine osm, high urine Na (more than 20 mmol/L), and usually other signs or labs consistent with renal disease (elevated BUN/Cr, proteinuria, hematuria); pts with DI will have low urine osm (less than 150; i.e., dilute urine even in the setting of severe dehydration) (Am Fam Phys 2000;61:3623).

In cases of DI, can use response to desmopressin to differentiate central from nephrogenic cause; administration of ADH analog will improve central DI.

Noninv: No routine testing necessary, but if acute neuro sx, consider brain imaging with CT or MRI to look for intracranial bleeding, cerebral edema, and r/o other causes.

Rx: Approach to the treatment of hypernatremia:

- Diagnose and assess severity of hypernatremia based on the following:
  - Serum Na level: most cases with Na less than 150 mmol/L do not require specific rx, other than rx of underlying cause
  - Symptoms, as described above: presence of severe neuro sx requires emergent eval and rx
  - Assessment of fluid volume and urine output; hemodynamic instability (i.e., severe hypotension) requires administration of isotonic saline (0.9% NS) for resuscitation, regardless of initial sodium levels
- Treat underlying disease/cause:
  - Reduce GI fluid losses with antiemetics, antidiarrheals; stop NG suction.

- Control fevers (sweat loss) with antipyretics.
- Treat underlying hypercalcemia or hypokalemia; see "Hypercalcemia" in Section 2.4 and "Hypokalemia" later in Section 8.2 for details.
- Remove iatrogenic causes; i.e., change IVF or feeding administration.
- In cases of severe hypernatremia associated with sx:
  - If pt can take oral replacement of free water, this may be adequate rx; however, most hospitalized pts in this setting require IV replacement.
  - Set goal for sodium correction rate (in mmol/hr); typically in cases of chronic (or unknown duration) hypernatremia, try to decrease serum sodium no more than 0.5 mmol/L/hr (or 8–12 mmol/L/d); in cases of acute hypernatremia or associated with severe neuro sx, can drop faster (1–2 mmol/L/hr); faster rates of repletion increase the risk of cerebral edema (Intensive Care Med 1979;5:27).
  - Use the equation proposed by Adrogue and Madias (NEJM 2000;342:1493) to calculate the change in serum sodium with 1 L of infusate:
    - Change in $Na_{serum} = ([Na_{infusate} - Na_{serum}] / [TBW + 1])$
    - TBW is total body water, calculated as weight (in kg) $\times$ 0.6 (in men); for women and elderly men, use 0.5; for elderly women, use 0.45.
    - Na concentrations of commonly used hypotonic solutions: D_5W 0 mmol/L; 0.2% NS (aka, ¼ NS) 34; 0.45% NS 77; D_5W or ¼ NS most commonly used, no difference in safety or efficacy (¼ NS will require more fluid infused or more time to correct).
  - Divide the Na correction goal (in mmol/hr) by the change in Na_{serum} per 1 L (1000 mL) of infusate to determine the total amount of fluid (in mL/hr) to give to correct the sodium.

- For example, a 50 kg 80-yo woman presents after a stroke at home with lethargy and a serum sodium of 165 mmol/L:
  - Set a goal correction rate of 0.5 mmol/hr
  - Calculate that 1 L of D_5W would be expected to decrease her Na_{serum} by 7 mmol ($[0 - 165] / ([50 \times 0.45] + 1)$)
  - Divide correction rate by the expected change with 1000 mL of fluid; (0.5 mmol/hr) / (7 mmol/1000 mL) = 71 mL/hr of D_5W; correction of serum sodium to less than 145 mmol/hr would be expected to require 3 L of D_5W given over 42 hr
  - A common mistake in this situation is to use ½ NS instead of D_5W; using the same calculations, ½ NS would require 135 mL/hr, and approximately 6 L of fluid over the same time frame
- If potassium is added to the fluid, must add potassium concentration to the $Na_{infusate}$ (e.g., ¼ NS with 40 mEq KCl has cation concentration of 74 mmol/L (34 + 40).
- Requires frequent assessment of serum electrolytes q 4–6 hr, with readjustment of goal and rates (and possibly change in infusate) based on response.
- If pt has evidence of fluid overload, can give IV furosemide, but this will also affect the rate of sodium correction.
- Watch for hyperglycemia with administration of IV dextrose.
- Treatment of DI (Arch IM 1997;157:1293):
  - Central DI requires replacement of ADH, usually with intranasal desmopressin (Ann IM 1985;103:228).
  - Nephrogenic DI should be treated by correction of cause (replete hypokalemia, rx severe hypercalcemia, remove offending drugs); long-term rx with adequate oral fluid intake, thiazide diuretics and low-salt diet; amiloride specifically for lithium-induced DI (NEJM 1985;312:408).

Hypokalemia

(NEJM 1998;339:451; J Am Soc Nephrol 1997;8:1179)

Cause: Defined as serum K less than 3.6 mmol/L.

Common causes of hypokalemia in hospitalized pts include:

- Drug-induced (by far, the most common etiology)
  - Intracellular K shift (does not reduce whole-body K, usually transient)
    - Insulin: clinically evident only with overdose; chronic therapeutic use does not generally cause hypokalemia; do not use IV bolus of insulin in pts with DKA until confirmed lack of hypokalemia; see "Diabetic Ketoacidosis" in Section 2.3 for details
    - Beta-agonists: vasopressors, decongestants, bronchodilators, tocolytics
    - Theophylline
    - Caffeine
  - Renal loss (does reduce whole-body K):
    - Diuretics (cause reduced K in up to 50% of pts) (J Clin Hypertens 1986;2:331): thiazide and loop diuretics
    - Steroids: fludrocortisone, high-dose glucocorticoids
  - Intestinal loss: potassium-bonding resins (Kayexalate); laxatives
- GI losses from diarrhea; also upper GI losses causing metabolic alkalosis with subsequent renal K loss
- Hypomagnesemia: commonly seen in alcoholics (although hyperadrenergic state from delirium tremens may also contribute) (NEJM 1998;339:451); will not be able to fully replete K until Mg repleted (Arch IM 1992;152:40); see "Hypomagnesemia" in Section 2.4 for details
- Malnutrition: rare cause, usually associated with severely reduced intake, as K found in large amounts in Western diets
- Hyperaldosteronism (primary, or secondary due to CHF, liver failure, nephrotic syndrome), Cushing's syndrome

- Hypokalemic periodic paralysis: severe hypoK associated with weakness and paralysis; autosomal dominant genetic disorder (Postgrad Med J 1999;75:193); associated with hyperthyroidism in pts of Asian descent (Mayo Clin Proc 2005;80:99)
- Other genetic disorders: Liddle's, Bartter's, Gitelman's syndromes

Epidem: Hypokalemia is present in up to 20% of hospitalized pts (Postgrad Med J 1986;62:187).

Pathophys: Normal serum K (3.5–5.0 mmol/L); serum levels account for only 2% of total body K (98% intracellular).

Serum and total body K controlled by numerous hormonal stimuli (NEJM 1998;339:451) as follows:

- Insulin: drives K into cells by stimulating Na/K-ATPase; neg feedback loop where hypokalemia inhibits insulin secretion from pancreatic islet cells
- Catecholamines (epinephrine, norepinephrine): drives K into cells by stimulating Na/K-ATPase; beta-agonists cause hypokalemia and beta-blockers cause hyperkalemia
- Thyroid hormone (T3, T4): stimulates synthesis of Na/K-ATPase
- Aldosterone: stimulates kidneys to preserve Na and dump K; neg feedback loop with hypokalemia inhibiting aldosterone release
- Serum pH: alkalinization drives K into cells, but effect is variable

Sx/Si: Most are asx, especially with mild to moderate deficiency (3.0–3.5 mmol/L).

Initial sx/si include lethargy, weakness, constipation, hyporeflexia.

Severe hypokalemia (less than 2.5 mmol/L) can lead to rhabdomyolysis, ascending paralysis.

Cmplc: Cardiac arrhythmias, including ventricular tachycardia and fibrillation, can occur; highest risk in elderly, pts with CAD, CHF,

LVH, on digoxin rx; increased risk of sudden cardiac death (Circ 1998;98:1510; J Hypertens 1995;13:1539).

Other cmplc include hypertension (JAMA 1997;277:1624); paralytic ileus, particularly if associated with hypomagnesemia; rhabdomyolysis with myoglobinuria and renal failure; nephrogenic diabetes insipidus (see "Hypernatremia" earlier in Section 8.2 for details).

Lab: After confirming low potassium, most causes can be determined based on hx, sx, review of meds; consider Mg level, TSH, screening for hyperaldosteronism and Cushing's.

Noninv: EKG changes include flattened T waves, ST depression, U waves.

Rx: Guidelines for treatment of hypokalemia (Arch IM 2000;160: 2429):

- For most pts, oral K supplementation is preferred and well tolerated.
- Goal K level is greater than 3.5 mmol/L; consider goal of 4 mmol/L in pts with heart disease or on digoxin due to concerns for arrhythmias.
- Difficult to assess response to oral supplements; usually start with KCl 20–40 mEq PO bid–tid, then assess response with daily labs; potassium phosphate can be used if concomitant hypophosphatemia.
- Make sure to replete Mg if low; usually magnesium oxide 400–800 mg PO qd–bid; if NPO, can use magnesium sulfate 1–4 gm IV.
- For IV potassium replacement, follow these guidelines:
  - In cases of life-threatening hypokalemia associated with arrhythmias, can use 5–10 mmol of KCl IV given over 15 min, with continuous EKG monitoring.
  - In all other circumstances, usually given at 10 mmol/hr (can go up to 20 mmol/hr, but often causes discomfort if given through peripheral IV); given at this rate, would

expect to increase serum K by 0.1 mmol/hr, but effect can be variable (Arch IM 1990;150:613).

- If adding KCl to other IVF, consider change to ½ NS to avoid hypertonic solution; ½ NS with 40 mEq KCl/L is cation equivalent of ¼ NS.
- Watch serum K closely, especially if underlying renal disease, on K-sparing diuretics, or receiving K in multiple forms (IV, PO, dietary).
- Assess meds and consider discontinuation or adjustment as necessary.
  - If continuing diuretic rx, will need ongoing replacement; also can consider addition of K-sparing diuretic (triamterene, spironolactone), but may contribute to hypovolemia or cause hyperkalemia, especially in pts with renal failure (see the discussion of CHF in Section 1.2 for details).
  - Counsel on reducing Na intake; high-salt diet can worsen diuretic-induced hypokalemia.
- Counsel on increased dietary K intake (bananas, oranges, meat, green vegetables, nuts).

Hyperkalemia

(Am Fam Phys 2006;73:283; Mayo Clin Proc 2007;82:1553)

Cause: Defined as serum K more than 5.0 mmol/L.

Common causes of hyperkalemia in hospitalized pts include:

- Acute or chronic renal failure: most hospitalized pts with severe hyperkalemia due to acute renal failure in the setting of ACEI/ARB/spironolactone use
- Drug-induced: ACE inhibitors and ARBs most commonly (about 1–2% in all pts, higher risk in pts with DM, CKD) (Am J Cardiol 1995;75:793); also, spironolactone, NSAIDs, beta-blockers, digoxin toxicity, succinylcholine (avoid use in rapid sequence intubation in pts with known or suspected hyperkalemia, or pts with chronic neurologic disease where massive neuromuscular depolarization might induce

severe hyperkalemia; use non-depolarizing paralytic agent
instead)
- Muscle damage due to rhabdomyolysis, burns, significant trauma
- Tumor lysis syndrome; acute or chronic hemolysis
- Excessive K intake, although unlikely to cause clinically significant hyperkalemia unless another factor present as well
- Adrenal insufficiency: Addison's disease, hypoaldosteronism
- Renal tubular acidosis
- Severe metabolic acidosis: causing K to translocate from intracellular space; seen in severe DKA, causing an initial hyperkalemia despite usual whole-body K depletion
- "Pseudo-hyperkalemia" from red cell lysis due to trauma with phlebotomy

Epidem: Present in up to 10% of hospitalized pts (Arch IM 1998;158: 917).

Pathophys: See "Hypokalemia" earlier in Section 8.2 for hormonal control of serum K levels.

Sx/Si: Most cases of mild hyperkalemia (less than 6 mmol/L) are asx.
As serum K rises, can develop weakness, hyperreflexia, parasthesias, paralysis.

Cmplc: Ventricular arrhythmias, as described under Rx below.

Lab: If clinical picture does not suggest hyperkalemia (normal EKG, prior normal K, no clear underlying cause), consider redrawing labs to r/o RBC lysis.
Once hyperkalemia is established, eval other electrolytes, renal function; consider CPK, LDH; aldosterone levels or screen for adrenal insufficiency if no other precipitating cause (especially if concomitant hyponatremia).

Noninv: EKG findings include peaked T waves, prolonged PR, widened QRS, loss of P waves, BBBs; severe hyperkalemia leads to "sine wave" configuration, VF (Crit Care Med 2008;36:3246);

EKG changes do correlate with severity of hyperkalemia (EKG changes only in ~40% of pts with K 6.0–6.8, ~50% of pts with K more than 6.8) (Arch IM 1998;158:917); normal EKG can be seen even with critically high serum K levels (more than 8–9 mmol/L) (Am J Kidney Dis 1986;7:461; J Electrocardiol 1999;32:45).

Rx: Approach to treatment of hyperkalemia (Crit Care Med 2008;36:3246) includes the following guidelines:

- Decision on whether to treat based on serum K and EKG changes; most pts with K less than 6.0 do not require aggressive rx other than monitoring and rx of underlying cause; if any EKG changes, or K greater than 6.0–6.5, should rx.
- Stabilize cell membrane to prevent arrhythmias.
  - Should be given to any pts with significant EKG changes (some exclude sole EKG finding of peaked T's as significant enough to warrant use); has no effect on serum or whole-body K; acts to protect the myocardium until other measures can reduce K.
  - 10% calcium gluconate, 10 mL (1000 mg) IV given over 10 min; if no change in EKG, can give additional dose (Crit Care Med 1994;22:697).
  - Calcium chloride can be used as well, but infusion painful through peripheral vein (should be given in central line).
  - Effect lasts 30–60 min, enough time to start other rx.
  - Minimal contraindications, but caution in pts with possible digoxin toxicity, which may be potentiated by Ca; if concern, give slower Ca infusion (20–30 min) or use Mg instead (Emerg Med J 2002;19:183).
- Drive serum K intracellularly.
  - Insulin:
    - Dose: 10 U of regular insulin IV.
    - Typically will reduce serum K by 0.5–1 mmol/L within 20 min, with duration of 4–6 hr.

- Main side effect is hypoglycemia; should give with 0.5–1 amp (25–50 gm) of D50 (50% dextrose) to prevent hypoglycemia, unless pt already hyperglycemic (BS more than 200); monitor BS closely over next 60–90 min and consider continuous dextrose infusion if needed.
- Can use repeat doses as necessary.
- Beta-agonist (Ann IM 1989;110:426):
  - Albuterol nebulizer 10–20 mg over 10 min; note higher dose than given for respiratory indications; IV rx also effective but not available in the United States.
  - Typically will reduce serum K by 0.6–1 mmol/L within 30 min, with duration of 1–2 hr.
  - Main side effect is tachycardia.
  - Effect may be blunted in pts on beta-blockers, and up to 40% of all other pts for unclear reasons; because of this, beta-agonist should not be used as monotherapy (Kidney Int 1993;43:212).
  - Sodium bicarbonate:
    - Not considered 1st-line therapy, as minimal K reduction seen with acute rx; can have small effect on reducing serum K with prolonged infusion (Am J Kidney Dis 1996;28:508).
    - Can be used for rx of hyperkalemia in pts with severe metabolic acidosis (e.g., DKA), although hyperkalemia in these pts usually resolves with IV fluid and insulin rx alone (Nephron 1996;72:476).
- Reduce whole-body K levels.
  - Loop diuretics:
    - Furosemide 20–80 mg IV; may need higher dose in pts with chronic use.
    - Can add a thiazide diuretic (e.g. HCTZ, metolazone) PO, but probably better for chronic reduction than acute.

- Watch for si/sx of hypovolemia; may require NS infusion in addition to diuretic rx.
- Reduction in serum K variable, but does have quick onset of action and lasts for 2–6 hr.
- Sodium polystyrene sulfonate (Kayexalate):
  - This drug is a cation-exchange resin that exchanges sodium for potassium in the colon.
  - Dose: 15–30 gm given in 15–30 mL of 70% sorbitol orally; in obtunded pt, can be given via NGT or enemas; sorbitol added to offset the constipation effect (and possibly some hypokalemic effect from loose stools).
  - Slow onset of action (2–4 hr), so need to stabilize K levels with other rx.
  - Can be used chronically to control hyperkalemia in pts with CKD.
  - Small risk (up to 2%) for colonic necrosis, especially among post-op pts (Am J Kidney Dis 1992;20:159; J Trauma 2001;51:395).
- Hemodialysis (HD):
  - Most effective method for reducing whole-body K, but usually reserved for severe cases, unresponsive to other rx, or in pts with hyperkalemia in setting of ESRD.
- Assess and rx underlying causes.
  - For CKD, consider indications for chronic HD; can also use chronic diuretic or Kayexalate rx in selected pts not on HD.
  - Rx adrenal insufficiency, hypoaldosteronism, with mineralocorticoid replacement (i.e., fludrocortisone).
  - For mild hyperkalemia (5.5 mmol/L or less) associated with ACEI/ARBs (NEJM 2004;351:585), follow these guidelines:
    - Many low-risk pts do not require rx, but should have ongoing K monitoring.

- Advise benefits of a low-potassium diet.
- Consider addition of thiazide or loop diuretic for chronic kaliuretic effect.
- Avoid concomitant use of spironolactone.

8.3   Acute Renal Failure

(JAMA 2003;289:747; Lancet 2005;365:417)

Cause: Definitions:

- Acute renal failure (ARF); aka acute kidney injury (AKI):
  - For a description of AKI and RIFLE criteria, see Crit Care Med 2008;36:S141.
  - Acute onset (less than 2 wk) of decline in renal function (GFR), which may be complicated by electrolyte abnormalities, fluid overload.
  - Characterized by increase in baseline serum Cr of 0.5 mg/dL or more for 2 wk or less; if baseline serum Cr is more than 2.5 mg/dL, may also use rise of more than 20% from baseline; usually called severe if Cr is more than 3.0 mg/dL.
  - May be categorized by measurement of urine output, as follows:
    - Nonoliguric: preserved urine output of more than 400 mL/d; most commonly seen in drug or contrast-induced ARF; common in CKD
    - Oliguric: urine output less than 400 mL/d; most cases of ARF
    - Anuric: urine output less than 100 mL/d; severe ARF and postrenal/obstructive causes
- Chronic kidney disease (CKD): Not specifically addressed here, but many of the topics are germane to the treatment of inpatients with CKD.
  - Staging of CKD (Ann IM 2003;139:137):
    - Stage I: normal GFR (more than 90) with proteinuria
    - Stage II: GFR 60–89 with proteinuria

- Stage III: GFR 30–59
- Stage IV: GFR 15–30
- Stage V: GFR less than 15, or on dialysis
- May be difficult to assess elevated BUN/Cr in pt with no prior labs available; findings that suggest CKD rather than ARF include long h/o constitutional sx (fatigue, weakness), anemia of chronic disease, hyperphosphatemia, hypocalcemia, abnormal kidneys seen on US (BMJ 2006;333:786).
- Uremia (NEJM 2007;357:1316): Specific illnesses related to acute or chronic kidney disease, due to accumulation of fluid or renally metabolized solutes.
- Azotemia: Elevated BUN and Cr from any cause; not a specific term and should be avoided.

  Causes of acute renal failure include the following:

- Prerenal: conditions that cause a decrease in renal perfusion (~40–50% of ARF cases)
  - Hypovolemia/hypotension: usually associated with MAP less than 70, but may be higher in elderly and those with chronic hypertension
    - Sepsis (NEJM 2004;351:159): spectrum of disease with ATN, as described below along with other intrarenal (or intrinsic) causes
    - Cardiac: cardiogenic shock, symptomatic hypotension due to a variety of causes (e.g., ACS/MI, valvular disease, severe CHF, pericardial effusion with tamponade)
    - Hemorrhage/blood loss
    - Dehydration due to GI losses, insensible losses (including sweating, tachypnea), renal losses with excessive diuretics, osmotic loss due to hyperglycemia
    - 3rd spacing of extracellular fluid in acute or chronic diseases (cirrhosis, nephrotic syndrome, CHF, postsurgical)
  - HRS: see "Hepatorenal Syndrome" in Section 3.7 for details

- Drug-induced: ACEIs (reduce glomerular blood flow by dilation of efferent arterioles); NSAIDs (reduce GFR by blocking prostaglandins)
- Vascular obstruction: renal artery stenosis, embolic disease from cardiac or other sources, aortic or renal artery dissection
- Intrarenal (or intrinsic): destruction of renal tissue, including glomeruli, renal tubules, interstitium, and renal vasculature (~40–50% of ARF cases)
  - Acute tubular necrosis (ATN) (Ann IM 2002;137:744): destruction of the renal tubules
    - Ischemia: spectrum of disease with prerenal hypotension; ATN represents actual destruction of tissue rather than effects of hypoperfusion; prerenal hypovolemia and ATN cause approximately 75% of ARF seen in hospitalized pts
    - Drug-induced (Crit Care Med 2008;36:S216): IV contrast dye; aminoglycosides (up to 20%), amphotericin B (up to 80%), vancomycin (up to 30%), methanol
    - Pigment nephropathy
      - Myoglobinuria due to rhabdomyolysis (NEJM 2009; 361:62): destruction of skeletal muscle, leading to massive elevations in CPK and serum myoglobin; causes include trauma, strenuous exertion, infections, malignant hyperthermia, neuroleptic malignant syndrome, drugs (including alcohol, cocaine, statins), severe hypokalemia; myoglobin excess causes ATN in 15–50% (Arch IM 1988;148:1553)
      - Hemoglobinuria: related to underlying hemolysis
    - Tubular obstruction from urate and calcium oxalate crystals, immunoglobulins (in myeloma), antiretroviral drugs
  - Acute interstitial nephritis (AIN) (Am Fam Phys 2003; 67:2527): inflammatory disease of renal tissue
    - Drug-induced: antibiotics (most classes, including penicillins, cephalosporins, fluoroquinolones, macrolides,

sulfonamides, tetracyclines), NSAIDs, loop and
thiazide diuretics, antihypertensives, anticonvulsants,
chemotherapeutics
- Infections: viral, bacterial, rickettsial, tuberculosis
- Immune-related: SLE, vasculitis, lymphoma, sarcoid
- Small vessel disease: due to malignant hypertension, atherosclerotic disease, thrombotic thrombocytopenic purpura (TTP), hemolytic uremic syndrome (HUS), DIC, HELLP syndrome (seen in pregnancy)
- Glomerulonephritis: various forms
- Vasculitis: see "Interstitial Lung Diseases" in Section 7.3 for discussion of pulmonary-renal syndromes
- Postrenal: obstruction of urinary flow from the kidneys or lower urinary tract (~5–10% of ARF cases)
  - Requires urethral/bladder obstruction, or bilateral ureteral obstruction, unless pt has solitary (or nonfunctional) kidney
  - Ureteral obstruction: kidney stones, tumor, in situ thrombosis (postprocedural or trauma); extrinsic compression from lymphadenopathy, large AAA
  - Bladder obstruction: prostatic hypertrophy (or cancer), neurogenic bladder, bladder cancer
  - Urethral obstruction: stricture, blocked Foley catheter; extrinsic compression from pelvic tumor

Epidem: Primary dx in approximately 1% of all hospital admissions, but cmplc in many more; up to 20% in ICU pts (Crit Care Med 1996;24:192), requiring hemodialysis in 5% (Crit Care Med 2002;30:2051).

ARF in sepsis: Approximately 20% in moderate to severe sepsis; about 50% in septic shock (NEJM 2004;351:159).

In hospitalized pts, most cases of ARF due to sepsis (40–50%), postsurgical ATN (20%), contrast nephropathy (10%) (Lancet 2005;365:417).

Pathophys: Based on underlying causes (for a comprehensive review, see J Clin Invest 2004;114:5).

Sx/Si: Mild cases may be asx; increased severity associated with lethargy, weakness, delirium, N/V.

In most hospitalized pts, sx will be related to underlying cause/disease or cmplc, as follows:

- Hypovolemia: orthostasis, tachycardia, dry mucous membranes; signs of 3rd spacing, hemorrhage
- Sepsis/SIRS: fever, tachycardia, delirium; sx related to specific infections
- Rhabdomyolysis: myalgias, edema, dark urine
- Glomerulonephritis: hematuria
- Vasculitis: palpable purpura, other skin lesions
- Interstitial nephritis: classic triad of fever, rash, joint pain (triad seen in only ~5%, but fever in more than 70% and rash in more than 30%) (Am Fam Phys 2003; 67:2527)
- Lower urinary obstruction: pelvic/abdominal pain, mass (tumor or bladder), prostatic hypertrophy on rectal exam

Specific sx/si of uremia can include delirium, peripheral neuropathy, anorexia, muscle cramping, pericarditis, pleurisy (NEJM 2007;357:1316).

Crs: Despite improved recognition and therapies for ARF, overall mortality has remained unchanged (~50%, composite of multiple studies of in-hospital and up to 60-day mortality), likely because of aging population and increased use of nephrotoxic drugs (Am J Med 2005;118:827).

Related to underlying cause; mortality in pts with ARF usually due to infection (75%) or cardiopulmonary disease (Am Fam Phys 2000;61:2077); mortality in isolated cases of ARF (without other concomitant disease) is approximately 15% (QJM 1990;74:83).

Cmplc: 5–16% of cases of ARF lead to CKD, especially in elderly (QJM 1996;89:415).

For a discussion of long-term outcomes and QOL issues, see Crit Care Med 2008;36:S193.

Lab: Initial dx of ARF is usually made based on elevated BUN and Cr in the w/u of sx or for other dx.

In cases of mild ARF, with obvious cause (e.g., dehydration), usually does not require further eval unless resistant to standard supportive therapy.

In moderate to severe cases or associated with sx that suggest intrinsic renal disease, initial w/u should include the following:

- Serum BUN and Cr: by definition, always elevated in acute renal failure (for a discussion of markers of kidney function, see Crit Care Med 2008;36:S152)
  - BUN/Cr ratio of more than 15:1 suggests prerenal cause (hypoperfusion leads to increased renal tubular absorption of urea), but not very specific or sensitive.
  - Low BUN seen with poor nutritional states and cirrhosis; high BUN also seen with sepsis, GI bleeding.
  - Sulfa drugs, some cephalosporins, and cimetidine may cause an elevation in serum Cr due to inhibition of renal tubular Cr secretion without causing kidney damage; may be difficult to initially distinguish from AIN, but should rapidly improve with drug discontinuation.
  - Serum Cr is used as a marker for GFR, but is only one factor in renal filtration (also includes age, ideal body weight [IBW]); because of variability in serum Cr, several formulas have been developed to estimate GFR (or CrCl):
    - Cockcroft-Gault equation (Nephron 1976;16:31):
      - $CrCl = ([140 - age(yr)] \times IBW[kg]) / (Cr_{serum} \times 72)$; in females, multiply result by 0.85
      - Preferred method for estimating CrCl by the FDA in controlled trials
      - Multiple online calculators available (e.g., www.mcw.edu/calculators/creatinine.htm)

- MDRD equation (NEJM 2006;354:2473):
  - GFR = 186 × Cr_{serum} × age(yr); in females, multiply result by 0.742; in African Americans, multiply by 1.210
- Please note that these measures are based on pts with stable renal function; use in pts with ARF is imperfect at best.
- Urinalysis: if possible, on first urine sample obtained, prior to any other therapies, including fluid administration, diuretics, etc.
  - Urine dipstick for the following:
    - Specific gravity: In most cases, urine will be concentrated, more than 1.025; dilute urine in setting of ARF suggests intrinsic renal disease with lack of concentrating ability, diabetes insipidus (see "Hypernatremia" in Section 8.2).
    - Blood: Pos test with Hgb (due to hematuria or hemoglobinuria) or myoglobin (in rhabdomyolysis, with absence of RBCs on microscopy).
    - Protein: Proteinuria seen in intrinsic kidney disease, especially diabetic nephropathy.
      - Nephrotic syndrome (Am Fam Phys 2009;80:1129): A group of renal diseases marked by massive proteinuria (more than 3 gm/d), edema, hypoalbuminemia, hyperlipidemia; common types include focal segmental glomerulosclerosis, membranous nephropathy, minimal change disease; underlying causes can include DM, hepatitis and HIV, connective tissue diseases, NSAID-induced; ARF is rarely seen (usually diagnosed based on sx and confirmed with proteinuria).
    - Bilirubin: Bilirubinuria seen in jaundice from liver disease, hemolysis; may be mildly positive in dehydration.
    - Nitrite, leukocyte esterase: Suggests UTI.

- Guidelines for microscopic eval of urinary sediment:
  - "Bland" sediment: no cells or casts seen in prerenal and postrenal ARF (although obstructive causes may produce hematuria as well)
  - Brownish granular casts, renal tubular cells suggest ATN
  - Hematuria and RBC casts suggest glomerulonephritis
  - Pyuria and WBC casts suggest infection, AIN
  - Eosinophils suggest AIN; but sensitivity (40%) and PPV (38%) are poor (Clin Nephrol 1994;41:163)
- Urine osmolality and electrolytes
  - High urine osm (greater than 400) suggests prerenal cause or glomerulonephritis; low osm suggests intrinsic renal disease.
  - Urine sodium and creatinine: low urine Na (less than 20 mmol/L) suggests prerenal, glomerulonephritis, or postrenal cause; high urine Na suggests intrinsic renal disease.
    - Can use to calculate fractional excretion of sodium (FE_{Na}), the percentage of filtered sodium excreted in the urine: $[(Na_{urine}/Na_{serum}) / (Cr_{urine}/Cr_{serum})] \times 100$
    - FE_{Na} less than 1% suggests prerenal or postrenal ARF; greater than 1% (usually 2–3%) suggests intrinsic disease
    - Exceptions (Am Fam Phys 2000;61:2077) include:
      - Intrinsic renal disease with FE_{Na} less than 1%: glomerulonephritis, pigment nephropathy (Arch IM 1984;144:981), contrast-induced nephropathy (Arch IM 1980;140:531), and early phase of ATN
      - Prerenal ARF with FE_{Na} greater than 1%: pts who have been on diuretic rx or with prior CKD

Based on concern for other causes of ARF, further lab eval can include the following:

- CBC with diff and plt: leukocytosis to suggest infection, eosinophilia in AIN; anemia to suggest hemolysis, chronic disease, blood loss; thrombocytopenia to suggest sepsis, DIC, TTP (or thrombocytosis with chronic inflammatory disease)

- Serum electrolytes: commonly have metabolic acidosis, hyperkalemia, hypermagnesemia, hyperphosphatemia, hypocalcemia
- PT/PTT: for underlying coagulopathy
- Liver function: for acute or chronic liver disease with concern for HRS
- CPK: elevated levels in rhabdomyolysis; usually ARF associated with CPK levels greater than 15–20K, but can be as low as 5K in setting of other precipitants of ARF (sepsis, dehydration) (Arch IM 1988;148:1553); serum and urine myoglobin will also be elevated, but unnecessary as ARF in the presence of CPK elevations and pos urine dipstick for blood (without hematuria on microscopy) is dx for rhabdo-induced ARF
- Urine toxicology screen: concern for illicit drug-induced AIN
- PSA: concern for prostate cancer as cause for obstructive nephropathy
- Immune profile: concern for inflammatory cause of AIN (elevated IgE levels), vasculitis; see "Interstitial Lung Diseases" in Section 7.3 for eval of pulmonary-renal syndromes
- Serum and urine protein electrophoresis: concern for myeloma (especially with associated hypercalcemia, elevated serum protein)

Noninv: Renal US is suggested in most cases of ARF; can safely r/o obstruction (based on bladder distension, hydronephrosis); appearance of kidneys (size, cortical thickness, echogenicity) may suggest duration and severity of renal disease (Am J Kidney Dis 2000;35:1021).

Abd/pelvic CT may be useful in setting of unknown cause of obstruction (if not obvious based on exam and US), but may need to wait until ARF resolved to allow for contrast administration.

Gallium (tagged WBC) scan may aid in dx of AIN (Clin Nephrol 1985;24:84).

Kidney bx in cases of persistent ARF with unknown cause; should be done based on nephrology consultation.

Rx: Treatment of ARF includes general measures, rx for specific causes, and prevention.

General rx of acute renal failure

(Am Fam Phys 2005;72:1739)

- Prompt recognition and determination of underlying cause of ARF is crucial to proper therapy.
- Initial rx based on assessment of volume status, with most pts assumed to have prerenal cause unless other etiology evident immediately.
  - Assess intravascular volume and treat hypovolemia/hypotension with IVF (and pressors if needed) to improve MAP to goal of 60–70 mmHg; isotonic saline (0.9% NS) preferred.
  - If evidence of severe volume overload, particularly pulmonary edema, rx with IV diuretics; usually furosemide 20–80 mg IV (higher doses required in severe disease and chronic diuretic use); prior to diuretics, consider the necessity of urine electrolytes in mgt (see Lab section above for details).
- Primary therapy early in course of disease (up to 72 hr) is IV hydration to reverse hypovolemia and maintain intravascular volume.
  - Little direct evidence exists to help determine proper infusions and rates.
  - Isotonic saline is probably the best solution, usually at 1–1.5 mg/kg/hr (once initial resuscitation completed); colloid solutions do not have any more benefit (SAFE study) (NEJM 2004;350:2247), possibly harm (VISEP study) (NEJM 2008;358:125).
  - Consider eval of prerenal vs intrinsic renal disease to direct aggressiveness of IVF therapy; if evidence of intrinsic renal disease (low urine osm [less than 400], high urine Na [more than 30 mmol/L], FE_{Na} more than 1%, abnormal

sediment), aggressive hydration, especially with ongoing oliguria, will only worsen fluid overload and not likely improve renal outcomes (this effect has been termed "pseudo-ARDS" in critically ill pts) (Hosp Pract [Minneap] 1995;30:19); consider maintenance therapies of IV/PO fluids and rx based on close eval of I/O.

- Assess and treat electrolyte disturbances (see "Hyperkalemia" in Section 8.2, "Hypermagnesemia" in Section 2.4, "Hyperphosphatemia," in Section 2.4, and the discussion of metabolic acidosis in Section 8.1).
- R/o obstruction based on hx, exam, and imaging (usually with renal US).
  - If obstruction present, rx based on type:
    - Urethral obstruction: placement of Foley catheter (or suprapubic if unable to get by obstruction)
    - Bladder/ureteral: usually requires cystoscopy for eval and rx
    - Urology consultation recommended
  - Watch for postobstructive diuresis with elimination of high quantity, low osm urine over the 24–48 hr after relief of obstruction.
- Detailed med hx; hold any potentially nephrotoxic drugs; adjust dosing of necessary meds based on best assessment of renal function (realizing that CrCl estimates are imperfect in ARF).
  - Common home meds to consider holding: ACEI/ARBs, spironolactone, digoxin, thiazide and loop diuretics, NSAIDs, glyburide, metformin.
  - If antimicrobial agents required, consider avoiding nephrotoxic drugs (Crit Care Med 2008;36:S216).
    - Aminoglycosides: Best to avoid if possible; if needed, use daily dosing (Antimicrob Agents Chemother 1999;43:1549) and monitor peak and trough levels closely.

- Amphotericin B: Other antifungals often used now; if required, consider lipid-based formulation (higher cost, but less nephrotoxic).
- Vancomycin: High rates of use due to MRSA; follow trough levels closely to maintain lower than 15 mcg/mL.
- Consultation with clinical pharmacist may be useful in critically ill pts (Crit Care Med 2008;36:S216).
- Diuretic therapy with the following recommendations:
  - The rationale for routine diuretic use is based on the idea that nonoliguric ARF has better outcomes than oliguric ARF (i.e., improving urine output leads to better outcomes).
  - However, there is little direct evidence that stimulating the kidneys to diurese in ARF improves outcome; in fact, studies of "forced" diuresis in ARF have shown no benefit and possibly harm.
    - Cohort study of 552 ICU pts with ARF; diuretic use was associated with increased risk of death and nonrecovery of renal function (OR 1.7), mainly driven by pts unresponsive to diuretics (JAMA 2002;288:2547).
    - RCT of 338 pts with ARF requiring dialysis; randomized to furosemide 25 mg/kg/d IV (or higher oral dose) vs placebo; diuresis improved urine output, but no difference in mortality, recovery of renal function, or need for dialysis (Am J Kidney Dis 2004;44:402).
    - Meta-analysis of nine trials (more than 800 pts) showed similar lack of benefit (BMJ 2006;333:420).
  - Probably best to reserve diuretic use for rx of symptomatic volume overload and hyperkalemia, and otherwise avoid routine use in ARF.
- No role for "renal dose" dopamine: Low-dose dopamine (less than 5 mcg/kg/min) to maintain renal blood flow and urine output has not been proven effective; ANZICS study group of 328 critically ill pts did not show any difference in acute renal

failure, need for dialysis, LOS, or mortality with low-dose dopamine vs placebo (Lancet 2000;356:2139).
- Hemodialysis guidelines:
  - Indications for hemodialysis in ARF are as follows:
    - Persistent severe metabolic acidosis
    - Severe hyperkalemia, resistant to other K-lowering therapies
    - Volume overload, without adequate response to diuretics
    - Severe uremic sx, including encephalopathy and pericarditis
    - ARF associated with toxic ingestion of methanol; see discussion of metabolic acidosis in Section 8.1 for details.
  - Most centers use intermittent hemodialysis (2–3 times per wk depending on clinical sx).
  - Continuous renal replacement therapy (CRRT) used in some ICU settings, particularly in pts with hemodynamic instability; no evidence to support CRRT in all pts (JAMA 2008;299:793).
- Nephrology consultation early in the course of ARF, especially in pts not likely to have prerenal or ischemic ATN cause; one study suggested that delayed nephrology consultation (more than 48 hr) in ICU pts with ARF may contribute to increased mortality, but results may have selection bias and confounders (Am J Med 2002;113:456).
- Adequate nutrition is crucial; PO intake preferred (enteral feeding in critically ill); should be on low protein (0.6 gm/kg/d, higher if pt on HD), low potassium diet (Am Fam Phys 2000;61:2077).

Therapy for specific causes of acute renal failure

- AIN (Am Fam Phys 2003;67:2527)
  - High index of suspicion based on med hx and presence of other sx (rash, fever, arthralgias)
  - Look for blood and urine eosinophils

- Discontinue potential offending drugs, if possible
- Consider glucocorticoid therapy, prednisone 1 mg/kg/d, in nonresponsive or severe cases
- Myoglobinuria rx (NEJM 2009;361:62):
  - Often have severe volume depletion due to underlying cause (e.g., fall at home and prolonged dehydration in elderly) and 3rd spacing of fluid in damaged skeletal muscle.
  - Requires aggressive IVF resuscitation, usually 500–1000 mL/hr of isotonic saline initially; continue IVF until myoglobinuria resolved (based on appearance of urine or dipstick for blood).
  - Some advocate for routine use of alkaline fluid (e.g., ½ NS with 1–2 amps of $NaHCO_3/L$), but studies have not shown benefit (J Trauma 2004;56:1191); consider in pts with concomitant metabolic acidosis.
  - In severe cases, can consider addition of mannitol, but routine use not supported by current evidence.
- HRS guidelines: See "Hepatorenal Syndrome" in Section 3.7 for rx details.

Prevention of contrast-induced ARF (CI-ARF)

(J Am Coll Cardiol 2008;51:1419)

- Controversial subject with mixed data
- Related to significant morbidity and mortality
  - Retrospective study of 16K hospital inpatients requiring contrast study showed low overall rate of ARF (1.1%), but associated with a fivefold increase in mortality (7% vs 34%) (JAMA 1996;275:1489).
  - Highest risk in pts with known CKD: 37% of pts with baseline Cr 1.8 mg/dL or more developed CI-ARF with increased mortality rate (15% vs 5% in matched controls) (J Am Coll Cardiol 2000;36:1542).
  - CI-ARF adds an estimated $10,000 to the cost of hospital stay (J Med Econ 2007;10:119).

- If possible, contrast studies (including CT scans and angiography) should be avoided in pts with GFR less than 60; other risk factors include DM, dehydration, other nephrotoxic drugs.
- If study felt to be necessary, consider the following:
  - Hold potentially nephrotoxic drugs prior to and after the procedure (for 48–72 hr): ACEI/ARBs, NSAIDs, high-dose diuretics, aminoglycosides; also should hold metformin, but due to concern for lactic acidosis, not ARF.
  - Volume expansion with IVF suggested in all pts.
    - PRINCE trial showed that forced diuresis with IVF, mannitol, furosemide, and low-dose dopamine did not have significantly better outcomes than IVF alone, but showed that pts in general did better with urine output more than 150 mL/hr after contrast study (J Am Coll Cardiol 1999;33:403).
    - Isotonic saline (0.9% NS) is preferred: RCT of 1620 pts with elective angiography; randomized to 0.9% NS vs 0.45% NS, starting the morning of the procedure; 0.9% NS administration reduced CI-ARF (0.7% vs 2.0%, NNT 77) with no difference in cmplc (Arch IM 2002; 162:329).
    - If pt can tolerate, should use 1–1.5 mL/kg/hr of 0.9% NS started 3–12 hr prior to procedure and continued up to 24 hr after.
  - Other meds considered for prevention of CI-ARF include:
    - N-acetylcysteine (NAC)
      - Theoretically, NAC reduces oxygen free radicals and reduces the nephrotoxic effect of contrast.
      - Most studies have been done in pts undergoing angiography.
      - Consensus panel reviewed 27 studies of NAC rx in CI-ARF (and nine meta-analyses of the data) and

concluded that the data did not support routine use for prophylaxis (Am J Cardiol 2006;98:59K).

- Possible that NAC may reduce serum Cr levels (by renal excretion and muscle metabolism) but not have appreciable effect on clinical outcomes (J Am Soc Nephrol 2004;15:407).
- Typical dose is 600 mg PO bid on the day of and day following contrast administration (some studies looked at 1200–1500 mg doses as well).

- Vitamin C
  - RCT of 231 pts with baseline Cr of 1.2 mg/dL or more and undergoing angiography; randomized to ascorbic acid 3 gm PO 2 hr prior to procedure, then 2 gm PO q 12 hr for 2 doses vs placebo; rx reduced CI-ARF (9% vs 20%, NNT 9) (Circ 2004;110:2837).
  - RCT of 212 pts with baseline Cr 1.1 mg/dL or more and undergoing angiography; randomized to ascorbic acid (same dosing as above) vs high-dose NAC rx (1200 mg bid for 4 doses); no difference in rates of CI-ARF, but NAC rx had lower rise in overall serum Cr (Am Heart J 2009;157:576).

- Studies of other therapies including fenoldapam, furosemide, dopamine, mannitol, CCBs have shown no benefit (Am J Cardiol 2006;98:59K).

- Routine postcontrast hemodialysis probably not useful for prophylaxis against CI-ARF (Am J Cardiol 2006;98:59K).

- Bottom line is that no therapies (other than IV fluids) have been proven consistently effective in reducing CI-ARF; some still advocate for routine use of NAC and/or vitamin C in high-risk pts (known CKD, DM) because of possible efficacy and lack of significant side effects.

8.4   Nephrolithiasis

(Ann IM 2009;151:ITC2; Am Fam Phys 2001;63:1329)

Cause: Types of kidney stones (Am Fam Phys 2006;74:86) are as follows:

- Calcium oxalate: most common (calcium stones ~80%) (Lancet 2006;367:333); radio-opaque stones seen on plain Xray
- Calcium phosphate: often associated with underlying diseases: renal tubular acidosis, hyperparathyroidism, sarcoidosis, Crohn's disease
- Uric acid: increased risk in pts with gout/hyperuricemia
- Struvite: aka triple phosphate stones with $Mg/NH_3/Ca$ phosphates; due to underlying infection with urease-positive organisms (*Proteus, Ureaplasma, Klebsiella, Staph. saprophyticus*); common cause of "staghorn" calculi
- Cystine

Epidem: Lifetime risk of kidney stones in the United States is approximately 10%; 2–3 times more common in men.

Risk factors include family hx, obesity, DM (JAMA 2005;293:455; Kidney Int 2005;68:1808), hot climate.

Pathophys: Precipitation of crystals in the urine forming stones; pain due to passage of stones with luminal distension of the ureters, urethra; obstruction can cause urinary stasis, which may lead to infection.

Stone formation depends on multiple factors including urine volume, electrolyte concentrations, and urinary pH (Semin Nephrol 1996;16:364).

Sx: Flank pain most commonly; renal stones may have costovertebral, back pain (although many are initially asx); as stones migrate, pain radiates to flanks, pelvis, groin; bladder and urethral stones may present with dysuria; N/V.

Sepsis/SIRS present if associated infection.

Si: Gross or microscopic hematuria; flank tenderness is often present.

Crs: Refer to discussion of abdominal pain in Section 3.1 for diff dx of flank/abdominal pain.

Probability of stone passage based on size and location; more proximal and larger stones are less likely to pass spontaneously; for stones seen at dx in distal ureter, 74% of stones smaller than 5 mm will pass, but only 25% of those larger than 5 mm (J Urol 1991;145:263).

High rate of recurrence: 14% within 1 yr, 52% within 10 yr (Ann IM 1989;111:1006).

Incidentally noted, asx renal stones do not usually require rx (but may become symptomatic within 5 yr in 50%) (J Urol 1992;147:319), unless large "staghorn" calculi, which are associated with high rates of future sx and infection.

Cmplc: Ureteral obstruction, causing infection, or postrenal acute/chronic renal failure (significant ARF requires bilateral obstruction or solitary functioning kidney).

High rates of malingering, opiate abuse: "Red flags" include stated allergy to contrast dye (less of an issue in the current era of noncontrast CT studies), allergy to specific NSAIDs or opiates, h/o leaving against medical advice (Urol 1997;50:858).

Lab: Initial labs to include CBC with diff, metabolic panel, renal and liver function tests; U/A to look for evidence of hematuria, infection; urine Cx if si/sx of infection or pyuria on microscopic eval.

In pts with recurrent stones (Urol Clin N Am 2007;34:315), consider:

- Stone collection and eval for type
- Serum bicarbonate, calcium, magnesium, phosphorus, uric acid levels
  - Low serum bicarbonate (non-anion gap metabolic acidosis) may suggest RTA.
  - Hypercalcemia suggests sarcoid, hyperparathyroidism.

- Hypophosphatemia is seen with renal phosphate losses.
- Hyperuricemia, especially with h/o gout, suggests urate stones.
- Serum PTH levels for hyperparathyroidism
- 24-hr urine collection for volume, creatinine, calcium, oxalate, citrate, sodium, uric acid; should have two samples and probably best done once stable after acute episode, as outpatient

Noninv: Review of imaging for kidney stones:

- Noncontrast CT of abdomen/pelvis is preferred initial test
  - Widely available, allows for quick assessment for stones, as well as cmplc (hydronephrosis, pyelonephritis, perinephric abscess, emphysematous changes) (Am J Roentgenol 1996;167:1109) and alternative causes of pain.
  - Comparison study of CT vs IVP in 106 pts with flank pain; CT had 100% spec and 97% sens, compared to 94% spec and 87% sens with IVP (Urol 1998;52:982).
  - Some centers using quicker, low radiation dose scans in this setting, with little lost in spec/sens, especially in non-obese (BMI less than 30) pts (Am J Roentgenol 2007;188:927).
- Ultrasound of kidneys
  - Highly sensitive for hydronephrosis, but poor visualization of ureteral stone (spec 97%, but sens only 19%) (Eur Radiol 1998;8:212).
  - Due to lack of radiation, safest test in pregnant pts (but pregnancy-related hydronephrosis may cause a false positive test).
- Intravenous pyelogram (IVP)
  - Now rarely performed due to lower dx capability and need for contrast administration, as compared to CT.
- Plain film radiography
  - Adequate only for visualization of radio-opaque stones (calcium, some struvite and cystine); many false positives,

including calcified lymph nodes, phleboliths (calcified pelvic veins), stool.

- Best reserved for f/u of known stones or eval for other possible dx (pneumoperitoneum, bowel obstruction).

Rx: Many cases of kidney stones can be treated as outpatients; consider hospitalization for the following:

- Severe pain, N/V unable to be controlled with oral meds
- Si/sx of infection associated with UTI
- Evidence of significant obstruction on imaging
- Large stones (more than 1 cm) that seem unlikely to pass spontaneously
- Elderly pts with exacerbation of comorbid diseases

Acute rx for kidney stones

- Pain control: NSAIDs (especially IV ketorolac) (Ann EM 2006;48:173) are as effective for pain control as opiates; avoid if renal failure, bleeding risks, or plan for emergent surgical intervention.
- Guidelines for IV hydration:
  - Aggressive, high-volume hydration may not facilitate stone passage; one small study of 43 pts with acute renal colic, randomized to 2 L IV fluid over 2 hr vs maintenance fluid rate showed no difference in pain control or stone passage rates (J Endourol 2006;20:713); in most pts, adequate PO fluids or maintenance IVF warranted.
  - IV fluids warranted in pts with N/V, dehydration; evidence of sepsis/shock from associated UTI.
  - Avoid fluid overload in pts with known CHF, CKD, cirrhosis.
- Meds to facilitate stone passage:
  - Guidelines recommend considering meds in pts with uncomplicated stones, smaller than 1 cm in diameter (J Urol 2007;178:2418).

- Smooth muscle relaxation presumably will facilitate ureteral dilation, improving pain and stone passage.
- Consider alpha-1-adrenergic antagonist: tamsulosin (Flomax) 0.4 mg PO qd; doxazosin, terazosin likely as effective (J Urol 2005;173:2010).
  - Meta-analysis of 11 trials (911 pts) showed rx with alpha-blocker increased rates of spontaneous passage of stones (J Urol 2007;177:983).
  - Main side effects are orthostasis, dizziness.
- Consider nifedipine (CCB) as alternative.
  - Study compared nifedipine to tamsulosin in 86 pts with ureteral stones smaller than 1 cm (all pts were also treated with oral steroid therapy); both CCB and alpha-blocker rx reduced time to stone passage and need for analgesics (J Urol 2004;172:568).
  - May have more hypotensive effect than alpha-blocker rx.
- Treatment of infection:
  - If si/sx of infection, abnormal urinalysis/urine Cx, start appropriate abx rx (see UTI discussion in Section 5.7 for details).
  - Prompt imaging and urology consultation for consideration of surgical therapy (may include percutaneous nephrostomy for relief of obstruction and drainage, or ureteroscopy in lower-risk cases).
- Surgical intervention:
  - Small (less than 5 mm), uncomplicated (no evidence of significant obstruction or infection) stones may be treated conservatively without the need for urology consultation, in most cases; 98% will pass within 2 wk spontaneously with adequate hydration and analgesia (J Urol 1997;158:1915); if not passed within 4 wk, consider urology consultation.

- Consult urology in larger stones, recurrent episodes, staghorn calculi (J Urol 1994;151:1648), or associated cmplc; possible interventions include:
  - Extracorporeal shock wave lithotripsy (ESWL): appropriate as 1st-line rx for ureteral stones smaller than 1 cm.
  - Ureteroscopy with stone removal and stenting
  - Percutaneous nephrolithotomy

Discharge therapy

- In stable pts with adequate pain control and taking PO, prompt discharge for outpatient f/u is warranted.
- Increased fluid intake will help prevent future stones.
  - Study of 300 pts with prior kidney stones; rx group was counseled to drink large amounts of fluid qd (with subsequent daily urine volumes of 2.6 L vs 1 L in control group); increased fluid intake reduced recurrent stones over 5 yr (12% vs 27%, NNT 7) and increased interval between recurrence (by 13 mo) (J Urol 1996;155:839).
- Dietary recommendations: Increase calcium intake (1200 mg/d), recommend low-protein and low-Na diet.
  - Old concerns for high-Ca diet precipitating kidney stones is incorrect; dietary Ca probably binds to intestinal oxalate and reduces stone formation (as well as pos effects of reducing osteoporosis); confirmed in study of Italian men (NEJM 1993;328:833).
- For pts with recurrent stones, consider urology consultation for determination of risk factors and prophylactic rx.
  - Prophylactic rx depends on stone type and urine/electrolyte eval.
  - Common therapies includes thiazide diuretics, potassium citrate, dietary changes, allopurinol.

Index

A

ABCD score, for TIA, 350
abdominal pain, 127–29
abdominal wall, pain from, 128
absence seizures, 360
absolute neutrophil count (ANC), 240–41
accelerated hypertension, 74
ACE inhibitors, 21, 34–35
acetaminophen overdose, 187–92
acid-base disorders, 437–43
acidosis, 108
  metabolic, 437–38, 440–42
  respiratory, 438–39
ACTH stimulation tests, 92
activated protein C therapy, 277, 285
ACTIVE trial, 61
acute coronary syndromes (ACS), 1–22
  angiography and revascularization, 19–20
  anti-ischemic therapy, 11, 14–15
  antiplatelet and anticoagulant therapies, 15–19
  GI bleed and, 132
  risk factors, 2–4
  secondary prevention, 21–22
  stress testing procedures, 8–9, 10
acute disseminated encephalomyelitis (ADEM), 346
acute eosinophilic pneumonia (AEP), 419
acute hypersensitivity pneumonitis, 419, 430
acute inflammatory demyelinating polyradiculopathy (AIDP), 367
acute interstitial nephritis (AIN), 466–67, 476–77

acute interstitial pneumonia, 419
acute liver failure, 187–92
acute lymphocytic myocarditis, 72
acute myocardial infarction (AMI), hyperglycemia and, 100
acute renal failure. See renal failure
acute respiratory distress syndrome (ARDS), 417–29
  definition, 417
  differential diagnosis, 418
ACUTE trial, 59
acute tubular necrosis (ATN), 466
Addison's disease, 90, 92
ADDRESS trial, 285
adenoma, toxic (thyroid), 96
adenosine, 48–49
adrenal disorders, 87–93
adrenal insufficiency, 90–93, 234, 460
AFFIRM trial, 53–54
A-HeFT, 39
airway diseases, 399–416
  asthma, 411–16
  chronic obstructive pulmonary disease, 399–411
albumin, 197–98, 205, 206
albumin cytologic dissociation, 368
albuterol, 406, 407, 414
alcohol
  alcoholic liver disease, 179–87
  metronidazole and, 263
  pancreatitis and, 149
  thrombocytopenia and, 225
  toxic ingestions, 442
  withdrawal, 186
aldosterone, 457
aldosterone antagonists, 37
alkaline phosphatase, 204

alkalosis
  metabolic, 438, 442–43
  respiratory, 439
allergic reactions, cellulitis and, 294
alpha-1-adrenergic antagonist, 484
alpha-1 antitrypsin deficiency, 180
alphaglucosidase inhibitors, 104
alteplase, 353, 381
ALVEOLI trial, 427
amantadine, 372
Amato study, 424–25
amikacin, 259
aminoglycosides, 259, 474
aminotransferases, 204
amiodarone, 54, 55, 56, 94, 180
ammonia, serum, 199
amphotericin B, 319, 322, 324, 475
ampicillin, 257
ampicillin-sulbactam, 257
amyloidosis, 248
anal causes, of gastrointestinal
      bleeding, 130
anemia,
  acute blood loss, 132, 136–37, 210,
      216
  chronic disease, of (ACD), 209, 210,
      217–18
  chronic kidney disease, of, 218
  critical illness, of, 210, 217–18
  hemolytic, 210, 218, 224, 258, 262
  iatrogenic, 209–10
  iron deficiency, 209, 212, 213–14,
      216–17
  macrocytic, 211, 215–16
  microcytic, 209
  multiple myeloma and, 250, 252
  normocytic, 209–10, 211, 214–15
  sepsis and, 286
  thrombocytopenia and, 227
  transfusion practices, 218–222
angiography, invasive versus
      conservative strategies for, 19–20

angiotensin II receptor blockers
      (ARBs), 34, 35–36
angiotensin converting enzyme
      (ACE) levels, 432. See also ACE
      inhibitors.
anion gap metabolic acidosis, 109, 112,
      437–38, 439
ankle-brachial index (ABI), 301
antiarrhythmic drugs, 34, 43, 49–50
antibiotic-impregnated catheters,
      291–92
anticholinergics, for Parkinson's
      disease, 372
anticoagulation
  acute coronary syndrome, 15–19
  atrial fibrillation, 59–61
  endocarditis, 67
  HIT, 237–240
  interstitial lung diseases, 434
  thyrotoxicosis, 99
  venous thromboembolism, 385–89
antiepileptic drug therapy, 362, 364–65
antifungal medications, 319–20
antigen testing, for pneumonia, 310
anti-glomerular basement membrane
      (GBM) antibodies, 432
anti-inflammatory therapy, for ILDs,
      434–35
anti-ischemic therapy, 11, 14–15
antimicrobial medications, 257–63
antineutrophilic cytoplasmic antibodies
      (ANCA), 432
anti-PF4 antibodies, 235
antiplatelet therapies
  acute coronary syndrome, acute
      therapy, 15–19
  acute coronary syndrome, prevention
      of, 21
  ischemic stroke, acute therapy,
      354–55
  ischemic stroke, prevention of,
      357–60

antispasmodics, for diarrhea, 266
aortic arch embolism, 351
APACHE-II scoring, 152
appendicitis, 163–66
    physical signs, 164
ARDSNet study, 422
argatroban, 238
ARMA study, 425
arrhythmias
    atrial fibrillation, 50–61
    supraventricular tachycardia, 46–50
    syncope, 80
    ventricular ectopy, 42–44
    ventricular tachycardia, 42–46
arterial embolism, 174, 351
arterial thrombosis, 174
ascending cholangitis, 144, 145
ascites, 192–98
ASCVD risk factors, 40
aspergillosis, 320–22
aspirin
    ACS, 16, 21
    ischemic stroke, 357
    pericarditis, 70
    VTE prophylaxis, 396–97
asterixis, 198
asthma, 411–16
    pregnancy and, 416
asymptomatic bacteriuria, 335–36
atherosclerosis, 1
Atlanta criteria, 152
atrial fibrillation, 50–61
    anticoagulation therapy, 59–61
    CHADS2 score for, 60
    CHF and, 24, 32
    definitions, 51
    hospitalization for, 53
    rate control versus rhythm control
        strategies, 53–59
Atrial Fibrillation and Congestive Heart
        Failure Investigators trial, 54
atrial flutter, 52

autoimmune hepatitis, 180
automated implantable
        cardiodefibrillator (AICD),
        31–32, 45–46, 73
azithromycin, 261
azoles, 319–20
azotemia, 465
aztreonam, 262

B

bacteremia, *Staph aureus*, 64, 65
bacteriuria, asymptomatic, 335
barium enema, 170
Bartter's syndrome, 457
beta-agonist therapy
    asthma exacerbation, 414
    COPD exacerbation, 406
    hyperkalemia, 462
    hypokalemia, 456
beta-blockers
    ACS, 14–15, 21
    atrial fibrillation, 54, 55
    CHF, 34, 36–37
    gastrointestinal bleeding, 140
    syncope, 84
    thyrotoxicosis, 98–99
bicarbonate therapy, sodium
    diabetic ketoacidosis, 111
    HHS, 113
    hyperkalemia, 462
    metabolic acidosis, 440–41
bile duct obstruction, 144, 148
biliary colic, 143, 144, 145
biliary tract disease, 143–48
bilirubin, 205
bipap therapy. *See* noninvasive positive
        pressure ventilation
bisphosphonate therapy, for
        hypercalcemia, 120, 121
bivalirudin, 239
bladder obstruction, 467
blastomycosis, 322–23

blood cultures
  C. diff colitis, 270
  candidiasis, 330
  cellulitis, 296
  CVC infection, 290
  meningitis, 339
  pneumonia, 308–9
  urinary tract infections, 334
blood pressure management, for
      ischemic stroke, 354, 356
blood transfusions
  anemia, 218–22
  sepsis, 286
BNP
  causes of elevated, 25
  levels in CHF, 25–26
  levels in COPD, 402
  levels in PE, 377, 381
  rx in CHF, 30
body weight, ideal, 426
bone lesions, multiple myeloma and,
      250, 252–53
bone marrow disorders, anemia and, 210
bortezomib, 254
bowel stimulants, 172
brain natriuretic peptide. See BNP
bradykinesia, 371
Breathing Not Properly (BNP) study,
      25–26
British Thoracic Society, stroke scoring
      system, 305
bronchiolitis obliterans, 419
bronchitis, chronic. See chronic
      obstructive pulmonary disease
bronchodilator therapy, 406–7, 414
Brudzinski's sign, 337
Brugada criteria, 43–44
Budd-Chiari syndrome, 192
BUN, serum, 469
bupropion therapy, 409
burns, hyperglycemia and, 100

C

calcitonin, 120–21
calcium channel blockers, 15–16, 34,
      54, 55
calcium disorders, 116–21
calcium oxalate kidney stones, 480
calcium phosphate kidney stones,
      480
calcium rx, 117–18, 461
calf-vein DVTs, 384
Cameron lesions, 130
cancer
  hypercalcemia and, 118
  pulmonary embolism and, 375–76
candidal UTI, 336
candidiasis. See systemic candidiasis
CAPRIE study, 16, 358
capsule endoscopy, 134
caput medusa, 132, 181
carbamazepine, 365
carbapenems, 259–60
carcinoid syndrome, 264, 266
cardiac resynchronization therapy
      (CRT), 40
cardiac tamponade, 69
cardiac transplants, 41
cardiogenic shock, 29
cardiogenic syncope, 80, 82
cardioversion, DC, 55
carotid bruit, 349
carotid dopplers, for ischemic stroke,
      352
carotid sinus stimulation, 80
carotid stenosis, 357
caspofungin, 320
CAST I study, 44
CAST II study, 44
catecholamines, and potassium, 457
catheter-associated UTI, 332
catheter-based therapy, for ischemic
      stroke, 354

catheters. *See also* central venous catheters.
  antibiotic-impregnated, 291–92
  tunneled, 288
Cat-scratch disease, 119
cefazolin, 258
cefotaxime, 196, 259
cefoxitin, 258
ceftazidime, 259
ceftizoxime, 259
ceftriaxone, 258–59
cefuroxime, 258
cellulitis, 292–99
central diabetes insipidus, 451
central nervous system infections
  encephalitis, 345–47
  meningitis, 336–44
central venous catheters, 287–92
cephalosporins, 258–59, 314
cerebral edema
  diabetic ketoacidosis and, 108
  HHS and, 112
  hypernatremia and, 453, 454
  hyponatremia and, 446, 447
cerebral salt-wasting syndrome
    (CSWS), 444, 445
cerebrospinal fluid (CSF), meningitis
    and, 339–41
CHADS2 score, 60
Chagas disease, 25, 71
CHARISMA trial, 358
chemoprophylaxis, for meningitis, 344
chemotherapy, for multiple myeloma,
    254–55
chemotherapy-induced
    thrombocytopenia, 230
chest pain, causes of, 1–2
Child-Pugh-Turcotte (CPT)
    classification, 182, 183
Chinese Acute Stroke Trial (CAST),
    355

chloramphenicol, 263
cholangitis, 144, 145
cholecystectomy, 147–48
cholecystitis, 144, 145, 146, 147–48,
    258
choledocholithiasis, 144, 145, 146
cholelithiasis, 143
cholestyramine, 271
chronic bronchitis. *See* chronic
    obstructive pulmonary disease
chronic kidney disease
  acute renal failure and, 464–65
  anemia of, 218
  thrombocytopenia and, 225–26
chronic mesenteric ischemia, 175
chronic obstructive pulmonary disease
    (COPD), 399–411
  hyperglycemia and, 100
chronic pancreatitis, treatment for,
    158–59. *See also* pancreatitis.
chronic thromboembolic pulmonary
    hypertension (CTPH), 376
Churg-Strauss syndrome, 431, 432
Chvostek's sign, 117
ciprofloxacin, 260
cirrhosis. *See* alcoholic liver disease,
    liver disease and complications
cisapride, 172
clindamycin, 263
clonidine, 79
clopidogrel, 16–17, 21, 61, 358
Clostridium difficile colitis, 263, 264–65,
    268–73
CLOT study, 389–88
coagulopathy, treatment of, 137, 189,
    287
coccidiomycosis (San Joaquin Valley
    fever), 119, 323–24
cochicine, 70–71
Cockcroft-Gault equation, 469
colic. *See* biliary colic

colitis. *See Clostridium difficile* colitis

collagen-vascular disease-related lung disease, 430

colloid solutions, 280–81, 473

colon, gastrointestinal bleeding and, 130

colonic pseudo-obstruction, 166, 173–74

colonoscopic decompression, 174

colonoscopy, 135, 177, 212, 266

colony-stimulating factors (CSFs), 247

COMMIT study, 14

common bile duct (CBD) obstruction, 144, 148

community-acquired pneumonia (CAP), 260, 302–3, 311, 312, 313, 314–15, 316

complicated urinary tract infections, 331–36

congestive heart failure, 22–41

  chronic therapy adjustments, 33–41

  discharge planning, 41

  perfusion assessment and therapy, 28–29

  volume status assessment and therapy, 29–31

conservative strategy, for angiography and revascularization, 19–20

contact dermatitis, 294

contraction alkalosis, 442

contrast barium enema, 170

contrast-induced acute renal failure (CI-ARF), 471, 477–79

Coomb's test, 215, 227

COPE trial, 71

core measures, CMS

  Acute MI, 15, 16, 21, 22

  CHF, 27, 35, 41

  pneumonia, 304, 309, 315, 317

coronary artery disease, atrial fibrillation and, 58

coronary syndromes. *See* acute coronary syndromes

corticosteroids. *See* steroids

CORTICUS study, 93

cortisol levels. *See* adrenal insufficiency; Cushing's syndrome

C-peptide, 114

cryptococcal meningitis, 325

cryptococcosis, 324–25

Cullen's sign, 150

CURB-65, 305

CURE study, 16–17

Cushing's syndrome, 87–90, 438, 451

  hypernatremia and, 451

cystine kidney stones, 480

D

dabigatran, 388

Dallas criteria, 72

dalteparin, 386

danaparoid, 239

DC cardioversion, 55

D-dimer testing, 376–77

deep venous thrombosis (DVT), 294, 382–84

  upper extremity, 384

dehydration

  diabetic ketoacidosis and, 108

  HHS and, 111

delayed-onset HIT, 233

dermatitis, 294

dexamethasone, 254

dexamethasone suppression test (DST), 89

diabetes insipidus (DI), 448, 451, 455, 458

diabetes mellitus. *See also* diabetic ketoacidosis.

  hyperglycemia and, 99–105, 106–7

  pancreatitis and, 158

diabetic and glucose disorders, 99–115

  diabetic ketoacidosis, 105, 108–11

hyperglycemia, 99–105, 106–7
hyperosmolar hyperglycemic state, 111–13
hypoglycemia, 113–15
diabetic foot ulcers, 299–302
diabetic ketoacidosis (DKA), 105–11
diarrhea
  acute, 263–68
  differential diagnosis, 264
  hospital-acquired, 264–65
  inflammatory, 265
  noninflammatory, 265
  traveler's, 264
diastolic dysfunction, 23–24
Dieulafoy's lesions, 130
diffuse alveolar hemorrhage (DAH), 419
DIG study group, 38–39
DIGAMI 1 study, 102
DIGAMI 2 study, 103
digestive enzymes, replacement of, 158
Digitalis Investigation Group study, 38
digoxin, 34, 37–39, 54, 55, 56, 94, 117–18, 119
diltiazem, 54, 56
discharge planning and therapy
  congestive heart failure, 41
  nephrolithiasis, 485
  pneumonia, 307
disopyramide, 57
disseminated intravascular coagulation (DIC), 223, 227, 230
  DIC score, 228
diuretic therapy
  acute renal failure, 475
  ascites, 194–95
  CHF, 29–30, 33
  hypertension, 79
diverticulitis, 159–63
diverticulosis, 159
dobutamine, 283–84
dofetilide, 57

dopamine, 281–82, 283, 284, 475–76
dopamine agonists, 372
doripenem, 260
doxycycline, 262
Dressler's syndrome, 5, 68
drug rashes, cellulitis and, 295
drug-induced AIN, 466–67
drug-induced ATN, 466
drug-induced hyperkalemia, 459–60
drug-induced hypokalemia, 456
drug-induced parkinsonism, 369–70
drug-induced thrombocytopenia, 223, 225, 230
Duke criteria, 66–67
Dunphy's sign, 164
duodenal causes, of gastrointestinal bleeding, 130

E

early goal-directed therapy (EGDT), 277–78
echinocandins, 320
echocardiography, 380
ECST study, 357
ectopy. See ventricular ectopy
effusion, parapneumonic, 307
EKG
  ACS, 6–7, 10
  acute pericarditis, 70
  arrhythmias, 43
  atrial fibrillation, 51–52
  CHF, 27
  hypercalcemia, 120
  hyperkalemia, 460–61
  hypermagnesemia, 123
  hypertensive crisis, 75
  hypocalcemia, 117
  hypomagnesemia, 122
  infective endocarditis, 66
  ischemic stroke, 352
  myocarditis, 72–73
  myxedema, 95

EKG (*cont.*)
  pulmonary embolism, 377
  supraventricular tachycardia, 47–48
  syncope, 82
ELATE trial, 387
electroencephalogram (EEG)
  encephalitis, 347
  epilepsy and seizure disorders, 361–62
  ischemic stroke, 353
electrolytes, diabetic ketoacidosis and, 109
electrophoresis
  serum protein (SPEP), 251
  urine protein (UPEP), 251
ELLDOPA study, 371
embolectomy, 381
embolism. *See also* venous thromboembolism.
  arterial, 174
  ischemic stroke and, 351
emphysema. *See* chronic obstructive pulmonary disease
emphysematous pyelonephritis, 333
empyema, parapneumonic, 307
enalaprilat, 78
encephalitis, 343, 345–47
encephalomyelitis, acute disseminated (ADEM), 346, 347
encephalopathies, 345
endocarditis, infective, 61–68
  causes, 62
  Duke criteria, 66–67
  physical findings, 63
  prophylaxis, 67–68
endoscopic evaluation and therapy, for UGIB, 133–34
endotracheal intubation, 405–6, 413
enoxaparin, 385, 398
enteroclysis, 171
epilepsy, 360–67
epinephrine, 283
ERCP, 148, 157–58

ertapenem, 260
erysipelas, 294
erythema chronicum migrans, 294
erythromycin, 172
erythropoiesis stimulators, 217
erythropoietin, 217, 286
esmolol, 76
esophagus, gastrointestinal bleeding and, 130
ESPRIT trial, 359
ESPS-2 trial, 358
essential tremor, 370
ethylene glycol, 441–42
euvolemic hyponatremia, 443–44, 448
exposure-related lung disease, 430

F
FACCT study, 423
factitious Cushing's syndrome, 87
factitious syndrome, hypoglycemic, 114
fasciitis, necrotizing, 292–99
febrile neutropenia, 243, 244–45
fecal enemas, for *C. diff.* colitis, 272
fenoldopam, 77
ferritin, 213–14
fetor hepaticus, 181
fever, neutropenia and, 243
fistula, colonic, 160–61
flecainide, 49, 57
fluconazole, 319, 324
flucytosine, 320
fludrocortisones, 84
fluorinated pyrimidines, 320
fluoroquinolones, 260–61
focal seizures, 360
FOCUS trial, 221
folate deficiency, 211, 215, 217
fomepizole, 441–42
fondaparinux, 18, 240, 240, 386, 398
foot ulcers, diabetic, 299–302

fosphenytoin, 366
fractional excretion of sodium (FENa), 471, 473
fulminant lymphocytic myocarditis, 72
functional adrenal insufficiency, 91
functional HIT assay, 235
fungal encephalitis, 345
fungal infections
  antifungal medications, 319–20
  aspergillosis, 320–22
  blastomycosis, 322–23
  cellulitis and, 293
  coccidiomycosis (San Joaquin Valley fever), 323–24
  cryptococcosis, 324–25
  histoplasmosis, 326–27
  Pneumocystis pneumonia, 327–29
  systemic candidiasis, 330–31
furosemide, 79, 194–95

G

G6PD deficiency, 210
galactomannan, serum, 321
gallium nitrate IV infusion, for hypercalcemia, 121
gallstones
  biliary tract disease and, 144, 145
  pancreatitis and, 148–49, 157–58
gas gangrene, 292–99
gastric acid suppression, 137–38
gastric antral vascular ectasia (GAVE), 130
gastric causes, of gastrointestinal bleeding, 130
gastroenteritis, 263–68
gastrograffin, 170
gastrointestinal bleeding, 129–43
  gastric acid suppression, 137–38
  stress ulcer prophylaxis, 141–43
  variceal bleeding, 139–41
gastrointestinal causes, of abdominal pain, 127

gastrointestinal infections
  acute diarrhea and gastroenteritis, 263–68
  Clostridium difficile colitis, 268–73
gatifloxacin, 261
Geneva score, 375
gentamicin, 259
gestational thrombocytopenia, 225
Gilbert's syndrome, 206
GISSI-HF trial, 40
Gitelman's syndrome, 457
Glasgow Coma Score (GCS), 337–38
glitazones, 104
glucagon, 179
glucocorticoids. *See also* steroids.
glucose
  diabetic ketoacidosis and, 109
  HHS and, 112
  hypoglycemia and, 114, 115
glucose control, for hyperglycemia, 101–4
glucose disorders. *See* diabetic and glucose disorders
glycoprotein IIb/IIIa inhibitor, 19, 223
goiter, multinodular, 96
gout, 295
GRACE risk model, 4
granulocyte colony-stimulating factors (G-CSFs), 247
granulocyte-macrophage colony-stimulating factors (GM-CSFs), 247
Grave's disease, 96, 97
Grey Turner's sign, 150
Guillain-Barre syndrome, 265, 367–69
gynecologic causes, of abdominal pain, 128

H

HACEK organisms, 61
haptoglobin, 215, 227

healthcare-associated pneumonia
(HCAP), 302–3, 311, 312, 313
heart failure. *See* congestive heart
failure
Helicobacter pylori, 131, 133, 139
HELLP syndrome, 224
hemodialysis, 206, 442, 463, 476
hemoglobinuria, 466
hemolytic anemia. *See* anemia,
hemolytic
hemolytic uremic syndrome, 265. *See
also* TTP.
heparin. *See also* LMWH.
ACS, 17–18
ischemic stroke, 355–56
VTE prophylaxis, 397
VTE therapy, 385–86, 389
heparin-induced thrombocytopenia
(HIT), 223, 231–37, 240, 376
HIT score, 233–34
hepatic causes, of abdominal pain, 127
hepatic encephalopathy, 198–201
hepatic hydrothorax, 193
hepatitis, 180. *See also* alcoholic liver
disease.
hepatitis, viral 180, 188–89
hepatorenal syndrome, 201–6
hereditary hemochromatosis (HH),
180
HIDA scan, for biliary tract disease,
146
Hinchey's criteria, 160
histoplasmosis, 326–27
holter monitoring, 52
hospital-acquired pneumonia (HAP),
302–3, 304, 306, 311, 311, 312,
313, 316
HSV encephalitis, 343, 345, 346
hydralazine, 39–40, 78
hyperaldosteronism, 438, 451, 456, 458
hypercalcemia, 118–21, 249, 252, 323,
481

hyperglycemia, 99–105, 106–7, 108,
111, 284–85
fluoroquinolones and, 261
stress, 99, 100, 102
hyperkalemia, 33, 459–64
hyperlipidemia, 40
hypermagnesemia, 122–23
hypernatremia, 451–55
Cushing's syndrome and, 451
iatrogenic, 451
hyperosmolar hyperglycemic state
(HHS), 111–13
hyperosmolar nonketotic coma. *See*
hyperosmolar hyperglycemic state
hyperparathyroidism, 118, 119, 482
hyperphosphatemia, 124–25
hypersensitivity pneumonitis, 419, 430
hypersplenia, 225
hypertension, 58
hypertensive crisis, 73–80
hypertensive emergency (HE), 73–74
hypertensive urgency (HU), 73
hyperthyroidism, 96–99
hypertonic hyponatremia, 444
hypertriglyceridemia, 149, 158
hypertrophy, left ventricular, 75
hyperviscosity syndrome, 250, 253
hypervolemic hyponatremia, 444
hypoalbuminemia, 116
hypocalcemia, 116–18
hypoglycemia, 113–15, 261, 440
hypoglycemic medications, oral, 104
hypokalemia, 32–33, 456–59
hypokalemic periodic paralysis, 456
hypomagnesemia, 116, 121–22, 456
hyponatremia, 96, 182, 443–51
euvolemic, 443–44, 448
hypervolemic, 444
hypotonic/dilutional, 443–44
hypovolemic, 443, 448–49
hypoparathyroidism, 116
hypophosphatemia, 123–24

hypotension, sepsis and, 280, 284
hypothalamic-pituitary-adrenal axis, 87
hypothalamic-pituitary-thyroid axis, 93
hypothermia, 96
hypothyroidism. *See* myxedema
hypotonic/dilutional hyponatremia,
        443–44
hypovolemic hyponatremia, 443,
        448–49
hypoxemia, 421

I

idiopathic interstitial pneumonias,
        430
idiopathic thrombocytopenic purpura
        (ITP), 223–24, 230–31
ileus, 166, 167, 168. *See also* intestinal
        obstruction.
imipenem-cilastatin, 259–60
immune-related AIN, 467
immunosuppressive drugs, for ILDs,
        434
induction therapy, for multiple
        myeloma, 254–55
infective endocarditis. *See* endocarditis
influenza vaccination, Guillain-Barre
        syndrome and, 367
ingestion-related metabolic acidosis,
        440–42
inotrope therapy, 40–41
inpatient hyperglycemia. *See*
        hyperglycemia
insulin, 105
    factitious syndrome due to, 114
    hyperkalemia and, 461–62
    hypokalemia and, 456, 457
insulin therapy, 101–4
    diabetic ketoacidosis and, 110
    HHS, 113
    hypoglycemia, 115
International Stroke Trial (IST),
        354–55

interstitial lung diseases (ILDs), 429–35
interstitial nephritis, acute (AIN),
        466–67, 476–77
interstitial pneumonia, acute, 419
intestinal ileus. *See* intestinal
        obstruction
intestinal ischemia, 174–79
intestinal obstruction, 166–74
    "closed loop" obstruction, 168, 175
intracranial hemorrhage, 353
intracranial vessels, imaging of, 352–53
intrarenal acute renal failure, 466
intravenous catheter (IVC) filter
        replacement, 390
intravenous immunoglobulin therapy
        (IVIG)
    C. diff. colitis, 272
    Guillain-Barre syndrome, 369
    thrombocytopenia, 229, 230, 231
intravenous pyelogram (IVP), 482
invasive strategy, for angiography and
        revascularization, 19–20
iodine rx, 98
ipratropium bromide, 406, 407, 414
iron deficiency anemia (IDA), 209,
        213–14, 216–17
iron rx, 216
irritant dermatitis, 294
ischemia, acute mesenteric, 174–75
ischemia, acute tubular necrosis and,
        466
ischemic stroke, 351–60
itraconazole, 319–20, 322, 324

K

Kernig's sign, 337
ketoacidosis. *See* diabetic ketoacidosis
ketoconazole, 320
ketones, 109
ketosis, 108
kidney stones, acute therapy for,
        483–85. *See also* nephrolithiasis.

L

labetalol, 76
lactulose therapy, 199, 201
lamotrigine, 364
large-volume paracentesis (LVP), 195–96
LBBB, 10
lead poisoning, 209
lenalidomide, 254, 255
lepirudin, 239
leukocytosis, 109
Leuven 1, 101–2
Leuven 2, 102, 113
levalbuterol, 406, 414
levetiracetam, 364
levodopa, 371–72
levofloxacin, 260
levothyroxine, 96
LFTs, abnormal, 204–5, 206–7
Liddle's syndrome, 457
linezolid, 245, 262
lipid management, for ACS, 21–22
lithotripsy, extracorporeal shock wave, 485
liver disease and complications, 179–207
  acute liver failure, 187–92
  alcoholic liver disease, 179–87
  ascites and spontaneous bacterial peritonitis, 192–98
  evaluation, 185, 206–7
  hepatic encephalopathy, 198–201
  hepatorenal syndrome, 201–6
liver enzymes, alcoholic liver disease and, 184
liver failure, acute, 187–92
liver function tests, abnormal, 204–5, 206–7
liver transplantation, 187
LMWH,
  ACS, 12, 17–18
  ischemic stroke, 352, 355
  VTE prophylaxis, 397–98
  VTE therapy 385, 387–88, 389
loop diuretics, 29–30, 462–63
lorazepam, 366
low-molecular-weight heparin (LMWH). See LMWH
low-tidal-volume ventilation, 425–26
lower gastrointestinal bleeding (LGIB), 129, 135–36, 141
LVH criteria, 75
lymphopenia, 241–42

M

macrocytic anemia, 211, 215–16
macrolides, 261
Maddrey's discriminant function, 182
magnesium, for asthma, 415, 416
magnesium disorders, 121–23
malignant hypertension, 74
Mallory-Weiss tears, 130
MAT trial, 20
MATCH trial, 358
McBurney's point, 163
MDRD equation, 470
mechanical ventilation
  ARDS patients, 424–29
  asthma, 413
  COPD, 405–6
  sepsis and, 287
  weaning, 428–29
Meckel's diverticulum, 130, 135
MEDENOX trial, 397
megacolon, toxic, 265, 269
meglitinides, 104
Meigs syndrome, 192
MELD score, 182
melphalan, 255
meningitis, 325, 326, 336–44
MERIT-HF study, 36
meropenem, 260
mesenteric angiography, 177
mesenteric ischemia, 174–75

mesenteric venous thrombosis, 175
metabolic acidosis, 437–38, 440–42
metabolic alkalosis, 438, 442–43
   contraction, 442
   posthypercapneic, 405, 438, 443
metastatic carcinoma, 248
metformin, 104
methanol, 441–42
methimazole, 98
methylmalonic acid levels, 216
methylnaltrexone, 172
metoclopramide, 172
metoprolol, 54, 56, 78
metronidazole, 263
micafungin, 320
microcytic anemia, 209
mid gastrointestinal bleeding, 129
midodrine, 84–85, 205
milk-alkali syndrome, 119, 438
monobactams, 262
monoclonal antibodies, for C. diff.
   colitis, 273
monoclonal gammopathy, 247–48
monomorphic VT, 42
morphine, for ACS, 14
motility agents, for postoperative ileus,
   172
moxifloxacin, 261
MRI
   biliary tract disease, 146
   intestinal obstruction, 171
   ischemic stroke, 352
multifocal atrial tachycardia, 52
multinodular goiter, 96
multiple myeloma, 247–55, 466
Murphy's sign, 145
myeloma. See multiple myeloma
myelophthistic disorders, 210
myocardial infarction (MI)
   definitions, 1
   gastrointestinal bleeding and, 132–33
   hyperglycemia and, 100

myocarditis, 71–73
myoglobinuria, 466, 477. See also
   pigment nephropathy;
   rhabdomyolysis.
myxedema (severe hypothyroidism),
   94–96, 211

N
N-acetylcysteine (NAC), 478–79
nafcillin, 257
NASCET study, 357
necrosis, acute tubular (ATN), 466
necrotizing fasciitis, 292–99
neomycin, 201
neostigmine, 173
nephritis, acute interstitial (AIN),
   466–67, 476–77
nephrogenic diabetes insipidus, 451,
   455
nephrolithiasis, 480–85
nesiritide, 30
neurogenic syncope, 81, 82–83
neutropenia, 240–47
   febrile, 243, 244–45
   sulfa drugs and, 262
neutrophils, 242
New York Heart Association (NYHA),
   CHF classification, 23
nicardipine, 77
nifedipine, 79, 484
NINDS study, 353
nitrates, 11, 39–40, 140
nitroglycerin, 30, 77
nitroprusside, 76–77
nonalcoholic fatty liver disease
   (NAFLD), 180, 262
non-heparin anticoagulants, 237–40
noninvasive positive pressure
   ventilation (NIPPV), 31, 404–5,
   413, 421
nonocclusive mesenteric ischemia,
   174–75

nonsecretory multiple myeloma, 248
norepinephrine, 206, 281, 282, 283, 284
normocytic anemia, 209–10, 211, 214–15
NSAIDs, 34, 70, 131, 139, 459, 466, 467, 474, 478, 481, 483

O

obesity, pancreatitis and, 152
obscure gastrointestinal bleeding, 129
obstruction. See intestinal obstruction
obturator sign, 164
occult gastrointestinal bleeding, 129
octreotide, 139–40, 205
Ogilvie's syndrome, 173–74
orthostatic syncope, 81, 82
osmolality, 446
osmolar gap, 440
oxacarbazepine, 365
oxacillin, 257
oxazolidinones, 262
oxygen administration
    ARDS, 427
    asthma, 413
    COPD, 403, 410

P

pancreaticobiliary causes, of abdominal pain, 127
pancreaticobiliary diseases
    biliary tract disease, 143–48
    pancreatitis, 148–59
pancreatitis
    acute, 148–57
    antibiotics, 156–57
    chronic, 148, 157–58
    nutritional support, 155–56
    scoring methods for, 150–51
papaverine, 179
paracentesis, large-volume (LVP), 195–96

paracoccidiomycosis, 322
paradoxical embolism, 351
parapneumonic effusion and empyema, 307
Parkinsonian syndromes, 370
parkinsonism, drug-induced, 369–70
Parkinson's disease, 369–72
paroxysmal supraventricular tachycardia, 47, 52
partial seizures, 360
peau d'orange, 294
penicillin, 257–58
pentoxifylline, for alcoholic liver disease, 186–87
peptic ulcers, 131, 138–39
pericardial constriction, 69
pericarditis, acute, 68–71
perinephric abscess, 333
peripheral blood smear findings, 213
peripherally inserted CVCs (PICC lines), 288
peripheral polyradiculopathy, 367
phenobarbital, 365, 366–67
phentolamine, 77
phenylephrine, 283
phenytoin, 362–63, 365, 366
phosphate
    diabetic ketoacidosis and, 109, 111
    HHS and, 112, 113
phosphorus disorders, 123–25
pigment nephropathy, 466, 471. See also myoglobinuria; rhabdomyolysis.
piperacillin, 258
piperacillin-tazobactam, 258
plasmapharesis, 231, 369
platelet transfusions, for thrombocytopenia, 229, 230, 237
Plavix. See clopidogrel
pleural effusion, 70
pneumococcal vaccination, 317
Pneumocystis pneumonia (PCP), 253, 327–29

pneumonia, 302–19
  acute eosinophilic (AEP), 419
  acute interstitial, 419
  hyperglycemia and, 100
  idiopathic interstitial, 430
Pneumonia Severity Index (PSI), 305
pneumonitis, acute hypersensitivity,
    419, 430
polymorphic VT, 42
polyradiculopathy
  acute inflammatory demyelinating
    (AIDP), 367
  peripheral, 367
PORT score, 305
portal hypertension, 181
postoperative hyponatremia, 444
postoperative ileus, therapies for,
    172–73. See also intestinal
    obstruction.
postransfusion purpura, 224
postrenal acute renal failure, 467
posture, Parkinson's disease and, 371
potassium
  diabetic ketoacidosis and, 109, 110
  HHS and, 112, 113
potassium disorders
  hyperkalemia, 459–64
  hypokalemia, 456–59
potassium metabolism, 32–33
prandial insulin, 105
prednisone. See steroids
pregabalin, 365
premature ventricular contraction
    (PVC), 42
prerenal acute renal failure, 465–66
pressure support ventilation (PSV),
    428–29
PREVENT trial, 398
primary adrenal insufficiency, 90–91
primary biliary cirrhosis (PBC), 180
primary sclerosing cholangitis (PSC),
    180

PRINCE trial, 478
probiotics, for C. diff. colitis, 271
procainamide, 56
PROFESS trial, 359
prolactin, serum, 361
prone positioning, in ARDS, 427
Pronovost study, 291
propafenone, 49, 57
prophylaxis, in hospitalized VTE
    patients, 240, 390–98. See also
    stress ulcer prophylaxis.
propofol, 367
propranolol, 56
propylthiouracil (PTU), 98
protein C, activated. See activated
    protein C therapy
PROWESS trial, 285
pseudo-Cushing's syndrome, 87
pseudo-cysts, pancreatic, 159
pseudo-hyperkalemia, 460
pseudo-hyponatremia, 444
pseudo-obstruction, colonic, 166–74
pseudo-thrombocytopenia, 222
psoas sign, 164
psychogenic polydipsia, 444
pulmonary angiography, 379
pulmonary artery catheter (Swan
    Ganz), 277, 284, 420
pulmonary causes, of abdominal pain,
    127
pulmonary embolism (PE), 373–81
  massive, treatment for, 380–81
  See venous thromboembolism
pulmonary hypertension, chronic
    thromboembolic (CTPH), 376
pulmonary rehab, 411
pulmonary vasculitis, 430, 467
pulsus paradoxus, 411
purpura
  idiopathic thrombocytopenic (ITP),
    223–24, 230–31
  postransfusion 224

purpura (*cont.*)
  thrombotic thrombocytopenic
    (TTP), 224, 231
pyelogram, intravenous (IVP), 482
pyelonephritis, 331–36
pyrimidines. *See* fluorinated
    pyrimidines

Q

Q waves, 7
QT interval, prolonged, 42, 43, 261
quinidine, 56
quinupristin-dalfopristin, 263

R

RACE trial, 53
RALES trial, 37
Ranson's criteria, 150, 152
rate control strategies, for atrial
    fibrillation, 53–59
rectal causes, of gastrointestinal
    bleeding, 130
rectal stimulants, 173
red man syndrome, 263
reflex-mediated syncope, 80, 82
refractory ascites, 196
refractory hypoxemia, 427–28
relative adrenal insufficiency, 91
renal causes, of abdominal pain, 128
renal dose dopamine, 475–76
renal failure
  acute, 464–79
  chronic, 459
  hyperkalemia and, 459
  multiple myeloma and, 249, 252
renal tubular acidosis, 438, 460
respiratory acidosis, 438–39
respiratory alkalosis, 439
respiratory failure, acute, due to CHF, 31
reticulocytosis, 211, 214
revascularization, invasive versus
    conservative strategies for, 19–20

rhabdomyolysis, 457, 466, 468, 472.
    See also myoglobinuria; pigment
    nephropathy.
rhythm control strategies, for atrial
    fibrillation, 53–59
rifampin, 272
rifaximin, 201, 272
rigidity, Parkinson's disease and, 370
risk stratification, for acute coronary
    syndromes, 3–4, 12–13
rivaroxaban, 388
Rovsing's sign, 164

S

SAFE study, 280
salicylate ingestions, 442
SALT trials, 449
San Joaquin Valley fever, 323–24
SANAD study, 362
sarcoidosis, 118, 121, 430
secondary adrenal insufficiency, 91
secondary prevention
  acute coronary syndromes, 21–22
  ischemic stroke, 356–60
seizure disorders, 360–67, 450
selective decontamination of digestive
    tract (SDD), 318
sepsis and septic shock, 273–287
  anemia and, 221
  SIRS criteria, 274
  thrombocytopenia, 222, 230
serum-ascites albumin gradient, 194
SHEP study, 356
shock
  cardiogenic, 6, 28–29
  septic, 273–87
shock bowel, 174–75
shock liver, 276
sickle cell disease, 210
sigmoid colon, gastrointestinal bleeding
    and, 130
Sinemet. *See* levodopa

sinus arrhythmia, 51
sinus rhythm, 51
sinus tachycardia, 46
situational syncope, 80
small bowel follow-through (SBFT), for
    obstruction, 170
small intestine, gastrointestinal
    bleeding and, 130
smoking cessation
  COPD, 409
  pneumonia, 317
SOAP study, 218
SOAP II trial, 282
sodium, HHS and, 112
sodium bicarbonate. *See* bicarbonate
    therapy
sodium disorders
  hypernatremia, 451–55
  hyponatremia, 443–51
sodium polystyrene sulfonate, 463
Somogyi phenomenon, 101
sotalol, 57
Spanish Lung Failure Collaborative
    study, 429
spherocytosis, hereditary, 210, 213
spirochetes, 345
spironolactone, 34, 37, 194
spontaneous bacterial peritonitis
    (SBP), 192–98
sputum Gram stains, for pneumonia,
    309–10
SSRIs, 85
Staph aureus bacteremia, 64, 65
status epilepticus, 363, 366–67
ST depressions, 7
ST elevations, 7, 10
steroids
  adrenal insufficiency and, 93
  alcoholic liver disease, 186
  ARDS, 421–22
  asthma, 415
  cellulitis and, 298

COPD, 408–9
Guillain-Barre syndrome, 369
hypercalcemia and, 121
hypokalemia and, 456
ILDs, 434, 435
meningitis, 344
myeloma, 255
pericarditis, 71
Pneumocystis pneumonia, 329
sepsis and, 284
stress dosing, 92
thrombocytopenia, 230, 231
thyrotoxicosis, 99
stress testing procedures
  ACS, 8–9, 10
  CHF, 27
stress ulcer prophylaxis, 141–43, 319
stroke
  ACS and, 6
  atrial fibrillation and, 60
  differential diagnosis, 350
  hyperglycemia and, 100
  ischemic stroke, 351–60
  transient ischemic attack, 349–50
struvite kidney stones, 480
sudden cardiac death, 31–33
sulfonamides, 262. *See also*
        trimethoprim-sulfamethoxazole.
sulfonylureas, 104, 114
superficial thrombophlebitis, 294, 384
superficial venous thrombosis (SVT).
        See superficial thrombophlebitis
supraventricular tachycardia, 46–50
surgical embolectomy, 381
surgical therapies
  cholecystitis, 147–48
  nephrolithiasis, 484–85
  pancreatitis, 157
  Parkinson's disease, 372
Surviving Sepsis Campaign, 277
Swan Ganz catheter. *See* pulmonary
    artery catheter

synchronous intermittent mandatory
	ventilation (SIMV), 429
syncope, 80–85
syndrome of inappropriate ADH
	secretion (SIADH), 443, 446,
	447, 448, 451
systemic candidiasis, 279, 330–31
systemic fungal infections. *See* fungal
	infections
systemic inflammatory response
	syndrome (SIRS). *See* sepsis and
	septic shock
systolic dysfunction, 23, 24

T
tachycardia
	multifocal atrial, 52
	sinus, 46
	supraventricular, 46–50
	ventricular, 5, 42–46, 80
	wide complex, differential dx of, 42,
		47–48
tagged RBC scan, 135
tamponade, cardiac, 69
tamsulosin, 484
terbutaline, 416
terlipressin, 203, 206
tetracyclines, 262
thalassemia, 209, 214
thalidomide, 254, 255
theophylline, 410
thiazolidinediones, 34, 104
thrombocytopenia, 222–40
	drug-induced, 223, 225, 230
	gestational, 225
	heparin-induced, 231–37, 240
	liver disease and, 184
	non-heparin anticoagulants, 237–40
thromboembolism. *See* venous
	thromboembolism
thrombolytic therapy
	ACS, 10, 20

DVT, 384
	ischemic stroke, 353–54
	pulmonary embolism, 381
thrombophlebitis, superficial, 294, 384
thrombotic thrombocytopenic purpura
	(TTP), 224, 231
thyroid disorders, 94–99
thyroid hormone, 457
thyroid hormone replacement, 96
thyroid radioiodine uptake, 97–98
thyroid storm, 96–99
thyroid ultrasound, 98
thyroiditis, 96
thyrotoxicosis, 96–99
thyroxine ingestion, 96
tiagabine, 365
ticarcillin-clavulanate, 258
tigecycline, 262, 298
TIMI IIIB, 20
TIMI Risk Score, 4
tinzaparin, 386
tiotropium, 410
TIPS, 141, 196, 198, 206
tobramycin, 259
tolvaptan, 449
topiramate, 364
torsades de pointes, 42
toxic adenoma, 96
toxin sequestrants, for *C. diff.* colitis,
	271
transfusion practices. *See* anemia
transfusion-related acute lung injury
	(TRALI), 219, 418
transient ischemic attack (TIA),
	349–50
trauma, hyperglycemia and, 100
traveler's diarrhea, 264
treadmill testing, 52
tremor, 370
TRICC study, 219, 221
trimethoprim-sulfamethoxazole (TMP-
	SMX), 262, 328, 329, 335

troponin, serum
  ACS, 6
  atrial fibrillation, 51
  CHF, 26
  PE, 377
  pericarditis, 70
Trousseau's sign, 117
T-tube, 429
tuberculosis, 118
tumor lysis syndrome, 250, 253, 460
tunneled catheters, 288

U

ulcers. *See* diabetic foot ulcers; peptic
      ulcers
ultrasound
  biliary tract disease, 146
  intestinal ischemia, 177
  intestinal obstruction, 170
  nephrolithiasis, 482
  pulmonary embolism, 379
unfractionated heparin (UFH), 17–18,
      397. *See also* heparin.
upper extremity DVT, 384
upper gastrointestinal bleeding
      (UGIB), 129
  endoscopic evaluation and therapy,
      133–34
  gastric acid suppression, 137–38
upper gastrointestinal study, for
      obstruction, 170
urease-producing organisms, 333–34
uremia, 465
ureteral obstruction, 467
urethral obstruction, 467
uric acid kidney stones, 480
urinalysis, for acute renal failure,
      470–71
urinary tract infections, 331–36
urine osmolality and electrolytes, 446,
      471
urologic causes, of abdominal pain, 128

V

vaccinations
  COPD and, 409–10
  Guillain-Barre syndrome and, 367
  pneumococcal, 317
vagal maneuvers, 48
valproate, 364
valsartan, 35–36
vancomycin, 245, 263, 273, 475
Van den Berghe MICU study, 101,
      113
Van den Berghe SICU study, 101
VANQWISH study, 20
variceal bleeding, 132, 139–41
varices, 131
vascular causes, of abdominal pain,
      127
vasculitis, 467
vasodilator therapy, for CHF, 30–31
vasopressin, 283
vasopressors
  cardiogenic shock, 28–29
  CHF, 40–41
  hepatorenal syndrome, 203, 206
  intestinal ischemia, 175, 178
  sepsis and, 281–84
vasovagal syncope, 80, 81
VASST trial, 283
venous insufficiency, 294
venous thromboembolism, 373–98
  anticoagulation for, 385–89
  deep venous thrombosis, 382–84
  HIT and, 234
  IVC filter replacement, 390
  prophylaxis in hospitalized patients,
      390–98
  pulmonary embolism, 373–81
  risk factors, 373–74
  stroke and, 352
ventilation. *See* mechanical ventilation
ventilation/perfusion (V/Q) scan,
      378–79

ventilator-associated pneumonia
    (VAP), 302–3, 304, 306, 311,
    312, 313, 316
ventilator weaning, 428–29
ventricular arrhythmias, 31–33, 460
ventricular-assist devices (VADs), 41
ventricular bigeminy/trigeminy, 42
ventricular ectopy, 42–44
ventricular tachycardia, 5, 42–46, 80
verapamil, 56
V-HeFT I, 39
V-HeFT II, 39
viral encephalitis, 345
viral hepatitis, chronic, 180
viral meningitis, 337
viral myocarditis, 71
Virchow's triad, 373
VISEP study, 103, 280
vitamin A intoxication, 180
vitamin B12 deficiency anemia, 211, 217
vitamin C, 216, 479
Von Willebrand disease, 226
voriconazole, 320, 322

W

Waldenstrom's macroglobulinemia
    (WM), 248

wandering pacemaker, 52
warfarin, 60
  ACS, 18–19
  heparin-induced thrombocytopenia
    and, 237, 238
  ischemic stroke, 359
  VTE, 387, 389, 398
WARSS trial, 359
WASID trial, 359
Waterhouse-Friderichsen syndrome,
    90, 234
weaning, ventilator, 428–29
Wegner's granulomatosis, 431
Well's criteria, 375, 382
Whipple's triad, 113
Wilson's disease, 91, 180, 188
Worcester DVT study, 390
wound infections (post-op),
    hyperglycemia and, 100

Z

zonisamide, 364

Other books in the Jones & Bartlett Learning LITTLE BLACK BOOK Series:

The Little Black Book of International Medicine,
William A. Alto

The Little Black Book of Emergency Medicine, Second Edition, Steven E. Diaz

The Little Black Book of Urology, Second Edition,
Pamela Ellsworth and Anthony Caldamone

The Little Black Book of Geriatrics, Fourth Edition,
Karen Gershman

The Little Black Book of Gastroenterology, Third Edition,
David W. Hay

The Little Black Book of Sports Medicine, Second Edition,
Thomas M. Howard and Janus D. Butcher

The Little Black Book of Nephrology and Hypertension,
Charles N. Jacobs and Dmitry Opolinsky

The Little Black Book of Rheumatology,
Marc L. Miller

The Little Black Book of Psychiatry, Third Edition,
David P. Moore

The Little Black Book of Primary Care, Sixth Edition,
Daniel K. Onion and James Glazer

The Little Black Book of Pulmonary Medicine,
Edward Ringel

The Little Black Book of Cardiology, Second Edition,
John A. Sutherland

CPSIA information can be obtained at www.ICGtesting.com
Printed in the USA
LVOW01s0103250315

431873LV00015B/260/P